Neurology of Infancy and Childhood

SIDNEY CARTER, M.D.

Dwight D. Eisenhower United Cerebral Palsy Professor of Neurology, and Chi
Division of Pediatric Neurology, Columbia University College of Physicians a
Surgeons; Attending Neurologist, Neurological Institute, and Columbia-Presbyteri
Medical Center, New York, New York

ARNOLD P. GOLD, M.D.

Associate Professor of Clinical Neurology, and Associate Professor of Clinic
Pediatrics, Columbia University College of Physicians and Surgeons; Associa
Attending Neurologist, and Associate Attending Pediatrician, Columbia-Presb
terian Medical Center, New York, New York

APPLETON-CENTURY-CROFTS/New York
A Publishing Division of Prentice-Hall, Inc.

Neurology of Infancy and Childhood

Library of Congress Cataloging in Publication Data

Carter, Sidney, 1912-
Neurology of infancy and childhood.

Includes bibliographies.
1. Pediatric neurology. I. Gold, Arnold P., 1925- joint author. II Title. [DNLM: 1. Nervous system diseases—In infancy and childhood. WS340 C325n 1974]
RJ486.C35 618.9′28 74-7135
ISBN 0-8385-6710-X

74 75 76 77 78 79 80/10 9 8 7 6 5 4 3 2 1

Library of Congress Catalog Card Number 74-7135

PRINTED IN THE UNITED STATES OF AMERICA
0-8385-6710-X

To Dr. Rustin McIntosh, Professor Emeritus of Pediatrics at the Columbia-Presbyterian Medical Center, and to the first Director of the National Institute of Neurological Diseases and Stroke (formerly Blindness), Dr. Pearce Bailey, whose farsightedness made pediatric neurology a reality.

Contributors

DORA CHAO, M.D.

Pediatrician, Houston, Texas

ABE M. CHUTORIAN, M.D.

Associate Professor of Clinical Neurology and Pediatrics, Columbia University College of Physicians and Surgeons; Associate Attending Neurologist, Columbia-Presbyterian Medical Center; Consultant in Neurology, Blythedale Children's Hospital; Consultant in Neurology, Harlem Hospital Medical Center, New York, New York

DAVID B. CLARK, Ph.D., M.D.

Professor and Chairman, Department of Neurology, University of Kentucky Medical Center, Lexington, Kentucky

HERBERT J. COHEN, M.D.

Associate Professor of Pediatrics and Rehabilitative Medicine, Albert Einstein College of Medicine; Director, Bronx Developmental Services, New York State Department of Mental Hygiene, New York, New York

WILLIAM DE MYER, M.D.

Professor of Child Neurology, Indiana University School of Medicine; Attending Physician, Riley Memorial Hospital for Children, Indianapolis, Indiana

ARTHUR L. DREW, M.D.

Professor of Neurology, and Director of Pediatric Neurology, Indiana University School of Medicine; Attending Physician, Riley Memorial Hospital for Children, Indianapolis, Indiana

FRED J. EPSTEIN, M.D.

Assistant Professor of Neurosurgery, New York University School of Medicine, New York, New York

MELVIN GREER, M.D.

Professor and Chairman, Department of Neurology, University of Florida College of Medicine, Gainesville, Florida

JAMES F. HAMMILL, M.D.

Professor of Clinical Neurology, Columbia University College of Physicians and Surgeons; Associate Attending Neurologist, Neurological Institute, Columbia-Presbyterian Medical Center, New York, New York

HORACE L. HODES, M.D.

Professor and Chairman, Department of Pediatrics, The Mt. Sinai School of Medicine; Pediatrician-in-Chief, The Mt. Sinai Hospital, New York, New York

NIELS L. LOW, M.D.

Associate Professor of Clinical Neurology and Associate Professor of Clinical Pediatrics, Columbia University College of Physicians and Surgeons; Associate Attending Neurologist, Columbia-Presbyterian Medical Center, New York, New York; Clinical Director, Blythedale Children's Hospital, Valhalla, New York

ERNEST S. MATHEWS, M.D.

Associate Professor of Clinical Neurosurgery; Chief, Pediatric Neurosurgery, Mt. Sinai School of Medicine of the City University of New York; Associate Attending Neurosurgeon, Mt. Sinai Hospital, New York, New York

J. GORDON MILLICHAP, M.D.

Professor, Departments of Neurology and Pediatrics, Northwestern University Medical College; Attending Neurologist and Pediatric Neurologist, Children's Memorial and Northwestern Medical Center Hospitals, Chicago, Illinois

RALPH E. MOLOSHOK, M.D.

Clinical Professor of Pediatrics, Mt. Sinai School of Medicine of the City University of New York; Attending Pediatrician, Mt. Sinai Hospital, New York, New York

JOSEPH RANSOHOFF, M.D.

Professor and Chairman, Department of Neurosurgery, New York University School of Medicine; Director, Neurosurgical Service, Bellevue Hospital Center, University Hospital, Veterans Administration Hospital, New York, New York

KENNETH SHULMAN, M.D.

Professor and Chairman, Department of Neurological Surgery, Albert Einstein College of Medicine, New York, New York

ALEX J. STEIGMAN, M.D.

Professor of Pediatrics, Mt. Sinai School of Medicine of City University of New York; Attending Pediatrician, Mt. Sinai Hospital, New York, New York

LAWRENCE T. TAFT, M.D.

Professor and Chairman, Department of Pediatrics, Rutgers Medical School, University Heights, Piscataway, New Jersey

STUART WEISS, M.D.

Assistant Professor of Clinical Neurology, Washington University School of Medicine, St. Louis, Missouri

Preface

Pediatric subspecialization has grown considerably in the past decade due to the rapid increase in knowledge of diseases of infants and children. The development of pediatric neurology is further evidence of this trend toward specialization.

The 14th and 15th editions of Barnett's *Pediatrics* departed from the 13 previous editions of Holt's original *Diseases of Infancy and Childhood* by establishing associate editors for various subspecialties. A section on pediatric neurology was developed with the assistance of some 19 contributors. It became clear that this section on care for children with disorders of the nervous system was of particular interest to many readers, necessitating the preparation of the pediatric neurology material as a separate monograph.

The contents of this monograph were organized for readability, information, and above all, application. The initial chapter deals with the general principles of neurologic diagnosis and concerns itself with an evaluation of presenting symptoms and signs. The techniques of the neurologic examination of the neonate, infant and older child were omitted, as there are existing excellent publications that deal directly with this subject. In the twelve additional chapters, the common, the uncommon and the rare disorders of the developing nervous system are described.

Hopefully, this book is only a beginning. Increasing knowledge in pediatric neurology will justify subsequent editions.

Contents

Neurology of Infancy and Childhood

Chapter 1
DIAGNOSIS OF NEUROLOGIC DISEASE

Children with neurologic disorders comprise a significant portion of pediatric practice. It has been estimated that approximately 30 percent of all children admitted to an active teaching hospital either have primary neurologic disease or suffer from nervous system involvement secondary to other systemic conditions. Consequently, it is of great benefit to the pediatrician to have a thorough understanding of the fundamentals of good neurologic diagnosis.

Neurologic diagnosis is dependent on the evaluation of the history, the performance of a careful and detailed neurologic examination, and the utilization of appropriate ancillary procedures. Through evaluation of data compiled in this manner it is possible to localize a lesion to one or more areas of the nervous system. This localization is of primary importance in the establishment of a correct etiologic diagnosis because neurologic disorders have a predilection for specific areas of the nervous system. The astute clinician, then, attempts to answer two simple but very important questions: "Where?" and "What?" Ideally, an answer should also be found to a third question: "Why?"

Compilation and Evaluation of the History

A proper history is the initial guide to localization and differential diagnosis. The historical data must be documented by asking the proper questions of the persons most intimately involved, obtaining this information in a chronologic manner, and evaluating the symptoms and signs thus derived.

OBTAINING THE HISTORICAL DATA. Historical data are best obtained from both parents and, when possible, the child. It is of interest that even preschool children may supply invaluable diagnostic information. However, the initial history must be obtained in the absence of the child. Infants may be a source of distraction to both parents and physician, while older children may understand but often misinterpret historical facts and, as a result, suffer emotional trauma. Also, the cognizant child may, by his presence, limit the ability of the parents to relate a detailed and accurate history.

THE IMPORTANCE OF CHRONOLOGIC DOCUMENTATION. Chronologic presentation of the clinical manifestations will frequently suggest localization and etiology. Thus, in obtaining the history, it is essential to record the rate of onset and whether the signs and symptoms are progressive, regressive, or static in nature.

The rate of onset is important; diagnosis may be suggested by the rapidity with which the symptoms become evident. Thus, vascular disease may be a valid diagnosis when hemiplegia appears suddenly, while a subacute or insidious evolution of the hemiparesis is more characteristic of neoplasia.

Diagnosis of progressive lesions is largely dependent on the age of onset and the rate of evolution. For example, infantile amaurotic familial idiocy (Tay-Sachs disease) characteristically has its onset in early infancy and rapidly progresses to death in two or three years, while Friedreich's ataxia usually appears between the ages of 5 and 10 and slowly evolves for many years.

In static lesions of the nervous system, which account for two-thirds of the neurologic disorders of childhood, diagnosis must not be obscured by the fact that, despite the nonprogressive nature of such lesions, maturation of the nervous system may cause either improvement or worsening. As a consequence, in some cases of cerebral palsy, ataxia improves with age, while the hydrocephalus secondary to aqueductal stenosis becomes more marked, even though the disease itself is nonprogressive.

Evaluation of Symptoms and Signs

Certain manifestations by themselves suggest neurologic involvement, while others incriminate the nervous system only indirectly. The more important symptoms and signs and their relationship to localization and etiologic diagnosis are described here.

GASTROINTESTINAL COMPLAINTS. Children may exhibit abnormal feeding patterns following enteral or parenteral disturbances. Although the physician's attention is most often focused on possible local causes, it is most important, and at times lifesaving, to be aware of the multiple neurologic entities which may be the basis for altered function. Feeding problems, vomiting, and abdominal pain may be symptomatic of neurologic disorders.

TABLE 1. *Normal Age for the Acquisition of Major Developmental Milestones*

Age	Motor	Language	Adaptive Behavior
4-6 wk	Head lifted from prone position and turned from side to side	Cries	Smiles
4 mo	No head lag when pulled to sitting from supine position Tries to grasp large objects	Sounds of pleasure	Smiles, laughs aloud, and shows pleasure to familiar objects or persons
5 mo	Voluntary grasp with both hands Plays with toes	Primitive sounds "ah goo"	Smiles at self in mirror
6 mo	Grasps with one hand Rolls prone to supine Sits with support	Range of sounds greater	Expresses displeasure and food preferences Holds arms out to be picked up
8 mo	Sits without support Transfers objects from hand to hand Rolls supine to prone	Combines syllables: "baba, dada, mama"	Responds to "No"
10 mo	Sits well Creeping Stands holding Finger-thumb opposition in picking up small objects		Waves "bye-bye," plays "patty cake" and "peek-a-boo"
12 mo	Stands holding Walks with support	Says 2 or 3 words with meaning	Understands names of objects Shows interest in pictures
15 mo	Walks alone	Several intelligible words	Requests by pointing Imitates
18 mo	Walks up and down stairs holding Removes clothes	Many intelligible words	Carries out simple commands
2 yr	Walks up and down stairs by self Runs	2- to 3-word phrases	Organized play Points to some parts of body

Feeding problems include difficulties with sucking and/or swallowing which result from brainstem (bulbar) dysfunction. Newborns, most commonly prematures, may exhibit these sucking and swallowing difficulties as a result of physiologic immaturity of the nervous system or because of maternal oversedation during delivery. However, lesions in the nervous system should always be suspected when these symptoms occur. If the child suffers diffuse involvement of the brain of the static type, as seen in the cerebral palsies, the earliest manifestation may be problems with sucking and swallowing. These symptoms frequently diminish and disappear with age. In all newborns with these problems, subdural hematoma and neonatal myasthenia gravis must be suspected and require prompt recognition. Difficulty with sucking and swallowing in the newborn is also symptomatic of congenital defects of the motor nuclei of the brainstem (Möbius' syndrome), familial dysautonomia, and myotonic dystrophy.

The appearance of sucking and swallowing problems in the older child usually implies a progressive disorder of the nervous system. In such cases consideration should be given to infectious processes such as bulbar poliomyelitis, brainstem tumors, and metabolic and/or degenerative disorders resulting from disorders of lipid and glycogen storage.

Vomiting in the form of minor rumination and regurgitation may be physiologic in nature. Pathologic vomiting, however, may be due to indirect or direct involvement of the vomiting center in the brainstem. Persistent vomiting in the absence of an overt cause should always raise the question of increased intracranial pressure. In the absence of increased pressure, tumors of the third and fourth ventricles, disease of the brainstem, seizure variants, and labyrinthitis should be suspected.

Abdominal pain which is acute and persistent may be the result of radicular involvement secondary to polyneuritis, spinal cord tumors, or a complication of a lumbar puncture, while chronic or recurrent abdominal pain, with or without vomiting, may be the sole manifestation of an epileptic state. Abdominal pain due to acute intermittent porphyria or to lead colic is very rarely observed in the pediatric age group.

DELAYED ACQUISITION OF DEVELOPMENTAL MILESTONES. Developmental milestones represent the achievement of an expected physiologic function and include motor performance, language development, and adaptive behavior. Studies of large numbers of normal children have established age levels at which these various functions should be attained. Individual variations are common, and it should be noted that Table 1 is only an approximation of normal development.

While delay in the acquisition of a specific function may imply an impaired nervous system, there is a chance that such a delay is normal. However, multiple or global delay in achieving these milestones almost always signifies an underlying nervous system disorder, usually of the static type. This delay in the acquisition of many or all of the milestones usually indicates diffuse involvement of the brain and may be diagnosed as mental retardation or one of the more severe forms of cerebral palsy.

Specific delay in any one of the three areas of development is indicative of the following disorders: If *motor function* is delayed, cerebral dysfunction or disorders of muscle, spinal cord, or peripheral nerves may be the answer. If *speech* fails to develop, the causative factor may be either a brain disorder or peripheral hearing loss. Poor *adaptive behavior* usually implies a diffuse disturbance of the brain. In rare instances, of course, such behavior may be related to maternal deprivation or rejection.

ABNORMAL ENLARGEMENT OF THE HEAD. Every examination *must* include a measurement of head circumference. This has added value when it is compared with previous measurement and there is accelerated increase in size beyond the anticipated norm.

It is true, of course, that a head circumference greater than normal may be a physiologic manifestation of a familial trait. Pathologically, it is the result of alterations in any of the four cranial compartments: (1) the ventricles; (2) the brain; (3) the meninges; and (4) the skull and scalp. Accordingly, abnormal head enlargement may be due to any condition in which the cerebrospinal fluid flow is obstructed, since this causes enlarged ventricles with resultant hydrocephalus. The head may be large due to the presence of either too much or too little brain substance. An increase in brain substance is seen as a congenital abnormality in megalencephaly or in some metabolic and degenerative disorders. Decrease in brain substance is observed in hydranencephaly and porencephaly. In addition, an abnormally enlarged head may result from accumulation of fluid in the subdural space. Changes in the membranous bone of the skull, such as cleidocranial dysostosis or achondroplasia, as well as scalp involvement by cephalhematoma may result in an enlarged head.

MOTOR DISTURBANCES. Disturbances in motor function may be manifested as muscle weakness, ataxia, or abnormal involuntary movements. Symptoms of motor disturbance may be evidenced from early infancy by a delay in the development of the motor milestones. At a later age they may appear as a loss of, or a disturbance in, voluntary motor activity.

Muscle weakness may be the result of upper motor neuron disturbances. Lesions of the brain involving the motor cortex or its outflow will cause total or partial spastic paralysis of the extremities of the opposite side. Such lesions may be either congenital, fixed defects, or acquired disturbances due to tumors, vascular insults, or degenerative diseases. With fixed lesions the weakness does not increase and actually may improve by compensatory mechanisms. In acquired lesions, the sudden appearance of a hemiparesis suggests vascular disease, while a slowly developing weakness implies a tumor or degenerative disorder. Additional clinical features indicative of upper motor neuron disease are exaggerated deep tendon reflexes and the pathologic extensor plantar sign (Babinski reflex) on the involved side.

Lower motor neuron disturbances also may be responsible for muscle weakness. These disorders are characterized by a flaccid weakness, and result from involvement of either muscle, peripheral nerve, or anterior horn cells. In primary muscle disorders, such as muscular dystrophy, the weakness is greatest in the large girdle muscles. Symmetric involvement of the nerve trunks, as in polyneuritis, causes diffuse weakness; however, in this instance, the distal musculature of the hands and feet is more involved than the proximal girdle musculature. In anterior horn cell disease, weakness may be symmetric or asymmetric, involving isolated muscle groups. Lower motor neuron disease is further characterized by atrophy, hypoactive to absent deep tendon reflexes, and the presence of a normal plantar response.

Ataxia results from involvement of the cerebellum and its pathways. This unsteadiness of voluntary movements may be due to a congenital defect of the cerebellum (ataxic form of cerebral palsy), which is characterized by poor sitting and standing balance and the development of unsteady gait and hand function.

Acquired forms of ataxia may be either acute or insidious in onset. The ataxia which appears acutely may follow intoxications, the exanthems (particularly varicella), and nonspecific infections (acute cerebellar ataxia), or it may be episodic in nature, as in vertiginous epilepsy or vestibular neuronitis. Slowly developing ataxia may be observed with increased intracranial pressure, cerebellar and brainstem tumors, heredodegenerative disorders, as in ataxia-telangiectasia and Friedreich's ataxia, and some inborn errors of metabolism, such as Hartnup disease.

Abnormal involuntary movements may be either psychogenic in origin, as in tics, or the result of extrapyramidal dysfunction, as manifested by chorea, athetosis, dystonia, tremor, and ballismus.

Tics or habit spasms are the most common of the abnormal movements. They are characterized by isolated repetitive movements, such as winking, blinking, grimacing, twisting the neck, and shrugging the shoulders. More complex tic phenomena may have associated vocalizations, such as coughing, barking, and clearing the throat. When the vocal component is manifested by the use of obscenities, it is called the syndrome of Gilles de la Tourette.

Chorea is characterized by irregular, sudden, and jerky movements involving any group of skeletal muscles, including the face. Such movements may be indicative of rheumatic fever (Sydenham's chorea), encephalitis, hypoparathyroidism, and, less commonly, lupus erythematosus.

The movements of *athetosis* are slow and writhing, involving primarily the distal musculature. They may be accompanied by choreiform movements and are then described as choreoathetosis. Athetosis is a manifestation of kernicterus and congenital defects of the brain.

Dystonia is characterized by involuntary sustained muscle spasms of the neck, trunk, and extremities, resulting in abnormal posture. Dystonic movements may be a manifestation of dystonia musculorum deformans, some forms of encephalitis, and birth defects. They may be associated with rigidity in hepatolenticular degeneration (Wilson's disease). Children most commonly demonstrate dystonic phenomena as a complication arising from an idiosyncrasy to the phenothiazines.

Tremor of the basal ganglia origin occurs at rest, while the cerebellar form of tremor becomes evident in volitional movements. It is seen in its most benign form as familial or essential tremor and may be dramatic in the wing-beating tremor of Wilson's disease.

DISTURBANCES IN SENSATION. Pain, burning, tingling, and numbness are manifestations of sensory disorders. Episodic disturbances of this nature may be the only manifestations of a focal seizure or may be symptoms of hypoparathyroidism. Persistent sensory phenomena are seen in the polyneuropathies. Dysautonomic children, interestingly, have a raised pain threshold. There are also a small number of other children who have a congenital indifference to pain.

VISUAL LOSS. Sudden loss of vision is the manifestation of retrobulbar or optic neuritis, while transient impairment in visual function may be seen in seizure disorders or migraine. It is difficult to detect the onset of gradual visual loss, since children tend to be uncomplaining and parents unobservant; however, it does become evident when the child is observed holding books closer to his face, sitting nearer to the television set, or bumping into objects. It is difficult to detect a decrease in the field of vision in young children.

OCULAR DISORDERS. *Diplopia* follows rapid development of extraocular muscle paresis and is rarely, if ever, mentioned by children with long-standing eye muscle dysfunction. Nonparalytic *strabismus* is seen with extraocular muscle imbalance and often is a manifestation of nonprogressive lesions of the brain. Paralytic squint, on the other hand, is most commonly the result of involvement of the third and sixth cranial nerves. The turning in of one or both eyes may be the nonspecific result of increased intracranial pressure. Brainstem gliomas and myasthenia gravis also give rise to a variety of extraocular muscle palsies.

Nystagmus, exhibited as rhythmical, wiggling, jerky, or pendular oscillations of the eyeball, is associated with disorders of the eye, brainstem, and cerebellum. A searching type of nystagmic movement is seen in the blind. Pendular oscillations are most often ocular in origin, as in spasmus nutans and congenital forms of nystagmus. Vertical nystagmus is almost always a manifestation of brainstem dysfunction while the horizontal variety may indicate either brainstem or cerebellar pathology. Nystagmus in both vertical and horizontal directions of gaze is frequently the result of drug intoxication with barbiturates or hydantoins. Opsoclonus, a bizarre type of nystagmus, is characterized by coarse, irregular, nonrhythmic but conjugate eye movements in all directions of gaze. It often occurs in the syndrome of acute cerebellar ataxia with an occult neoplasm.

Ptosis may be permanent or intermittent and in some forms may be altered by the movements of the jaw (Marcus Gunn phenomenon). Permanent ptosis is seen congenitally and follows lesions of the third cranial nerve. The ptosis of myasthenia gravis is intermittent and is least evident on awakening; it increases with fatigue, and is most marked at the end of the day. When associated with miosis and enophthalmos (Horner's syndrome), ptosis is a manifestation of impaired sympathetic function.

Exophthalmos, when bilateral, usually signifies an endocrinopathy, while unilateral protrusions are most often secondary to retrobulbar tumors, optic nerve gliomas, or disease of the cavernous sinus.

HEARING LOSS. Defective hearing of peripheral origin may be secondary to kernicterus, trauma, exanthems (most commonly, mumps), tumors of the brainstem, drugs, or otologic disorders. Some children with intact peripheral pathways have apparent hearing loss. It is assumed that such children have impairment of the central connections of hearing (receptive aphasia). Often the first clue of an early hearing loss is the failure to develop normal speech patterns.

SPEECH DISORDERS. Defective speech may arise from impaired hearing or expressive difficulties. Delay in the acquisition and faulty development of speech patterns may be the first sign of fixed or progressive lesions of the brain, while loss of previously acquired speech is indicative of hearing disorders or degenerative disease of the brain.

POOR SCHOOL PERFORMANCE. Problems in learning are often related to visual or hearing defects. They may also be the result of unrecognized seizure states, particularly petit mal, or of progressive degenerative diseases. Specific learning disabilities, most commonly reading difficulties, are often seen in children with the syndrome of minimal cerebral dysfunction. Poor school performance may be the first indication of mild mental retardation.

PERSONALITY CHANGES. Personality changes often develop at some time during the course of neoplastic diseases, especially when the tumor involves the temporal lobe. The same is true of infectious, degenerative, or metabolic disorders. Hyperactivity and, less commonly, apathy are frequent manifestations of nonprogressive brain lesions.

HEAD TILT. Most commonly, this type of abnormal carriage of the head is related to tumors of the cerebellum or brainstem. Head tilt may also arise from local irritation of the cervical musculature, or it may be a manifestation of ocular and central nervous system pathology.

FACIAL WEAKNESS. Asymmetry of the face during crying or a complete lack of facial expression in a child is an indication of facial weakness. In the neonatal period this condition may be secondary to congenital anomalies, such as facial nuclear aplasia (Möbius' syndrome) and partial muscular hypoplasia (Hofnagel syndrome), or it may be acquired as the result of facial nerve compression. The older child, like adults, may demonstrate a peripheral facial weakness during the course of Bell's palsy, polyneuritis, brainstem gliomas, or mastoid disease. Rarely, there may be a progressive hemiatrophy of the face, which includes the facial muscles. Facial weakness limited to the lower half of the face (upper motor neuron paresis) may accompany a hemiparesis secondary to a brain lesion.

CONVULSIONS. In the newborn, convulsions may be due either to developmental or acquired lesions of the brain or to such metabolic disorders as hypoglycemia, hypocalcemia, hypomagnesemia, or pyridoxine dependency. Rarely, they may be a manifestation of maple syrup urine disease. Seizures taking place during this neonatal period may be confused with apneic or cyanotic spells of cardiac origin.

In children less than 2 years of age, seizures unassociated with fever are most often related to structural defects of the brain. Febrile convulsions, on the other hand, may be the only manifestation of meningitis or may be associated with extracranial infections. Breath-holding spells are common in this age group and, in some children, may be accompanied by convulsive phenomena. Focal motor seizures in children of this age group do not have the same significance as in adults. Often these focal spells will vary from side to side and, unless they persistently recur on one side, are usually not related to a specific brain lesion. Petit mal rarely occurs before 2 years of age.

HEADACHES. Headaches are relatively common in childhood. Undue irritability in young children may be an indication of recurrent or persistent headaches. Older children may have headaches which are related to increased intracranial pressure from any cause, or to migraine, tension, trauma, or systemic disease. These painful episodes may precede, follow, or be the only manifestation of convulsions.

VERTIGO. Evaluation of vertigo is very difficult and is dependent largely upon the ability of the child to describe this subjective phenomenon. Vestibular neuronitis results in paroxysmal episodes of vertigo, and seizures may be manifested only as vertiginous attacks. Vertigo may also be a symptom of Ménière's disease, which is rare in childhood.

COMA. Often a threat to life, coma in any age group is a perplexing problem. A careful history is invaluable in ascertaining the underlying pathology. Drug intoxication, trauma, and postictal states are common causes of coma. Less frequently, meningitis, encephalitis, cerebrovascular accidents, and metabolic disorders are accompanied by coma.

The Neurologic Examination

The neurologic examination is essential to the establishment both of nervous system involvement and of the site at which the pathologic process has occurred. Specific etiologic diagnosis may be possible when a detailed history is combined and evaluated with a thorough neurologic examination. For example, localization of a lesion to the brainstem is determined by the presence of multiple cranial nerve palsies, ataxia, and pyramidal tract signs. If the history shows slow progression, the lesion may be diagnosed as a probable tumor.

The *general pediatric examination* is of vital importance in providing data of significance in neurologic diagnosis. The head should be carefully measured and auscultated for intracranial bruits. Transillumination of the skull may indicate the presence of a subdural fluid collection, porencephaly, or hydranencephaly. Certain types of skin lesions are of significant value in neurologic diagnosis. For instance, depigmented nevi may be the initial cutaneous manifestation of tuberous sclerosis; later the child may develop the more classical adenoma sebaceum. Café-au-lait spots suggest neurofibromatosis, and port-wine facial hemangiomas often signify encephalotrigeminal angiomatosis (Sturge-Weber-Dimitri syndrome). Midline skin defects, patches of hair, or hemangioma may be associated with underlying defects of the spinal cord and brain.

In the *neurologic examination,* observation of the child is essential, since it may provide many clues to disturbed neurologic function. Successful observation depends upon the ingenuity of the examiner in obtaining the cooperation of the child. Ideally, the evaluation should be performed in a leisurely manner, and at all times a nonthreatening atmosphere should be carefully staged, perhaps with the child seated in his mother's lap. At some time during the examination the child must be completely undressed. Painful or difficult parts should be reserved until the end.

Examination of the newborn is difficult because the highly desired cooperation on the part of the patient is rarely available. In addition, it is difficult to determine whether the abnormal findings demonstrated in some newborns are a reflection of an immature nervous system or whether they represent transient or permanent defects.

The neonatal neurologic examination becomes significant when any of the following are demonstrated:

1. Alteration of the state of consciousness (lethargy, stupor, coma)
2. High-pitched, feeble, or absent cry
3. Manifestation of increased intracranial pressure
    a. Bulging fontanel
    b. Opisthotonus

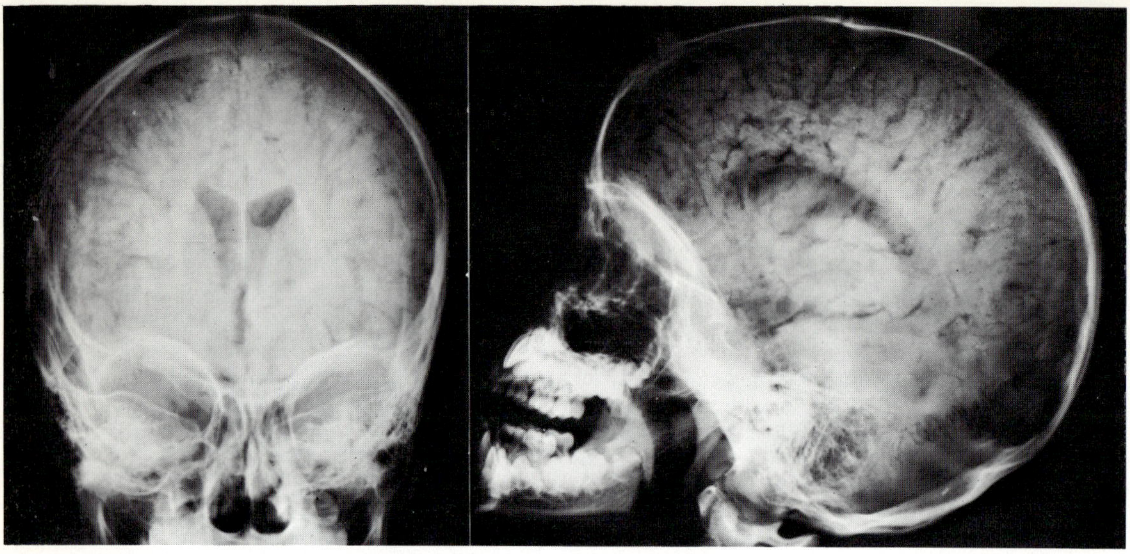

Fig. 1. Normal pneumoencephalogram in a girl 5 years of age.

   c. Setting-sun sign of eyes
   d. Dilated and unresponsive pupils
4. Abnormal or asymmetric positioning of extremities
5. Reduced spontaneous movements of extremity
6. Abnormalities in muscle tone (flaccid or spastic)
7. Abnormal reflex responses: Absent or delayed acquisition of neonatal reflexes
   a. Moro
   b. Root and suck
   c. Grasp
   d. Head control in vertical position
8. Abnormalities of the cranial nerves
   a. Failure to blink in response to light or sound
   b. Unequal or fixed pupils
   c. Facial asymmetry on crying
   d. Difficulties in sucking or swallowing
   e. Funduscopic abnormalities
9. Impaired response to pinprick, suggesting a spinal cord lesion

Evaluation of the older infant can be quite informative except that detailed sensory testing is usually not reliable. Neurologic examination of older children differs little from that of adults.

At the conclusion of the examination the physician should have evaluated the child's mental capacities, cranial nerve functioning, motor power, coordination, sensation and reflex phenomena. The findings of such an examination, plus the evaluation of the history, should lead to the performance of appropriate ancillary studies.

Ancillary Procedures

Additional diagnostic procedures must be carefully planned, and maximum information should be obtained from each study. Increasing knowledge in the field of electrophysiology, and improved radiologic techniques have made available a variety of new diagnostic aids. Many of these tests are highly specialized, and their value is dependent upon expert interpretation.

RADIOGRAPHIC STUDIES. ***Skull.*** Plain radiographs of the skull are indicated in all children with suspected intracranial disease and head trauma. Routine films include anteroposterior, posteroanterior, stereolateral, and base views. In special circumstances films of the optic foramina, mastoids, and laminograms may be necessary.

Significant findings on plain radiographs of the skull include evidence of increased intracranial pressure, premature closure of sutures, fractures, tumors of the skull, intracranial calcifications, and unilateral cerebral atrophy (Dyke-Davidoff-Masson syndrome).

Signs of increased intracranial pressure include suture diastasis, erosion of the posterior clinoids, and deepening of the sella turcica. The so-called beaten-silver appearance may be a normal finding and, by itself, is not evidence of increased intracranial pressure.

The presence of intracranial calcifications is usually abnormal and may be seen after infections with toxoplasmosis, cytomegalic inclusion disease, and chronic brain abscesses. Calcifications can also be found in association with tumors, vascular malformations, neuroectodermal dysplasias, and metabolic disorders. Calcification of the pineal gland is rare in childhood.

Spine. Radiographs of the spine are indicated following trauma and when there is a suggestion of an underlying congenital anomaly or a suspected tumor. They may also have diagnostic significance in certain metabolic disorders, such as Morquio's or Hurler's disease. Anteroposterior and lateral views should be taken routinely.

Contrast Studies. These radiographic procedures

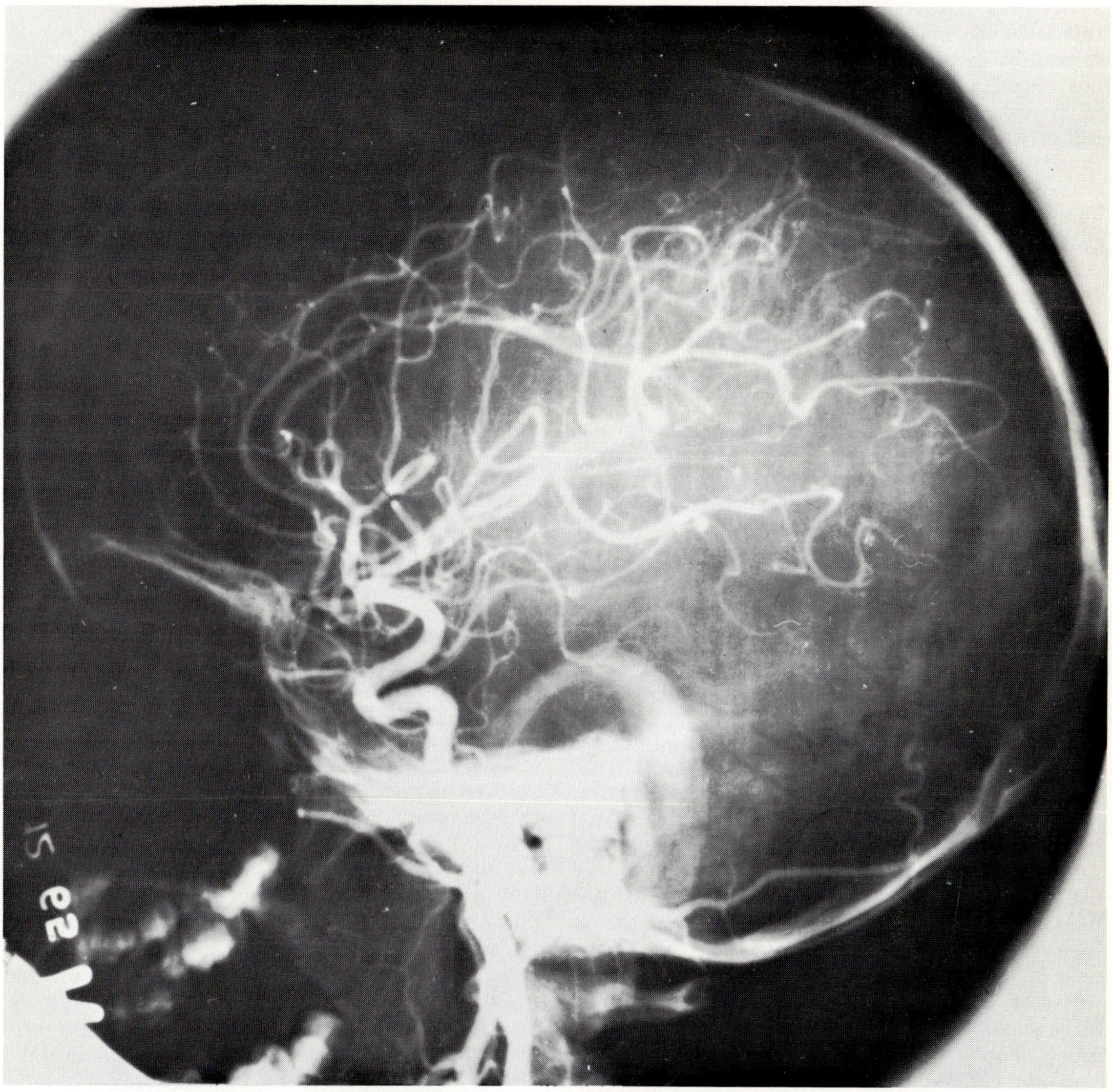

Fig. 2. Normal carotid arteriogram.

should only be performed in the presence of specific indications; their value is dependent upon proper performance and expert interpretation of the films. Contrast studies include air encephalography, cerebral arteriography, and myelography.

Air encephalography (Fig. 1) is primarily indicated in children with suspected mass lesions or with progressive neurologic disorders associated with increased intracranial pressure. Most epileptic children and those with nonprogressive conditions, including mental retardation, cerebral palsy, and abnormal behavior accompanied by learning disabilities, should not be subjected to this procedure. In the case of increased intracranial pressure, air is introduced directly into the ventricles (ventriculography). In most situations, however, air introduced via the lumbar subarachnoid space (pneumoencephalography) is adequate and is preferable for suspected brainstem and optic chiasm tumors.

Cerebral arteriography (Fig. 2) is a method of visualizing the vessels of the brain after injecting a major artery with a radiopaque substance; it is best utilized when there is evidence of a focal rather than a diffuse cerebral lesion. The primary indications for cerebral angiography include suspected vascular malformations, subdural hematoma, cerebral hemisphere tumors, and pseudotumor cerebri.

Myelography is a method of visualizing the spinal canal after the introduction of a radiopaque substance into the spinal subarachnoid space. The prime indication for this procedure is in cases of suspected intraspinal tumors.

LUMBAR PUNCTURE. Examination of the *cerebrospinal fluid* is the single most useful ancillary procedure in the evaluation of neurologic disease; it is mandatory in suspected infection of the central nervous system, and it may give considerable information in the evaluation of undiagnosed disease of the central nervous system. Lumbar puncture is also justified in all children with increased intracranial pressure when there is suggestive evidence of bacterial or viral infection of the central nervous system; it is contraindicated in the presence of increased intracranial pressure unrelated to infection, or when there is cutaneous infection at the site of the projected lumbar puncture.

Maximum information is obtained when the pressure of the cerebrospinal fluid is measured, the fluid is analyzed for its cellular, protein, and sugar contents, and a serologic examination is performed. Sedation and local anesthesia are important adjuncts, since reliable pressure measurements can be obtained only when the child is in a relaxed state and placed in a lateral recumbent position.

The pressure normally varies between 50 and 180 mm of water and is accurate only when measured with a water manometer. Rate of flow is a crude and often misleading method of estimating pressure. Jugular compression or formal cuff manometrics should be utilized when a spinal cord lesion is suspected.

Normal fluid is clear and colorless, but in the newborn, xanthochromic coloring is common. Hemorrhagic fluid may signify either a traumatic lumbar puncture or antecedent hemorrhage in the central nervous system. Differentiation is possible by the collection of fluid in three tubes and examination of the supernatant after centrifugation. Hemorrhagic fluid due to a traumatic lumbar puncture shows a progressive decrease in the number of red blood cells in the three consecutive tubes, and the supernatant is colorless; that due to antecedent hemorrhage shows no change in the three tubes, and the supernatant is xanthochromic.

The cell count of the fluid must be determined immediately; normally it does not exceed five white blood cells per cubic millimeter. If more than this number are present, a disorder in the central nervous system is suspected. Crenated red blood cells by themselves do not necessarily indicate previous hemorrhage.

Protein content has a normal range of from 10 to 15 mg per 100 ml in the lateral ventricles to a maximum of approximately 40 mg in the lumbar subarachnoid space. Newborns of both low and full birth weight have, normally, concentrations of protein in the range of 75 to 125 mg per 100 ml.

Sugar content is generally two-thirds of the blood sugar and its diagnostic value is enhanced when simultaneous determinations are performed. Significant decrease in glucose concentration is seen in hypoglycemic states, bacterial and fungal infections of the central nervous system, and neoplastic meningeal infiltrations.

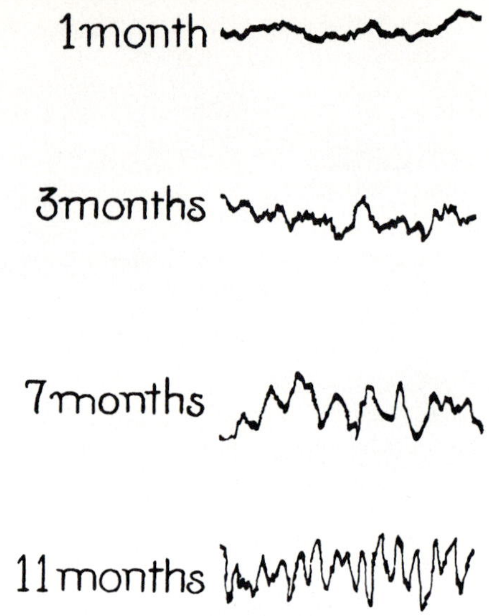

Fig. 3. Electroencephalogram in a normal infant at various ages, illustrating development of the fundamental rhythm. (From Lindsay. *J. Gen. Psychol.*, 19:285, 1938.)

When indicated, the fluid can be analyzed for its gamma globulin or enzyme concentrations. Millipore techniques for obtaining and identifying cells may be invaluable in the identification of some intracranial tumors.

SUBDURAL PUNCTURE. This technique, an important diagnostic and occasionally therapeutic procedure, should be employed in all infants with suspected subdural hematoma or effusions and in those with unexplained macrocephaly; it is contraindicated in the presence of scalp infections. Cerebrospinal fluid may be inadvertently obtained at the time of the puncture and misinterpreted as a subdural fluid collection. True subdural fluid has either a xanthochromic discoloration or, when colorless, a protein content considerably higher than that of the lumbar subarachnoid fluid.

ELECTRODIAGNOSTIC PROCEDURES. *Electroencephalography* (EEG) is a relatively simple and innocuous method of obtaining additional information about the central nervous system. Pediatric electroencephalography requires familiarity with developmental changes in order to interpret properly deviations from the norm (Fig. 3). Electroencephalography has its greatest use as a diagnostic aid in seizure disorders and suspected space-occupying lesions. It is also useful in monitoring the progress of encephalitis and head injury.

Electromyography and nerve conduction studies are useful in determining the site of pathology in neuromuscular disorders. Electromyography aids in differentiating between primary muscle disease and disorders of neural origin. Nerve conduction studies may be of value in differentiating peripheral nerve from anterior horn cell disorders.

MISCELLANEOUS. *Echoencephalography* is a procedure in which high-frequency sound recordings are used to establish the shift of midline structures secondary to subdural hematomas and hemispheric mass lesions. More recently it has been useful in the determination of ventricular size (echoventriculography).

Radioisotope brain scans utilize iodinated albumin, mercury, or technetium radioisotopes in the localization of intracranial lesions, including neoplasms, abscesses, and vascular malformations.

Psychologic tests, when properly performed, can be of considerable diagnostic value in the documentation of organic brain dysfunction and in the delineation of intellectual potential. Projective tests may show evidence of personality disturbances. The results of these procedures are less reliable when repeated too frequently.

References

André-Thomas, Chesni, Y., and Saint-Anne Dargassies, S. The neurological examination of the infant. Little Club Clinics in Developmental Medicine, No. 1. London, National Spastics Society, 1960.

Egan, D., Illingworth, R. S., and MacKeith, R. C. Developmental screening 0-5 years. Clinics in Developmental Medicine, No. 30. London, Spastics International Medical Publications, 1969.

Illingworth, R. S. An introduction to developmental assessment in the first year. Little Club Clinics in Developmental Medicine, No. 3. London, National Spastics Society, 1962.

Mayo Clinic. Clinical Examinations in Neurology. Philadelphia, W. B. Saunders Co., 1956.

Mealey, J., Jr. Brain scanning in childhood. J. Pediat., 69:399, 1966.

Paine, R. S. The immediate value of the neonatal neurological examination. Little Club Clinics in Developmental Medicine, No. 2, 62. London, National Spastics Society, 1960.

——— and Oppe, E. Neurological examination of children. Clinics in Developmental Medicine, No. 20, 21. London, National Spastics Society, 1966.

Prechtl, H., and Beintema, D. The neurological examination of the full term newborn infant. Little Club Clinics in Developmental Medicine, No. 12. London, National Spastics Society, 1964.

Schlagenhauff, R. E., Mazurowski, J., and Smith, B. H. Echoencephalography in neurologic diagnosis. New York J. Med., 67:1035, 1967.

Chapter 2
PRENATAL AND DEVELOPMENTAL DEFECTS

WILLIAM E. DeMYER

Brain

Microcephaly and Megalocephaly

An abnormal head size warns of an abnormal brain. To evaluate head size, the maximum occipitofrontal circumference (OFC) should be measured. Any OFC ± 2 standard deviations from the mean for the age raises strong suspicion of a brain disorder (Fig. 4A and B). Any OFC ± 3 standard deviations almost certainly means an abnormal brain. A significantly small head is termed *microcephaly;* one that is too large, *megalocephaly* (*macrocephaly*). Microcephaly necessitates *micrencephaly,* a small brain. In megalocephaly, the brain actually may be very small, or it may be huge and heavy, a condition termed *megalencephaly*.

Early recognition of abnormal head size depends on serial OFC measurements of every infant from the time of birth. For accuracy, a thin, flexible steel tape is decidedly superior to cloth or paper tapes. Accurate serial measurements, plotted against the normal curve, show the rate of change of the OFC with time, providing clear evidence of a head that is going to be too large or too small. Since microcephaly and macrocephaly are statistical concepts, some neurologically normal subjects will be incorrectly stigmatized if the physician relies only on the OFC. The patient's weight at birth, his somatotype and chest circumference, and the somatotype and OFC of the parents and siblings must all be considered.

Once microcephaly or macrocephaly has been identified, therapy, prognosis, and family counseling must depend on diagnosing the *type* of cerebral lesion and its *cause*. First the history, genealogy, and physical examination must be evaluated for diagnostic clues to distinct entities such as Down's syndrome. Then diagnostic tests must be done in proper sequence, innocuous procedures being performed first. In the course of every infant's examination, the head should be transilluminated. In a completely dark closet, an ordinary flashlight equipped with a rubber adapter is placed against the infant's head. If the cerebrum is absent or greatly thinned, as from increased intracranial pressure, the entire cranium lights up (Fig. 5). Focal lesions such as subdural fluid accumulations, encephaloceles, porencephaly, or

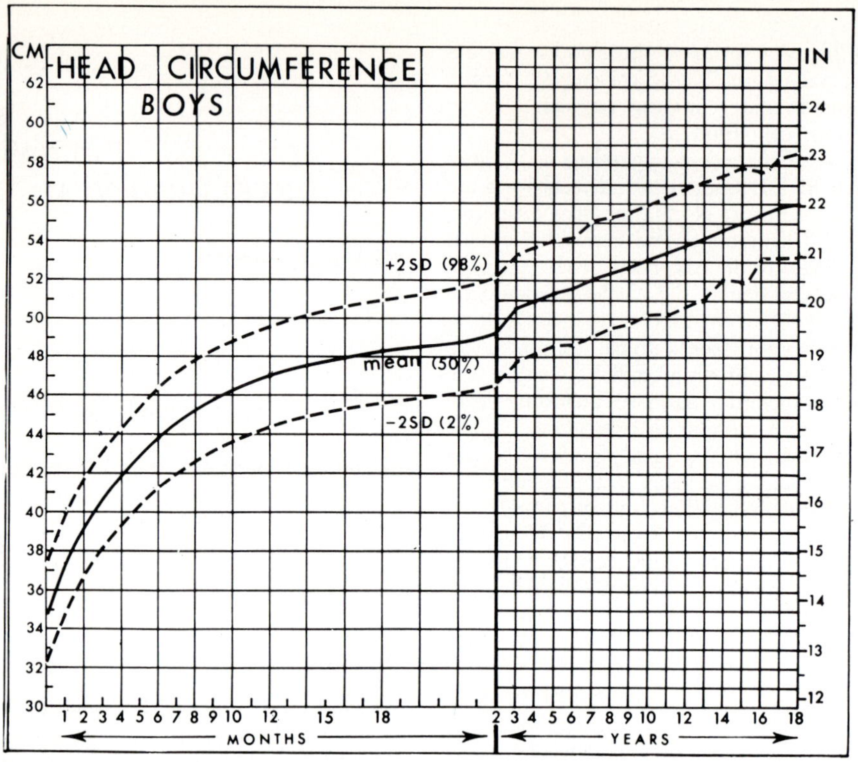

Fig. 4A. Graph of head circumference in boys from birth to 18 years of age. (From Nellhaus. *Pediatrics,* 41:106, 1968.)

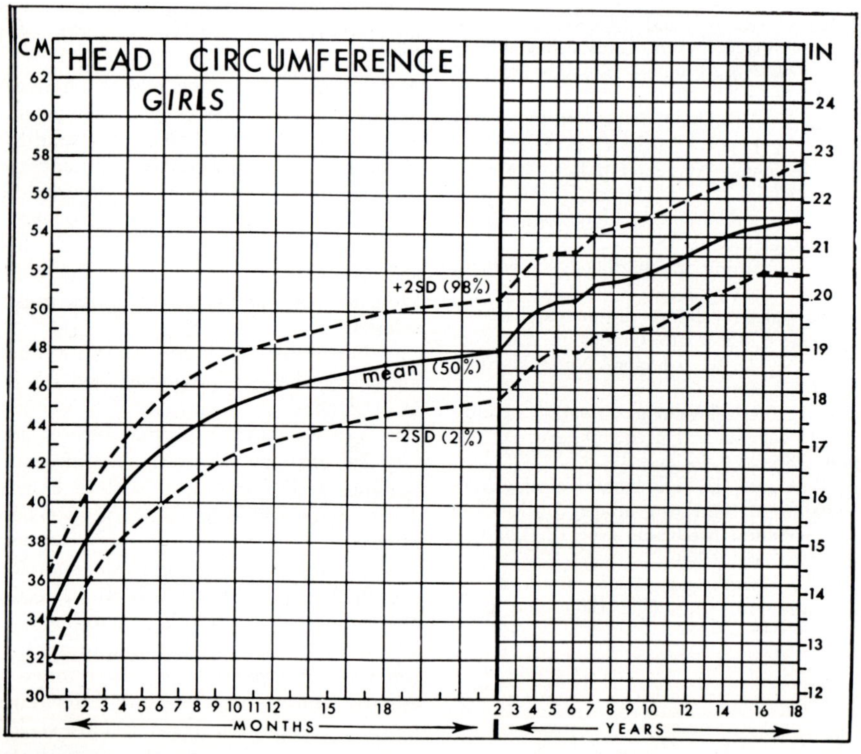

Fig. 4B. Graph of head circumference in girls from birth to 18 years of age. (From Nellhaus. *Pediatrics,* 41:106, 1968).

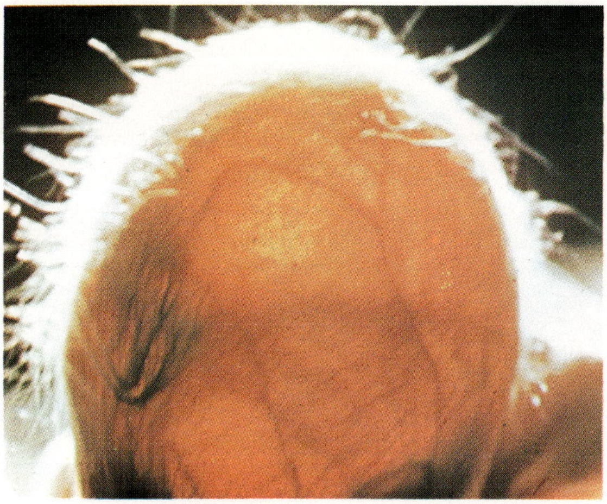

Fig. 5. Transillumination of skull in hydranencephaly.

atrophic defects in the cerebrum transilluminate more restrictedly.

Every infant with an abnormal OFC should next have skull radiographs and usually an electroencephalogram (EEG). Chromosome studies, nuclear sexing, and dermatoglyphic prints are useful if the patient has multiple somatic anomalies or if an intersex syndrome is suspected. If a degenerative, biochemical, or heredofamilial disorder is suspected, the chemistry of blood, urine, and cerebrospinal fluid should be examined. (See p. 856.)

Unless they have increased pressure and require ventriculography, most patients with an abnormal OFC should then have a lumbar puncture, the cerebrospinal fluid being examined for pressure, cell count, glucose, total protein, and protein electrophoresis. In some patients with microcephaly and in most with megalocephaly, air contrast studies, either pneumoencephalograms or ventriculograms, are necessary. In some instances cerebral angiograms are also required.

MICROCEPHALY. Aside from craniosynostosis, *microcephaly* is always secondary to micrencephaly. Any disorder which reduces brain size before maturation is complete may be responsible. A severe degree of micrencephaly implies a prenatal or early postnatal lesion. Common causes are malformations, prenatal or postnatal infections, hypoxia, and maternal disease. In experimental teratology, microcephaly may result from almost any teratogen, such as vitamin deficiency, drugs, or irradiation. Thus microcephaly, by itself, provides no clue as to its cause. The mother should be asked about the perinatal period, illnesses, and drug ingestion during the pregnancy. A history of infertility is common. Some cases are familial and follow a mendelian pattern.

In some microcephalics, the brain, although small, has a fairly normal internal and external configuration. Others may have malformation or destructive lesion, with symmetrically or asymmetrically dilated ventricles.

Microcephalics are usually mentally defective and may have cerebral palsy and seizures. In many instances, the combination of microcephaly with other clinical or laboratory findings permits a specific etiologic diagnosis.

Skull radiographs usually show a thickened calvarium and early closure of fontanels and sutures. Periventricular calcification suggests cytomegalic inclusion disease as the cause. Occasionally microcephaly is caused by craniosynostosis rather than primary micrencephaly. Although the sutures close prematurely in microcephaly, they usually are open at birth and in early infancy. In contrast, in craniosynostosis, the fontanels and sutures usually are obliterated at birth or during early infancy. Surgical opening of the sutures may be required in craniosynostosis but not in microcephaly.

MEGALOCEPHALY AND MEGALENCEPHALY. The most common cause of megalocephaly (an enlarged head) is increased intracranial pressure with hydrocephalus. The cerebral wall thins as the head enlarges. The brain weight, exclusive of intraventricular fluid, is normal or reduced. A much rarer cause of megal*ocephaly* is megal*encephaly,* an abnormally large and heavy brain.

Megalencephaly may be a primary malformation with huge gyri, often of simple pattern or with micropolygyria. It may be sporadic or associated with neurofibromatosis, tuberous sclerosis, myelomeningocele (Chiari malformation), and achondroplasia. The brain is large in pituitary gigantism but not in acromegaly; it is also large in the syndrome of "cerebral gigantism," in which no endocrine defects have been identified. Patients with primary megalencephaly are often mentally deficient and may have motor deficits and seizures.

In secondary megalencephaly, abnormal metabolic products accumulate in the brain. Included here are the infantile form of amaurotic idiocy, gargoylism, spongy degeneration of the white matter, and some of the leucodystrophies such as metachromatic leucodystrophy and Krabbe's disease. A large brain from cerebral edema or from neoplasms does not qualify as megalencephaly.

In hydrocephalus with increased pressure, the head enlarges rapidly, the fontanels bulge, the sutures split, and there may be papilledema. These features usually are absent in primary megalencephaly, but may occur in secondary megalencephaly. If the megalocephalic patient has none of the aforementioned features of increased pressure and no neurologic deficits, the most important step is to measure the OFC of siblings and parents. If other family members have enlarged heads without neurologic deficits, the patient, in all probability, has benign familial megalencephaly, and no further diagnostic procedures are necessary. If a simple familial large-headedness is excluded, the megalocephalic patient requires prompt, thorough investigation, including

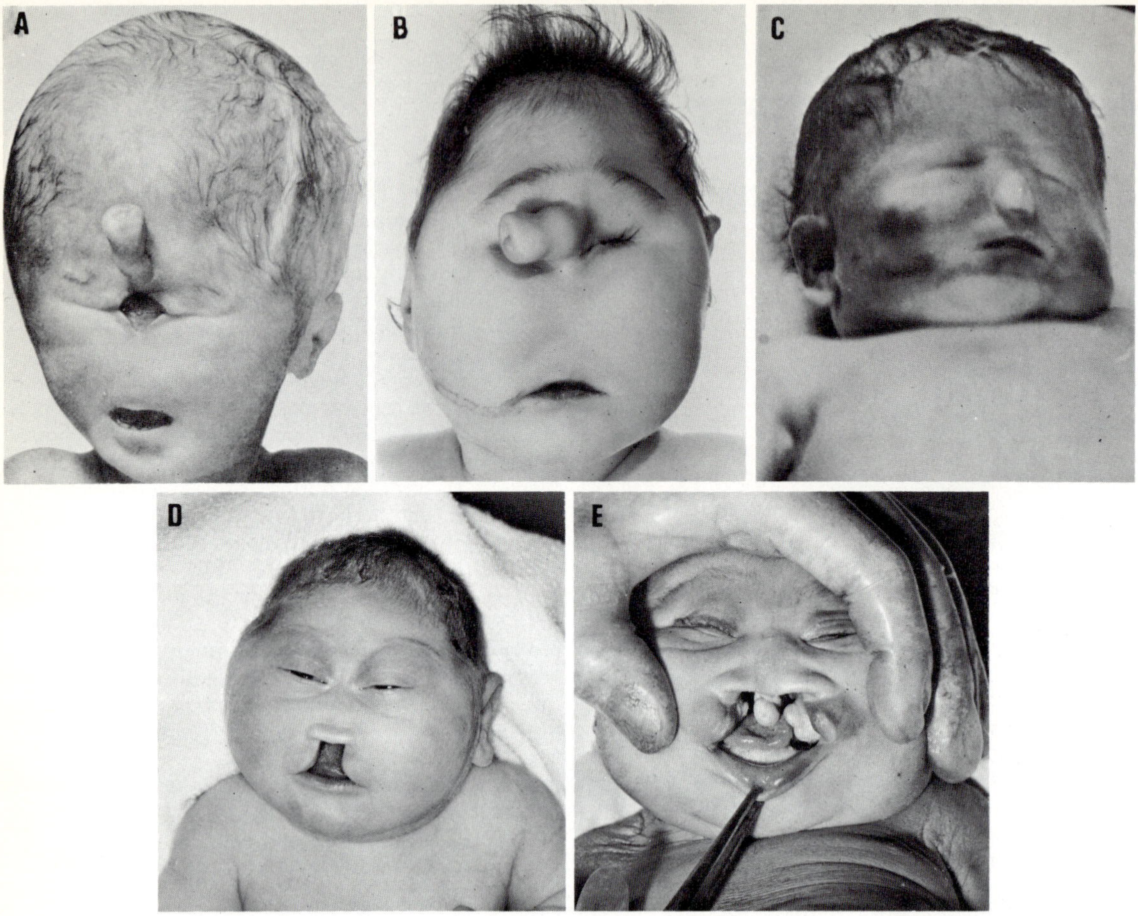

Fig. 6. Diagnostic facies of holoprosencephaly. *A*. Cyclopia. Notice the proboscis attached above the orbit. (From Potter. *Pathology of the Fetus and Newborn*. Courtesy of Year Book Medical Publishers, Inc.). *B*. Ethmocephaly. (Courtesy of Dr. P. Fluery.) The proboscis has migrated down between the orbits, which are separated but show hypotelorism, as do *C, D,* and *E*. *C*. Cebocephaly. The proboscis has migrated to the normal location for the nose. The single nostril leads into a cul-de-sac. *D*. With median cleft lip. Rudimentary nares and a nasal cavity are present. The nasal septum is lacking. *E*. With hypoplastic intermaxillary segment (philtrum-premaxillary anlage). A rudimentary nasal septum is present.

transillumination, skull radiography, and electroencephalography. Subdural taps for subdural hematomas or hygromas should be done in many cases. Air contrast studies are virtually mandatory. Pneumoencephalography is more informative than ventriculography, but ventriculography is often preferred when intracranial pressure is increased. Cerebrospinal fluid examination often should be deferred until it can be combined with the definitive air contrast procedure. Cerebral angiograms are less useful than air contrast studies in megalocephaly, but the "peeling away" of the cerebral vessels from the skull may disclose subdural fluid accumulations, particularly those missed by subdural taps.

Median Facial Defects and Holoprosencephaly (Arhinencephaly)

The holoprosencephalies are a teratologic series of graded severity, characterized by median malformations of the face and brain (Fig. 6). The unifying factor in this series is that the prosencephalon fails, in whole or in part, to undergo median cleavage into cerebral hemispheres or to form lobes. This holistic or *holo*-prosencephalon has a single-chambered ventricle and usually lacks olfactory bulbs and tracts.

Median facial anomalies consist of orbital hypotelorism in combination with a flat nose or proboscis, and oral deformities, such as a median cleft of the lip and palate. Some have trigonocephaly (a sharply pointed, keel-shaped forehead), and almost all are microcephalic. The crista galli, ethmoid, vomer, nasal, and premaxillary bones are absent or hypoplastic.

The unity of the median faciocerebral defects is explained by the role of prechordal mesoderm. This mesoderm normally gives rise to the median facial bones which are absent or hypoplastic in holoprosencephaly. Furthermore, by embryonic induction, this mesoderm determines not only the differentiation of the ectoderm as neural tissue but also its morphogenesis into lobated hemispheres.

According to the severity and pattern of median facial anomalies, at least five types of facies can be recognized which are pathognomonic of and predict the malformed brain. The facies are shown in Figure 6 arranged in order of decreasing severity. At the less severe end of the spectrum, when absence of the olfactory bulbs and tracts is the only brain abnormality, the face may have no obvious median defects; some of these subjects are eunuchoids.

The clinical diagnosis can be made from the pathognomonic facies, which are strikingly similar from patient to patient. Indispensable to the clinical diagnosis is orbital hypotelorism, as measured on posteroanterior skull radiographs, but one or more of the other median facial defects as detected clinically or radiographically must be present to distinguish the hypotelorism of holoprosencephaly from other conditions with *microcrania*. In categories A through D, the brain volume often is much smaller than the intracranial space, permitting transillumination of the head. The EEG records little or no electrical activity over the areas of transillumination but elsewhere shows repetitive seizure discharges.

The cause of holoprosencephaly is unknown. Most reported cases are regarded as sporadic, but familial cases occur. Some holoprosencephalics have 13/15 trisomy, others a 46-chromosome karyotype. The 13/15 trisomy patients usually have multiple extracephalic malformations, such as polydactyly, while the patients with 46 chromosomes usually have few or no extracephalic anomalies, although exceptions occur. The face predicts the malformed brain irrespective of karyotype or extracephalic anomalies.

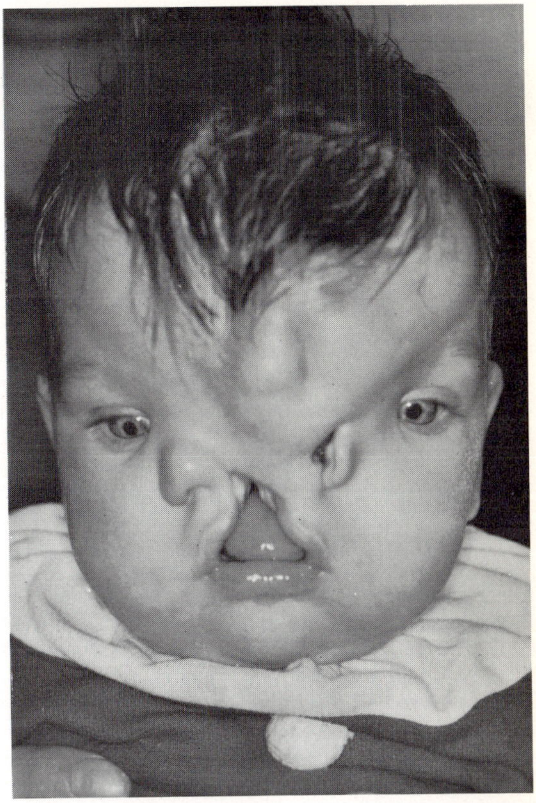

Fig. 7. Typical facies of median cleft face syndrome, consisting of median cleft lip, bifid nose, hypertelorism, and frontal encephalocele.

Median Cleft Face Syndrome: Hypertelorism, Median Cleft Lip, and Frontal Encephalocele

The stereotyped, stylized facies of holoprosencephaly should not be confused with another pattern of median facial defects consisting of frontal meningoencephalocele, orbital *hyper*telorism, a bifid nose, and a median cleft of the lip (Fig. 7). In spite of the grotesque facies, these patients often are mentally normal or only mildly retarded. As in holoprosencephaly these patients also can be arranged into a teratologic series of graded severity. The least severe degree of this defect is a simple median notch in the nose or upper lip. As listed by Waardenburg, hypertelorism is associated with a number of other syndromes.

Hydranencephaly

In this congenital malformation, the cerebral hemispheres are missing or have huge, complete, symmetric defects in the cerebral wall because of either intrauterine destruction, malformation, or possibly severe increased intracranial pressure which has run its course before birth. The skull and scalp are well formed, distinguishing hydranencephaly from anencephaly, encephaloceles, and other dysraphic lesions. Most cases are sporadic.

In contrast to holoprosencephaly, most patients have no facial or extracephalic malformations pointing to the brain defect. The disorder may not be suspected in the young infant until he fails to show psychomotor progress, has seizures, or has spastic quadriplegia. Most patients die in infancy, but some survive for years.

The head may be small, normal, or, in some instances, may enlarge rapidly. In young infants, the head always transilluminates brightly, as in Figure 5. An air bubble placed through the anterior fontanel can be traced around the inner table of the skull on radiographs. Angiograms show attenuated vessels. In hydranencephaly the EEG shows little or no electrical activity, except over local remnants of cortex. In hydrocephalus with preserved cortex, where the head transilluminates brightly because of the extremely thin cerebral wall, the EEG shows generalized activity.

Agenesis of the Corpus Callosum

The corpus callosum is a large bundle of nerve fibers which connect the cortex of one cerebral hemisphere with the other. It is formed as the axons from cortical neurons of each cerebral hemisphere reach the midline, decussate, and grow to the opposite cerebral cortex. There the fibers synapse with the cortical areas which are a mirror image of their own area of origin. As these fibers accumulate at the midline, they form the corpus callosum. Agenesis or hypoplasia of the corpus callosum occurs if the fibers fail to grow out, are destroyed, or are prevented from crossing. When the fibers have reached the midline and fail to decussate, they pile up along the ventricular wall.

Although experimental studies show that the corpus callosum normally mediates interhemispheric transfer of information (and also may mediate interhemispheric propagation of some seizure discharges), there is no characteristic neurologic deficit or bedside test for agenesis. Air encephalography is the only way to make the diagnosis. If simple nondecussation of the corpus callosum fibers is the sole brain lesion, the individual may lead an apparently normal life. More commonly, agenesis of the corpus callosum is associated with other malformations, such as heterotopias, holoprosencephaly, or destructive lesions. In these patients, the neurologic deficits reflect the associated brain lesions.

Most cases of agenesis of the corpus callosum are discovered incidentally when air contrast procedures are done to elucidate a neurologic problem such as mental deficiency, epilepsy, or cerebral palsy. In the pure cases of agenesis of the corpus callosum, the ventricular shadows in posteroanterior pneumoencephalograms have a pathognomonic "bat-wing" outline. In other cases of agenesis or hypoplasia of the corpus callosum, the cerebrum may have only a single ventricle.

Hydrocephalus

ERNEST S. MATHEWS, JOSEPH RANSOHOFF, and FRED J. EPSTEIN

Hydrocephalus is a pathologic condition characterized by an increased volume of cerebrospinal fluid (CSF) which is or has been under increased pressure. Almost without exception the fluid accumulates in the ventricular system as a result of distal obstruction in the normal cerebrospinal fluid circulation. When the condition develops prior to fusion of the cranial sutures, it produces enlargement of the head which may reach extreme proportions.

Hydrocephalus attracted the attention of early physicians and was well described by Hippocrates. Although modern theories are based largely on the classical studies of Dandy and Blackfan, concepts of the physiology of the cerebrospinal fluid have undergone considerable modifications.

CEREBROSPINAL FLUID CIRCULATION. The anatomy of the CSF pathways can be divided into the ventricular system and the subarachnoid spaces. The paired lateral ventricles lie within each cerebral hemisphere and connect via the foramina of Monro to the midline third ventricle. This in turn connects via the aqueduct of Sylvius with the midline fourth ventricle of the posterior fossa. Along the floor of each lateral ventricle, in the roof of the third ventricle and in the roof and lateral recesses of the fourth ventricle, lies an outpouching of highly vascularized pia with a modified ependymal covering called the choroid plexus.

The subarachnoid space lies between the arachnoid membrane, which follows the inner surface of the dura mater, and the pial membrane, which hugs the contours of the brain and spinal cord surfaces. In certain areas, especially at the base of the brain, the subarachnoid space is enlarged into lakes or cisterns (cisterna magna, basalis, chiasmaticus). The ventricular system connects with the subarachnoid spaces via the medial foramen of Magendie at the outlet of the fourth ventricle and the lateral foramina of Luschka. Along the large venous sinuses in the dura, outpouchings of arachnoid villi form a unidirectional valvar system being composed of a labyrinth of small tubules which establish open connections between the subarachnoid spaces and the venous channels.

It is generally accepted that the CSF is formed mainly within the ventricular system, approximately 50 percent from the choroid plexus and 50 percent from the cerebral capillaries. The choroid plexus actively secretes a hypertonic sodium solution which is followed by a diffusion of water into the ventricles, maintaining a normal osmotic pressure. The equilibrium maintained for other electrolytes and solutes, however, involves active and passive transport systems at many sites throughout the entire central nervous system. Penetration across the blood-cerebrospinal fluid barrier is highly specific for the substance involved and in disease states may vary considerably from the normal.

In an overall sense, the circulation of CSF is a unidirectional flow from the ventricular system to the posterior fossa foramina into the cisterns and subarachnoid spaces. A significant percentage of the fluid is reabsorbed into the bloodstream via the arachnoid villi in the venous sinuses. The generating force for this flow is in part derived from the arterial pulsation of the choroid plexuses and perhaps that of other large arteries at the base of the brain. In addition, absorption is probably also dependent on the CSF pressure being greater than the intracranial venous pressure.

PATHOGENESIS. There are three possible mechanisms for the development of hydrocephalus. One is an obstruction of the cerebrospinal fluid pathways within the ventricular system (e.g., foramen of Monro or aqueduct of Sylvius) or in the subarachnoid pathways (e.g., tentorial incisura) with secondary dilation of the channels proximal to the site of obstruction. The second is defective absorption of the cerebrospinal fluid at the subarachnoid level, especially over the convexities of the brain at the level of the arachnoid villi. A third but rare contributing factor is the occurrence of a choroid plexus tumor which results in the overproduction of cerebrospinal fluid with secondary dilation of the ventricular system and all associated subarachnoid pathways.

When the block is within the ventricular system, the process has been designated as "obstructive hydrocephalus"; the term "communicating hydrocephalus" is applied to cases in which the site of blockage is in the subarachnoid pathways. Strictly speaking, however, all hydrocephalus is obstructive. It would seem preferable to discard the older terms in favor of more accurate descriptions of the site and nature of the obstruction, such as intraventricular or extraventricular.

ETIOLOGY. The three major causes of hydrocephalus are neoplasms, congenital malformations, and posttraumatic or postinflammatory lesions.

Neoplasms are seldom encountered in the neonatal period but may develop at any time thereafter. The most common sites of neoplasms of infancy and childhood which produce hydrocephalus are gliomas located in the third ventricle, in the periaqueductal region, or in the fourth ventricle and the cerebellum.

Developmental anomalies are present in a number of children with hydrocephalus. Spina bifida with meningomyelocele is often associated with Arnold-Chiari type II hindbrain malformation. In this type of malformation there are elongation of the lower brainstem and caudal displacement of the fourth ventricle into the upper cervical canal, and at the inferior tip of the fourth ventricle there is a small knuckle of medulla suggesting a buckling effect at this site. This impaction of the posterior fossa structures down through the foramen magnum with associated adhesive arachnoidal thickening and subsequent blockage of the cerebrospinal fluid pathways may finally result in ventricular dilation.

Stenosis of the aqueduct of Sylvius or "forking" of the aqueduct produces early, severe hydrocephalus (Fig. 8), resulting from the inability of this narrowed structure to carry the amount of cerebrospinal fluid which is normally produced. It can also appear secondary to progressive periaqueductal gliosis, with symptoms and signs occurring at any age during childhood, in adolescence, or even in adult life. These patients experience an overgrowth of fibrillary subependymal neurolgia which constricts or even occludes what apparently was once a normal aqueduct. Some cases follow obstruction of the aqueduct by a blood clot, with subsequent organization.

Occasionally described are congenital septa or membranes occluding the outlets of the fourth ventricle (Dandy-Walker syndrome). When these outlets of the fourth ventricle are obstructed, a huge cyst develops in the posterior fossa displacing the cerebellar hemispheres to either side and resulting in a dysgenesis of the cerebellar vermis and associated elevation of the tentorium. This condition may not be truly congenital but may be the result of inflammatory processes, as suggested by the fact that these patients often have obliterated basilar cisterns as well; hence, simple opening of this membranous cavity into the subarachnoid pathways of the spinal canal does not always relieve the hydrocephalus. However, opening of the septa which may occur at the rostral end of the fourth ventricle usually results in the relief of hydrocephalus.

Probably the most frequent cause of hydrocephalus is postinflammatory or posttraumatic obstruction of the basilar cisterns and associated subarachnoid pathways, particularly in the region of the tentorium. There may be intracranial bleeding at the time of birth or episodes of meningitis in the perinatal or neonatal period which go unrecognized. These processes lead to progressive fibrosis of the arachnoidal pathways at the base of the brain, which eventually obliterate the routes of the extraventricular circulation and absorption of the cerebrospinal fluid. Cysticercosis, toxoplasmosis, and other parasitic infections may produce ventricular or subarachnoid obstruction. Gradual arrest of the hydrocephalic picture theoretically results from the reopening of these channels when they have not been irreversibly obliterated.

Apart from the lesions responsible for the obstruction, there are secondary changes in the brain. Pressure from the distended ventricles leads to progressive thinning of the brain, the white matter suffering greater loss or demyelinization than the gray. The layer of brain surrounding the ventricles or the "cortical mantle" is sometimes no more than 5 or 6 mm in thickness and at times the ependyma of the ventricle and the pia are actually in contact. When the ventricular system has dilated to such as extent, there is often rupture of the septum pellucidum. This extensive ventricular enlargement resembles a large sac, and at times there are areas that have ruptured into the subarachnoid space forming external cerebrospinal fluid fistulas. Attenuation of the dural venous sinuses as well as atrophy of the choroid plexuses has been seen in these extensive pathologic states. In less marked cases there is only flattening of the convolutions. Atrophic changes in ganglion cells may be observed microscopically. With this degree of enlargement of the head, the bones are often thinned, the fontanels are enlarged, and the suture margins widely separated.

CLINICAL MANIFESTATIONS. In many cases of congenital hydrocephalus the infant dies in utero. In others the process may be so far advanced before birth that cesarean section or craniotomy may be necessary before delivery is possible. In the majority of cases nothing unusual is observed at birth, or the head is only slightly larger than the normal. In

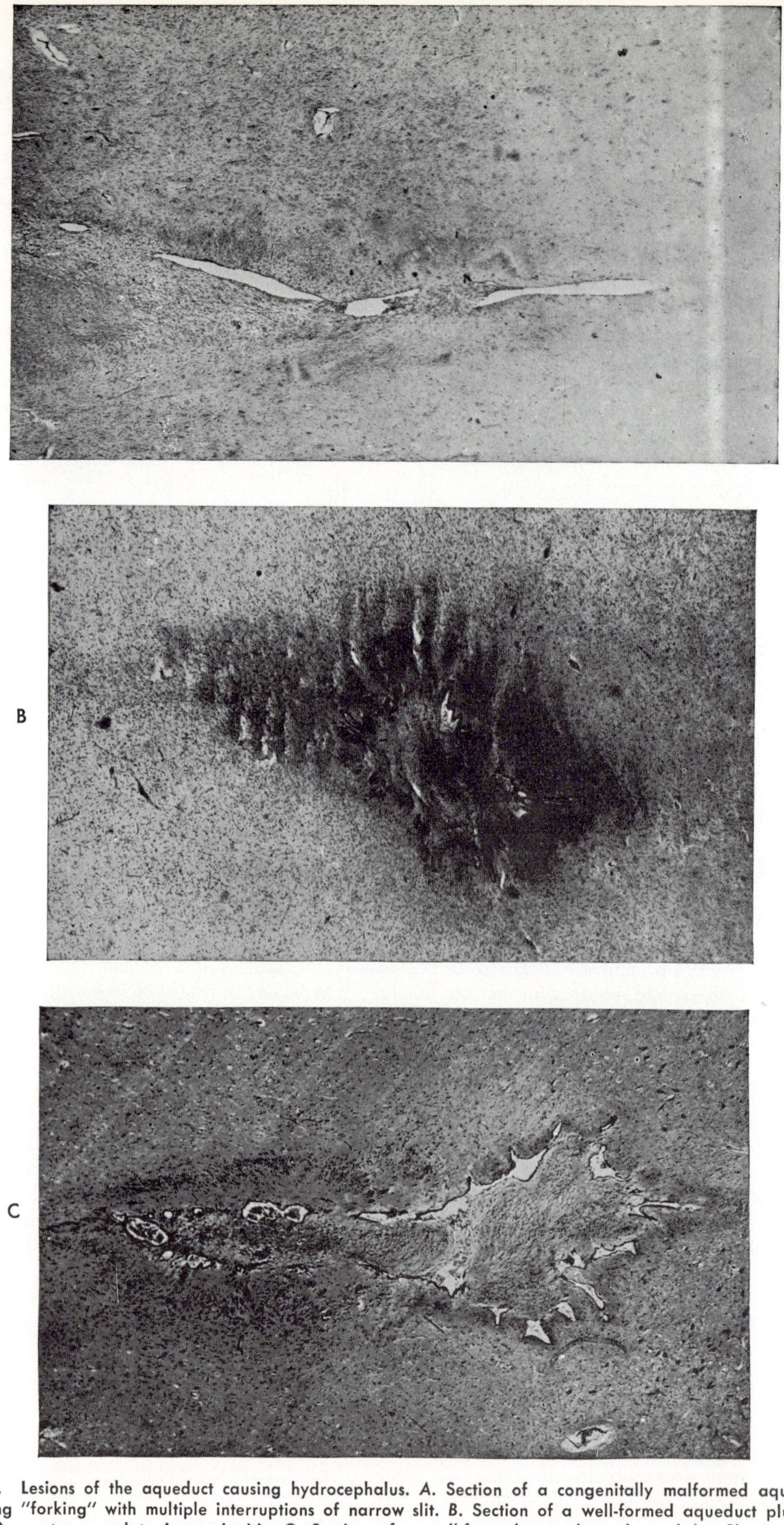

A

B

C

Fig. 8. Lesions of the aqueduct causing hydrocephalus. *A.* Section of a congenitally malformed aqueduct showing "forking" with multiple interruptions of narrow slit. *B.* Section of a well-formed aqueduct plugged by inflammatory exudate in meningitis. C. Section of a well-formed aqueduct plugged by fibrous tissue probably representing organization of an old intraventricular blood clot. (Courtesy of Dr. F. R. Ford.)

the early weeks of life, it may be discovered that the head is increasing in size at an abnormal rate and the fontanels are enlarging. The eyes may assume a staring expression, with sclera visible above the cornea (sunset sign), and the infant may have difficulty in holding up his head. Scalp veins are prominent, and the forehead becomes overhanging in appearance. There is a disproportion in size between the large cranial vault and the normal face. As a rule the capacity of the head to expand with increased intracranial pressure protects the eyes. Although the orbits may be shallow and the globes depressed in relation to the slits, vision usually remains unimpaired, and the eyegrounds fail to show evidence of papilledema. In severe, chronic cases optic atrophy may be found. Strabismus when observed is secondary to sixth nerve paresis. Neurologic examination may show no abnormalities except for delayed ability to hold up the head and other developmental limitations which can be explained entirely by the abnormal weight of the cranium. In some children spasticity with confirmatory pyramidal tract signs may be observed while others may show ataxic phenomena.

In the child with decompensating hydrocephalus, signs of increased intracranial pressure may be observed, with vomiting, lethargy, and inability to gain weight.

DIAGNOSIS. In the classical case of far-advanced hydrocephalus, characterized by a large head, distended scalp veins, downward deviation of the eyes, and retarded motor milestones, one has no need for reference to charts of head circumference or other aids, for the diagnosis is obvious. In earlier cases, however, the diagnosis may be more difficult to establish.

Although the head size (occipitofrontal circumference) in comparison with the normal is of importance, repeated observations of the rate of head growth done carefully at the same level by a nonelastic steel tape are of paramount importance. Additional information can be obtained from measurements of the anterior fontanel, since active hydrocephalus does not occur in conjunction with a closing fontanel. On the other hand, if the fontanel is enlarging from month to month, additional investigations are warranted. Roentgenograms of the skull confirm the disproportion between the facial bones and the enlarged vault and may show thinning of the bone and widening of the cranial sutures.

Careful transillumination of the head carried out in a darkened room may be of value in disclosing the presence of porencephalic cysts, hydranencephaly, or elevation of the tentorium secondary to a posterior fossa cyst (Dandy-Walker syndrome). A large subdural effusion with an enlarging head must always be considered; it can be ruled out by careful subdural taps. Toxoplasmosis and rarely cytomegalic inclusion disease may result in hydrocephalus. Toxoplasma dye test on mother and child and a urine examination for cytomegalic inclusion disease should be performed routinely. The presence of bloody cerebrospinal fluid may be indicative of a vascular malformation or a choroid plexus papilloma. Papilledema suggests a neoplastic cause for the hydrocephalus. Macrocephaly may result from conditions other than hydrocephalus (p. 3).

The final diagnosis of hydrocephalus rests on ventriculography or pneumoencephalography. These studies also give some indication as to the thickness of the cortical shell. If the ventricle is not tapped at a depth of 4 cm, hydrocephalus if present is not sufficiently advanced to require treatment. It is often helpful to inject neutral phenosulfonphthalein into the ventricles and check its appearance time in the lumbar subarachnoid space by spinal puncture. If no dye appears within 20 minutes, a block may be assumed to be present between the ventricles and the spinal subarachnoid space. This condition has been referred to usually as noncommunicating hydrocephalus.

Forty to 60 cm^3 of air injected into one ventricle and subsequent "bubble" ventriculographic studies will demonstrate: (1) whether the ventricles communicate via the foramina of Monro, (2) the thickness of the cortical mantle, (3) whether there is an unsuspected midline neoplasm, and (4) whether communication exists between the ventricular system and the subarachnoid spaces (Figs. 9 and 10). At times, air injected via the lumbar route will be helpful in confirming a suspected aqueductal insufficiency. CSF obtained at the time of contrast study should be routinely examined for cells, protein, sugar, and serology.

TREATMENT. Evaluation of any medical or surgical therapy must be made against the background of the rate of spontaneous arrest and the physical and mental state of the survivors. Although some children with hydrocephalus do arrest spontaneously, with active and progressive hydrocephalus, surgery offers a better prognosis for survival and intellectual function. In the final analysis, therapeutic success would seem to depend on the careful individualized treatment of each hydrocephalic infant.

Surgical treatment for hydrocephalus is directed toward either reducing the amount of spinal fluid produced or rerouting fluid around an obstruction by a shunting procedure. Rerouting may conduct the fluid from one part of the central nervous system to another or to other body areas or cavities, where fluid is either reabsorbed or diverted to the ureter and excreted.

In 1918 Dandy proposed removal of the choroid plexus of the lateral ventricles, later modifying the operation to endoscopic electrocoagulation for the treatment of hydrocephalus. Both an open procedure, with direct exposure of the plexus through a transcortical incision, and endoscopic coagulation of the plexus are employed currently. Results with this treatment indicate an arrest in 65 to 70 percent, a case fatality rate of 10 percent, and a yield of normal children of about 25 to 30 percent. Choroid plexectomy when successful is the most satisfactory thera-

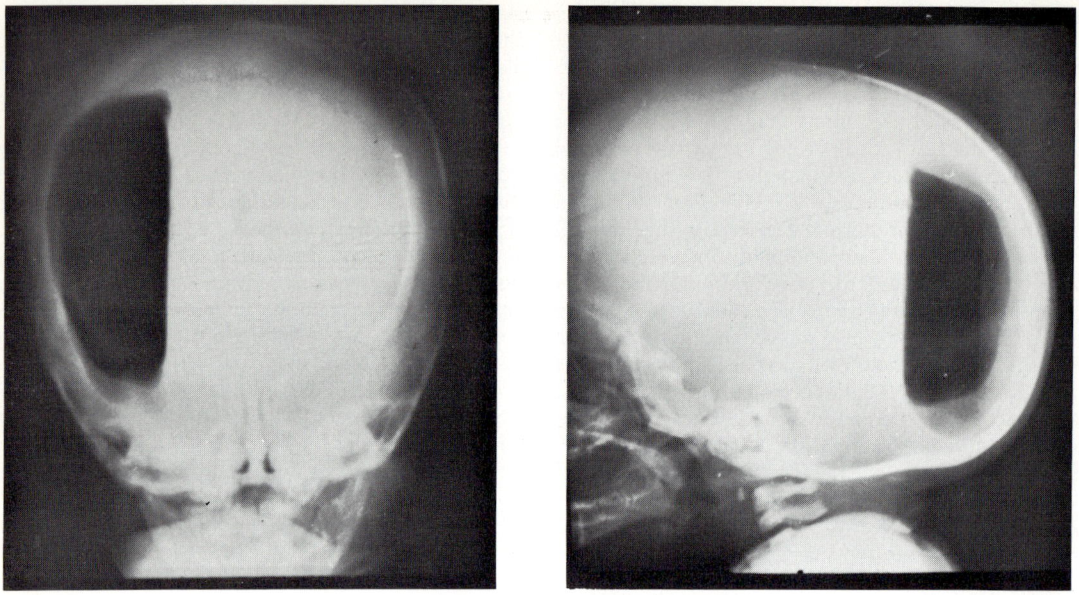

A B

Fig. 9. Bubble ventriculogram demonstrating advanced hydrocephalus. *A.* Anteroposterior view with left side of head down, showing fluid level in dilated right ventricle. *B.* Lateral view with brow down, showing posterior extent of lateral ventricles.

peutic physiologic procedure; it avoids mechanical devices, such as tubes and valves, which are prone to block, slip out of place, or separate at joints, and also secondary infection, a frequent complication.

With the advent of antibiotics and the development of the inert plastics well tolerated by the body, shunting procedures have achieved great popularity. While no single shunt is invariably successful or applicable to all patients, satisfactory results are frequently obtained. The so-called universal shunting procedures drain the lateral ventricles and are applicable to all types of hydrocephalus; draining the lumbar subarachnoid space is helpful only when the ventricles communicate with the spinal subarachnoid space.

If the obstruction is in the third ventricle, aqueduct, or fourth ventricle, the procedure described by Torkildsen in 1939 is often employed. Depending upon the patency of the foramina of Monro, a catheter is carried from one or both lateral ventricles over the occiput into the cisterna magna. No large series of ventriculocisternostomies in infants or children is available for study. The theoretical objection has been offered that the surface subarachnoid spaces are not sufficiently opened or developed in the hydrocephalic infant and therefore the procedure merely changes a noncommunicating hydrocephalus to a communicating one. In addition it is technically difficult to institute such drainage in the infant's posterior fossa because of the extreme venous vascularization of the dura in this region.

As early as 1908, attempts were made to channel cerebrospinal fluid into the great veins and into the heart. Development of competent silicone valves allowing one-way flow has finally led to a successful bypass from the ventricle into the right atrium via the jugular vein. The valve is placed either along the course of the tube system or in the cardiac end. Experience shows that, in order to avoid thrombosis, the vascular end of the shunt must lie freely in the large moving pool of blood. Therefore in this type of shunt, periodic follow-up visualization of the cardiac end of the tubing must be carried out in the growing infant to prevent retraction of the shunt from the right atrium and thrombosis of the jugular vein. It may be reasonable to carry out elective revisions in hopes of maintaining function rather than to wait for signs of active hydrocephalus and then attempt revision. This type of shunt mechanism is not without complications. Infection seems to be the most frequent complication, and the bacterium that is often involved is *Staphylococcus albus*. It is of interest to note that there may be no evidence of infection in any other part of the body. Children who have chronically been infected with the *Staphylococcus albus* organism may also show associated hepatosplenomegaly and anemia. A low-grade fever is also not an uncommon finding and despite all methods of parental antibiotic therapy, including intrathecal injection, this bacteremia can almost never be cleared unless the entire shunt is removed and replaced with a new, sterile shunt mechanism. Pulmonary hypertension may also be encountered; it is believed that microemboli arising from the right atrium embolize to the pulmonary parenchyma and occlude the smaller ramifications of the major pulmonary arteries, resulting in this pathologic condition. When the silastic tubing breaks off into the vascular pathways, the

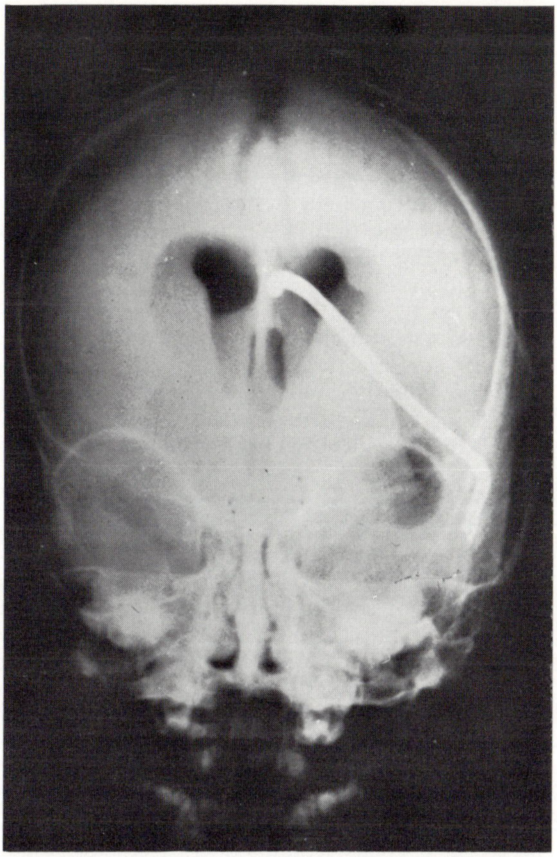

Fig. 10. Ventriculogram four months following shunting operation. The patient is the same as the one illustrated in Figure 9. Note thickening of cortical mantle in response to decompression and growth.

fragments may lodge in the ventricular wall of the heart or pass into the parenchyma of the lung. The silastic tubing may also become disconnected and migrate into the cerebral ventricle. This is not a serious complication, and the "lost" tubing can remain intraventricularly without producing any neurologic deficit.

If a kidney is sacrificed, the ureter can be used to accept a plastic or silicone rubber tube to drain the cerebrospinal fluid from the ventricle or subarachnoid space, which is then excreted with the urine. As the fluid is lost to the body economy, salt depletion may become a problem; urinary infection may, of course, lead to secondary meningitis.

The peritoneal and pleural cavities have been used as sites into which cerebrospinal fluid may be shunted, both having the advantage of being relatively sterile areas from which the fluid can be absorbed into the general circulation. Difficulties have arisen because of occlusion of the tubing due to pleural or omental reaction or due to the inability of the cavity to absorb the fluid as rapidly as it accumulates. On the other hand, these procedures have been successfully employed in a large series of patients.

As a rule, a child who has an open myelomeningocele at birth and associated hydrocephalus is not shunted primarily into the vascular system in spite of negative cultures from his ventricular fluid. A peritoneal shunt is first employed; if necessary, this can be converted later in life to a vascular or pleural shunt.

Thus, many procedures are currently utilized in the treatment of hydrocephalus. The choice of operation depends on the site of obstruction to the flow of cerebrospinal fluid as well as the experience of the group undertaking therapy. No operation is foolproof, and all require meticulous follow-up care for the life of the child.

LOW-PRESSURE HYDROCEPHALUS. In the past decade a series of reports has appeared defining a syndrome of occult or low-pressure hydrocephalus. The characteristic picture occurs in adults whose findings are those of disabling dementia with psychomotor retardation, often associated with ataxia and incontinence. This syndrome is rarely observed in children and is most frequently encountered as a complication of posterior fossa surgery. These chronically symptomatic patients have "a normal cerebrospinal fluid pressure" (180 mm or less). Pneumoencephalography reveals a communicating type of hydrocephalus without air being found over the convexities of the brain. Radioiodinated serum albumin (RISA) cisternography also confirms the diagnosis of an incisural block and probably is even more definitive in establishing the correct diagnosis. The underlying mechanism may be trauma, subarachnoid hemorrhage, or arachnoiditis secondary to infection. Shunting procedures utilizing low-pressure valves have often resulted in remarkable restoration of neurologic functions. This has also been the experience in most clinics, where the best results have been in patients in whom an episode of subarachnoid bleeding has occurred with secondary fibrosis of the subarachnoid space resulting in hydrocephalus.

Melanosis

In the normal state melanin-containing cells are present in most parts of the pia mater but are most numerous on the ventral aspect of the brain and upper cervical cord. In melanosis these cells undergo neoplastic changes and infiltrate the adjacent basal cisterna and cerebellum. Further extension may occur as a diffuse process with infiltration along the perivascular spaces of the brain and spinal cord, or rarely the melanoma cells cluster into tumor masses giving rise to localizing symptoms and signs.

CLINICAL MANIFESTATIONS. With diffuse leptomeningeal involvement, cerebrospinal fluid pathways are blocked, producing signs and symptoms of increased intracranial pressure. Irritability, nausea, vomiting, headache, papilledema, or cranial nerve palsy may be present. The spinal canal extension may be accompanied by a myeloradiculopathy. Other clinical manifestations include those of progressive

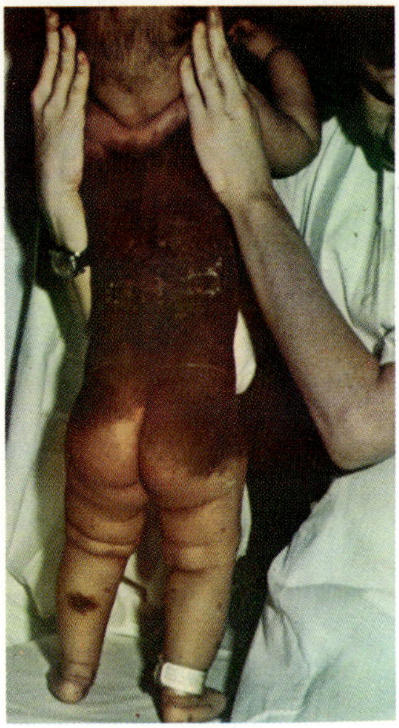

Fig. 11. Melanosis. The typical "bathing suit" nevus.

communicating hydrocephalus, posterior fossa tumor, or afebrile meningeal carcinomatous meningitis. This pathologic condition has been found in a hydrocephalic stillborn infant but may be present in any age group. Although commonly associated with giant hairy cutaneous nevi, melanosis should be regarded as a separate pathologic entity. On the other hand, when giant hairy nevi are seen in infancy, one should be alerted to the fact that the child may indeed be harboring melanosis of the leptomeninges (Fig. 11).

LABORATORY DATA. The lumbar puncture usually reveals xanthochromic spinal fluid with an elevated protein. There is an increase of white cells of various types, and in one single instance the spinal fluid was found to be "coal black" during myelography. It is not uncommon, when cytologic studies of the spinal fluid are done, to see clumps of large pleomorphic cells showing early mitosis and containing melanin.

DIAGNOSIS. The diagnosis should be suspected in the presence of the typical cutaneous nevi. Contrast air encephalography or ventriculography reveals an enlarged ventricular system secondary to a communicating hydrocephalus. When a posterior fossa tumor has been suspected and the posterior fossa explored, the typical involvement of the meninges by the process has been found.

The clinical course is usually rapid and progressive; the length of survival is greater when the spinal cord is primarily involved. The prognosis is poor, most therapy being unavailing. It is of interest that melanomas of the central nervous system, like other tumors of the central nervous system, rarely metastasize out of the confines of the cerebrospinal fluid axis, whereas malignant melanomas of the skin commonly metastasize to the brain.

Choroid Plexus Papilloma

This rare tumor has been found in the newborn but occurs most frequently in the first 2 years of life. It arises most commonly in the lateral ventricle, rarely in the third, but occasionally in the fourth ventricle with extension into the cerebellar pontine angle.

Its clinical course is insidious but may be sudden in onset, with intraventricular hemorrhage or with associated, sudden increase in intracranial pressure due to obstruction of one of the intraventricular foramina. The intraventricular location of this tumor results in the overproduction of cerebrospinal fluid with subsequent enlargement of the ventricular system as well as the subarachnoid pathways.

The tumor is histologically benign with a characteristic papillary architecture, its stroma being composed of vascularized connective tissue; it must be distinguished from the papillary ependymoma that also presents as an intraventricular tumor, but whose stroma is mainly composed of fibrillary neuroglia. It is rarely malignant but will invade local neural structures, losing the normal papillary architecture and showing obvious mitosis. The diagnosis is made from the clinical picture as well as by careful complete ventriculography in which all aspects of the ventricular system are well seen.

When the benign tumor is totally removed, the prognosis is excellent and the hydrocephalic condition arrested.

Defects of the Closure of the Neural Plate

KENNETH SHULMAN

Cranial Anomalies

ANENCEPHALY. The incidence of this catastrophic malformation ranges from 0.1 to 6.7 per thousand births, making it the most common central nervous system malformation incompatible with life. Female fetuses predominate, especially among prematures, with a ratio of between 3 and 7 to 1. The concordance rate in twins is low, identical twins approaching the incidence in fraternal twins. There is often an associated hydramnios in the mother, and the diagnosis of anencephaly can and should be made prepartum by x-ray of the hydramniotic abdomen. The fetus is either stillborn or dies a few minutes after birth, although rare instances of life lasting a few days are known.

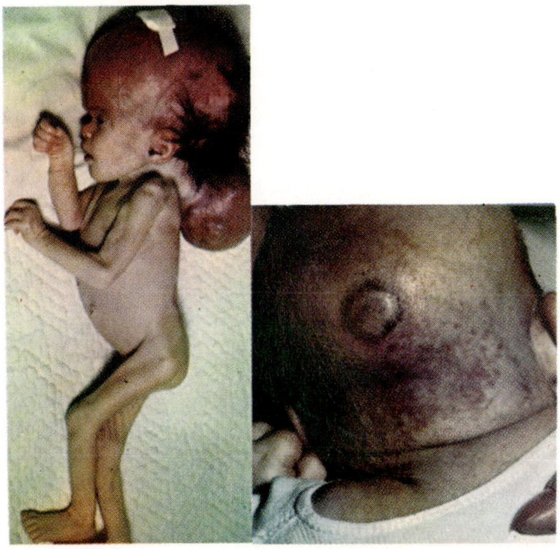

Fig. 12. ***A.*** **Large occipital encephalocele with associated hydrocephalus.** ***B.*** **Small occipital encephalocele with surrounding hemangioma.**

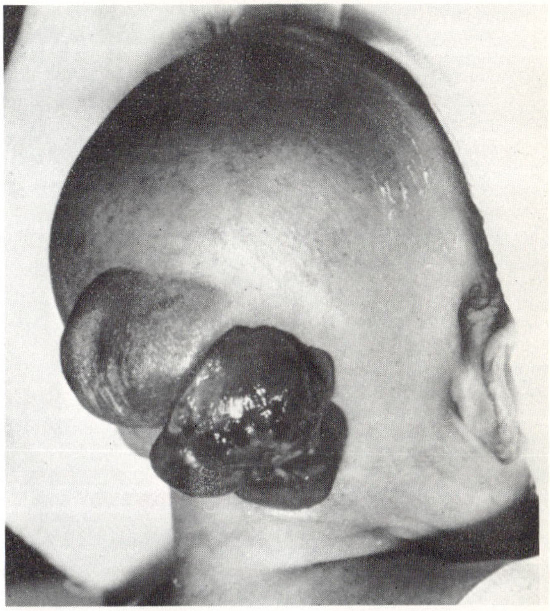

Fig. 13*A*. Newborn in posterior for surgical repair of poorly covered encephalocele containing brain tissue.

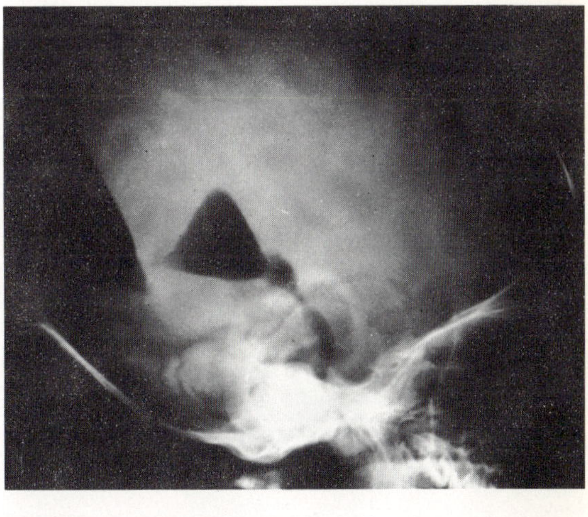

Fig. 13*B*. Ventriculogram in same child at one week after repair of encephalocele showing marked ventricular dilatation.

The pathology ranges from complete absence of the central nervous system associated with open cranium and vertebral canal, all bones of the skull vault and vertebral lamina being unfused, to the less severe defect known as hemicrania, in which the bones of the posterior skull vault, the brainstem, and the cerebellum are present. The brain remnant is pervaded with a highly vascularized stroma and covered with a thin membrane, continuous with hair-bearing skin. Choroid plexus and ependyma are usually found in the brain remnant. With poor development of the central nervous tissue, the posterior lobe of the pituitary is also absent, as are the ganglion cells of the retina. The anterior pituitary may be present, but the adrenals are usually small. Other abnormalities commonly found with anencephalus are poorly lobated lungs, a large thymus, and a high arched palate.

That the brain vesicles may develop and undergo secondary infarction due to insufficient blood during the third to fifth week of fetal life is suggested by the findings that the major arteries do not penetrate the areas of the cerebral malformation but rather are replaced by a number of abnormal branches arising from the internal carotid arteries. Experimentally, the teratogenic agent must be applied early, shortly after gastrulation, to cause anencephaly in the mouse. The cephalic end of the neuropore remains open, but the cerebral hemispheres and striatum develop and then necrose before histogenesis of the cortex has occurred.

The management of the condition involves suspicion of the disease in the hydramniotic abdomen, so that destructive procedures can be carried out if birth is delayed. Usually, the anencephalic fetus is born prematurely and presents no obstetric difficulties. Neurosurgical treatment, of course, is not indicated.

CRANIUM BIFIDUM—ENCEPHALOCELE. The term encephalocele has found wide neurosurgical usage in the description of all cystic masses associated with midline cranial closure defects (cranium bifidum); the term encompasses cranial meningocele and cranial meningoencephalocele. Whether or not brain is present within a cystic enlargement is not apparent before surgery, and more precise terminology is, therefore, not desirable. The occult form of closure defect, which is rare and not of major surgical interest, could

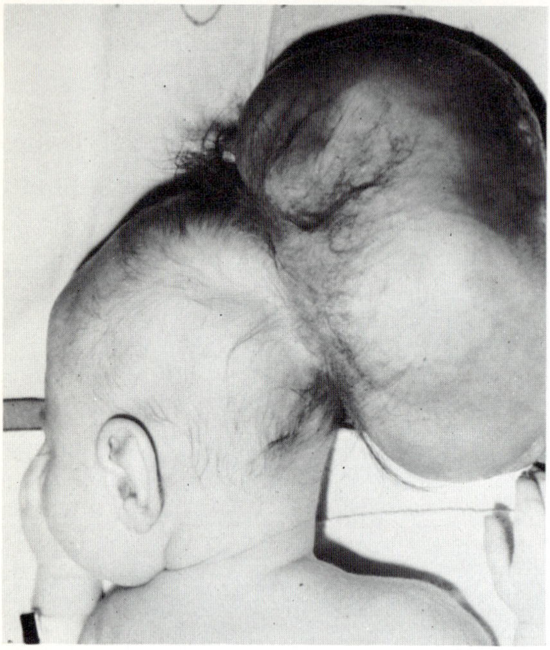

Fig. 14A. Large occipital encephalocele at 2 months of age. Because of size, surgery was inappropriately not done earlier, and contents of sac became infected with abscess formation.

be termed "cranium bifidum occulta." In the author's personal series of cases referred for neurosurgical care, encephaloceles have occurred with one-tenth the frequency of spina bifida cystica. The incidence of encephalocele has been estimated at one in every 3,000 to 10,000 live births. Occurring with greatest frequency in the occipital regions of the skull, the encephalocele is in the midline or slightly removed to one side. Those found at the anterior extreme of the skull present as nasal, nasopharyngeal, or naso-orbital masses.

Occipital Encephaloceles. Occipital encephaloceles vary in size from small pedunculated masses to those equal in size to the cranial cavity (Fig. 12). The base is usually small and well covered with non-hair-bearing skin. Those lesions with wider bases are more apt to contain significant amounts of brain tissue; and in the posterior encephaloceles there is a correlation between the amount of brain tissue within the sac and the associated anomalies of the brain residual in the cranial cavity, in a general way making overall prognosis less favorable. The most frequently associated secondary condition is hydrocephalus. Hence with sizable occipital encephaloceles one may perform a "bubble" ventriculogram prior to encephalocele repair, or before discharge after encephalocele repair, to assess the cerebrospinal fluid pathways (Fig. 13A and B). No exact relationship

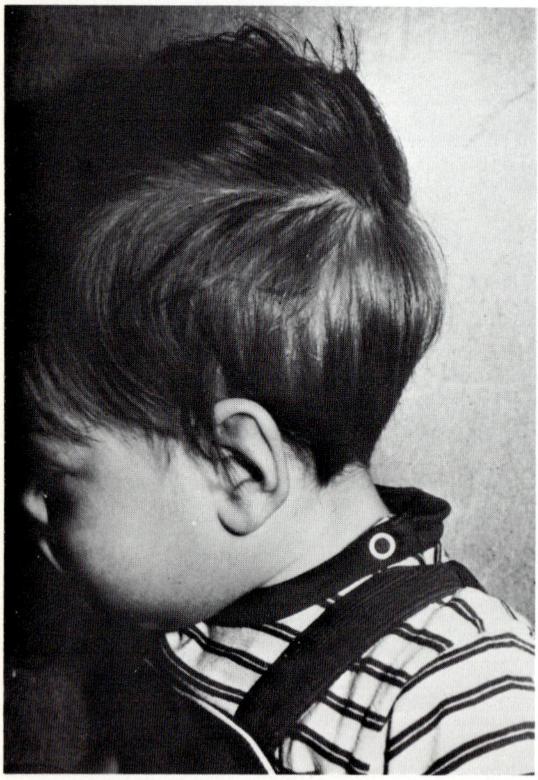

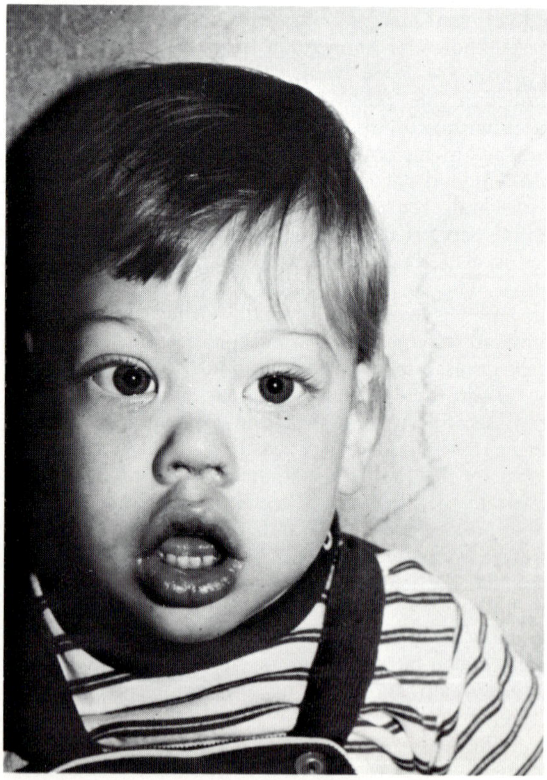

Fig. 14B and C. Same child at age 2 years. A ventriculo-atrial shunt is in place. Child has developed normally without neurologic deficit.

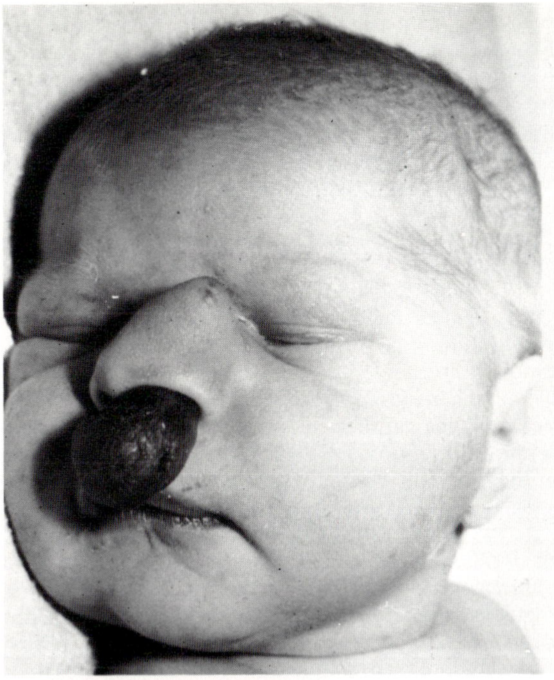

Fig. 15. Large nasal encephalocele in a newborn prior to repair by craniotomy plus nasal excision.

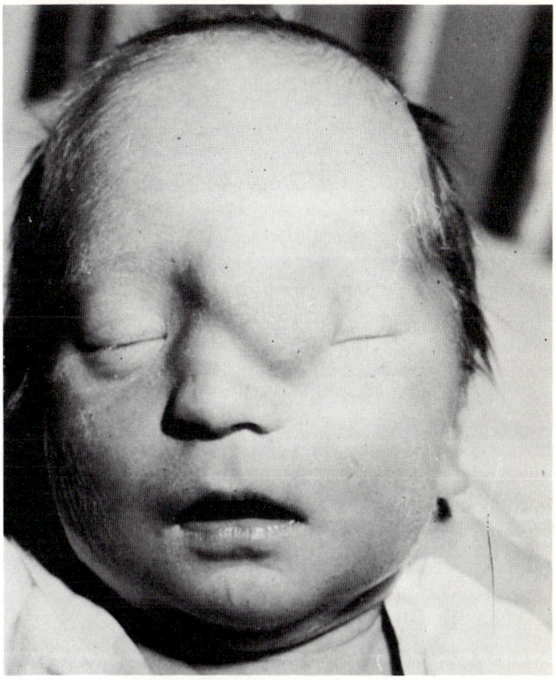

Fig. 16. Naso-orbital encephalocele in the newborn.

exists, however, between size of encephalocele and its contents. Adequate skin may cover the entire sac, or exposed brain or dura may occur at the tip of the lesion, making repair of the encephalocele an urgent matter.

Transillumination with a four-cell flashlight or a special electric lamp will often be useful in showing the contents of the sac. Skull x-rays will show the bone defect and its relation to cranial sutures and major intracranial venous sinuses.

Surgical repair of nearly all posterior encephaloceles in the newborn period is indicated in order to: (1) close over any communication through a skin defect with brain and meninges; (2) remove the mass so the child can be handled by nurses and the mother; (3) move the contents into more normal surroundings; and (4) prevent secondary skin breakdown over large encephaloceles, leading to infection and death. Surgery is well tolerated in the face-down position if care is taken to maintain the infant's temperature and replace proper amounts of blood during the procedure (Fig. 14, A, B, and C).

Because of the high incidence of hydrocephalus in infants with occipital encephaloceles, the child should be carefully observed for the signs of cerebrospinal fluid malabsorption and treated by shunting when this is diagnosed. The long-range care and prognosis will depend largely upon the success or failure in treating the hydrocephalus effectively. Moreover, a number of children will have more specific neurologic defects after encephalocele repair, especially those

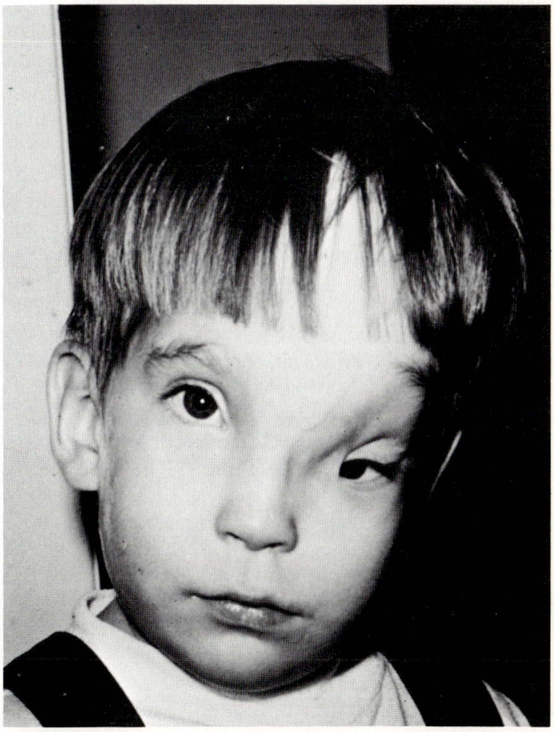

Fig. 17. Same child as in Figure 16 at 4 years of age after multiple surgical procedures with residual deformity. Left eye, however, is functional.

with a large amount of brain tissue within the sac. These deficits include blindness (occipital cortex) and incoordination (cerebellum).

Anterior Encephaloceles. Anterior encephaloceles are uncommon and comprise those that are nasofrontal, naso-orbital, or basal. The diagnosis is often quite difficult, particularly when the lesions extend into the nose and may be called polyps and biopsied, leading to catastrophic intracranial infection (Fig. 15). Encephaloceles at the nasal-orbital-cranial junction are obvious (Fig. 16) but their technical repair is often difficult. Compared with the occipital encephaloceles, the incidence of either hydrocephalus or significant associated brain anomalies is less with the anterior lesions.

Nasofrontal encephaloceles should be treated by frontal craniotomy with excision or replacement of intracranial contents, dural repair, and an attempt to fill the bony defect. Naso-orbital lesions, in which there is less risk of infection, should be repaired during the first year of life to obtain the best possible orbital alignment and cosmetic result (Fig. 17).

Spinal Anomalies

SPINA BIFIDA. Embryologically, the spinal cord develops from a thickening of the neural ectoderm, referred to as a medullary plate, in the midline of the embryo dorsally. With the proliferation of cells, the medullary plate invaginates to produce the medullary tube, which begins to close in the midline, first in the middorsal region, then at the anterior and posterior neuropores, with closure completed by the end of the fourth week. Segmentation of the medullary tube is accompanied by a separation into somites of the surrounding mesoderm, which comes to lie completely around the neural ectoderm and separates it from the ectoderm, which becomes the skin. The mesodermal segments give rise to the vertebral column, as well as the meninges and blood vessels of the spinal cord. In all forms of spina bifida, whether occulta or cystica, some part of the above process is deranged (Fig. 18). Spina bifida occulta is a condition which is fairly common and will be found in 10 percent of routine x-rays of the spine of children and adults. Although many names, such as myelodysplasia, myeloschisis, spinal dysraphism, meningocele, and meningomyelocele have been applied to the cystic form of spina bifida, it would seem that only the last two terms need be employed.

Spina Bifida Occulta. This form of spina bifida is rarely symptomatic. In a small number of children with the defect, neurologic difficulty will occur when the child is rapidly growing and the spinal cord is called upon to ascend. In such children there will be an underlying cord abnormality as the basis for the symptoms, such as dilation of the central canal (hydromyelia), a splitting of the cord (diastematomyelia, see below), or an associated congenital tumor, such as a lipoma or dermoid at the end of the cord, fixing it in the infantile position. A neurologic deficit resulting from such lesions will be noted as muscle weakness, leading to a gait disturbance, or sensory loss, resulting in trophic ulcers. Sphincter loss is not uncommon, and a child who was once toilet-trained may begin to become incontinent. Pain is usually not a feature. It is most important to investigate children who have progressive loss in these spheres by radiographs of the spine and myelography, if the former shows a defect. When progressive neurologic loss is demonstrated and a cause can be seen by the above studies, a good neurosurgical result may be expected if the lesion causing the loss can be explored and removed early or if the nerve roots of the cauda equina can be released from tension by section of the filum terminale. Aggressive preventive surgery in these lesions is usually not indicated, except when associated with a low spinal diastematomyelia.

Spina Bifida Cystica (Meningocele and Meningomyelocele). Like anencephaly, the geographic distribution and incidence varies widely in countries populated by Caucasians of similar backgrounds, with a reported incidence of 4.2 per thousand live births in Ireland, 2.8 per thousand in Buckinghamshire, and 1.5 per thousand in southeastern England. The lower socioeconomic groups seem to be more affected. Etiologic inquiries were made in 179 families and no evidence of any abnormal exogenous influence on pregnancy, such as infection, x-rays, drugs, or diet, could be elicited. It is possible, however, in all such studies that a prenatal insult sustained by the mother during her first month of gestation, and forgotten, could be of importance and not obtained by history. It has been shown in most series that the incidence of meningomyelocele in a second sib within the same family approaches 7.8 percent; and to this could be added the incidence of other congenital anomalies in siblings, a further 2.4 percent, making the risk taken by such a family in having another abnormal child considerable.

Meningocele. This is considered to be a cystic lesion in the midline of the back, containing only meninges or perhaps meninges and nerve roots, free of all central nervous tissue, well covered with skin, and unassociated with neurologic deficit. If this definition is subscribed to, meningocele comprises perhaps 10 percent of all cases of spina bifida cystica. This number may even be less, for if one excises such a lesion and examines the sac pathologically, a number that on clinical and gross pathologic examination were felt to be meningoceles will be found to contain nerve roots and spinal cord and would have to be classified as meningomyeloceles. The frequency of meningocele is about equal in the cervical, thoracic, and lumbar areas of the spine, although the incidence of spina bifida cystica is much higher in the lumbar region; thus, the chance of a lesion in the cervical or thoracic region being a meningocele is greater. As mentioned above, there may also be

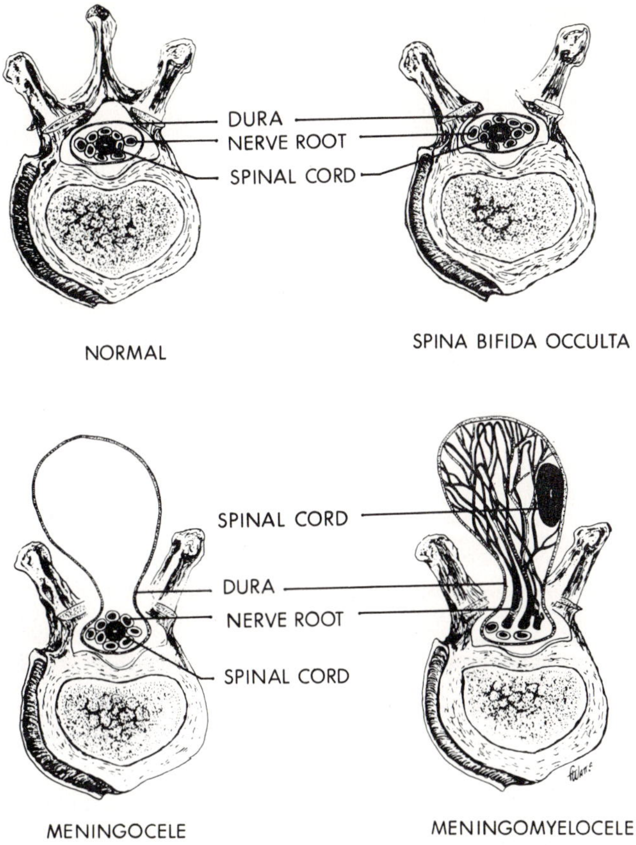

Fig. 18. The varieties of spina bifida.

associated cord abnormalities giving rise to neurologic deficit, but it is implied in the concept of meningocele that there will be no progressive neurologic symptomatology; therefore, it is advocated that the sac be closed sometime electively after the age of 3 months. By this time, a child who is destined to develop hydrocephalus will have done so, and it may be elected to treat the head enlargement prior to repair of the meningocele.

Meningomyelocele. In the meningomyelocele variety of spina bifida cystica, the neural ectoderm developing into the spinal cord and nerve roots appears to have failed to separate from the epithelium, leading to a sac containing cerebrospinal fluid, incompletely formed meninges, and malformed spinal cord. Most often, the neural plate which has failed to close is exposed in the center of the sac as a reddened, weeping area, the stroking of which may

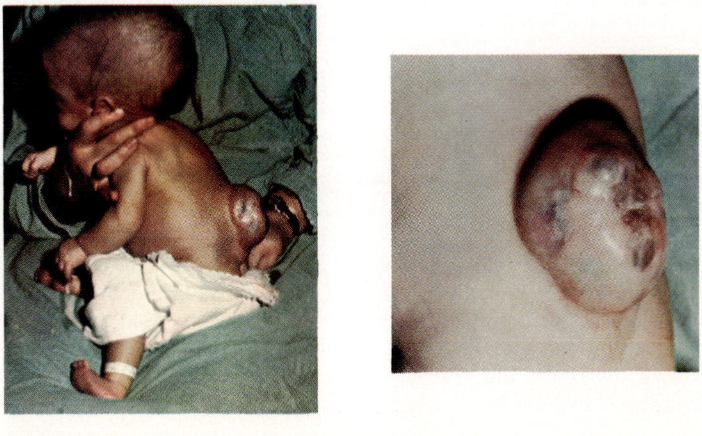

Fig. 19. ***A.*** **Meningomyelocele in lumbosacral region. Note paretic lower extremities and associated hydrocephalus.** ***B.*** **Same child. Detailed view of lesion.**

TABLE 2. *Rehabilitation Potential of the Child with Spina Bifida According to the Neurologic Level of the Defect**

Segmental Level	Motor Power	Most Frequent Acquired Deformities Due to		Prognosis for Ambulation After Growth Period	
		Muscle Imbalance	Malposition	Minimum Function	Maximum Function
T_6 to T_{12}	Upper extremities Thorax (upper trunk extensors) Abdominals (trunk flexors)		Hip flexion Hip adduction Hip abduction Knee flexion Scoliosis	Wheelchair: dependent or bedridden Needs help for transfer Gait: none	Wheelchair: partial use Transfers independently Gait: swing to or drag to Elevation: limited to low steps
L_1	Hip flexion		Hip flexion Hip adduction	Wheelchair: dependent or bedridden	Wheelchair: not needed
L_2	Hip adduction	Early hip dislocation	Hip abduction Knee flexion	Needs help for transfer	Gait: four point and swing through
L_3	Knee extension		Scoliosis Lumbar lordosis	Gait: none	Elevation: standard steps
L_4	Knee flexion Foot dorsiflexion	Hip flexion Hip adduction	Lumbar lordosis Late hip dislocation	Wheelchair: dependent Gait: limited drag to or four point	Wheelchair: not needed Gait: four point and swing through
L_5	Ankle eversion	Ankle valgus		Elevation: none	Elevation: with handrail
S_1	Plantar flexion Ankle inversion	Foot and ankle: varus	—	Wheelchair: not needed Gait: four points or alternate	Wheelchair: not needed Gait: independent walking
S_2	Hip extension	Equinus calcaneous		Elevation: independent with handrail	Elevation: independent
S_3 to S_5	Perineal musculature Sphincters			Independent	Independent

*Modified from Badell Ribera and Swinyard. 1964.

provoke involuntary movements of the legs. The sac often leaks in utero or ruptures at birth, so that cerebrospinal fluid drains freely; and it is distinctly unusual to have anything resembling normal skin covering the mass. The leakage of the cerebrospinal fluid with a threat of ascending meningitis makes immediate surgical closure of the defect the treatment of choice. Meningomyelocele is distinctly most common in the lumbosacral region (Fig. 19, A and B). In addition to the exposed, dysplastic neural plate, the spinal cord above often shows abnormalities, such as hydromyelia, diastematomyelia, or syrinx formation. Rarely, meningomyelocele may present ventral to the vertebra, as a pelvic mass which gives rise to symptoms of bowel obstruction.

By definition, some neurologic deficit will be present in the limbs and cutaneous areas below the mass. It is only in the sacral meningomyeloceles below the exit of the lumbosacral plexus that the lower extremities may be normal, with the loss being in the saddle area and in the sphincters. Such loss is detected in the newborn by dribbling of urine during crying and the inability to initiate a urinary stream in the male. A child with a lumbosacral meningomyelocele will most commonly present with reasonably good movements at the hips and knees with paralyzed ankles, the feet inverted and held in the position of equinovarus. Finally, if the mass is thoracolumbar, the legs may be flaccid, the lower abdominal musculature poorly developed so that the abdomen is protruberant, the hips will be congenitally dislocated, and there will be cutaneous and sphincter involvement.

The leaking meningomyelocele sac has certain

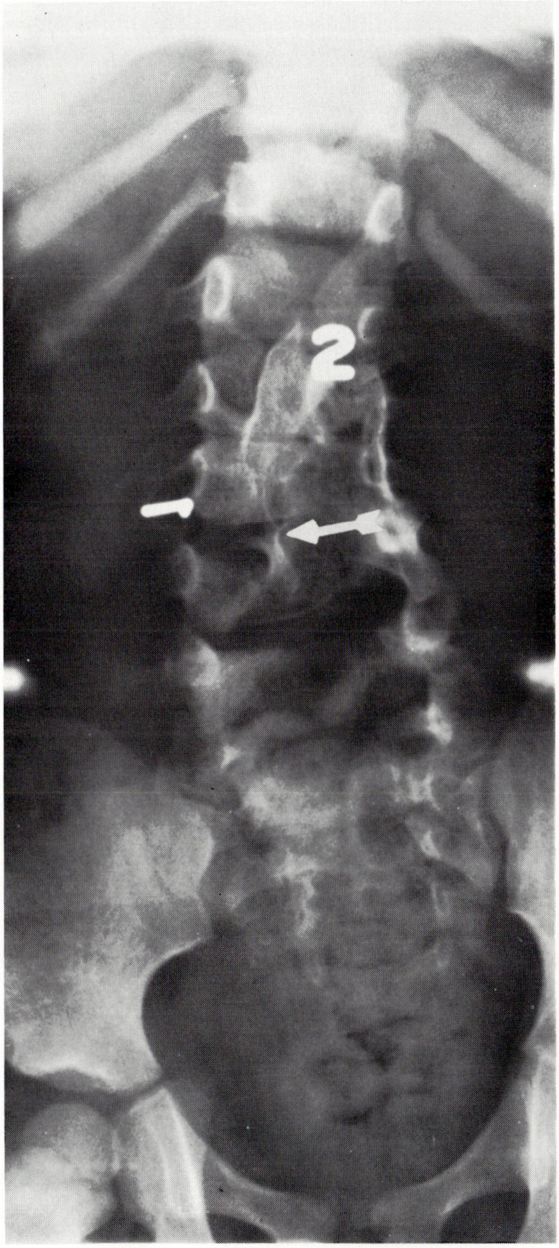

Fig. 20. Diastematomyelia. Plain radiograph showing bony spicule (arrow).

powers of recovery and repair, stimulated partly, at least, by granulation tissue response to infection. This inflammatory fibrosis leads to scarring and permanent loss of neural function. This threat to function, plus the possibility of ascending infection if the sac is not closed, suggests that ideal treatment is closure as soon after birth as possible. If, indeed, it can be shown that neurologic function can be improved by such early closure, such surgery would be

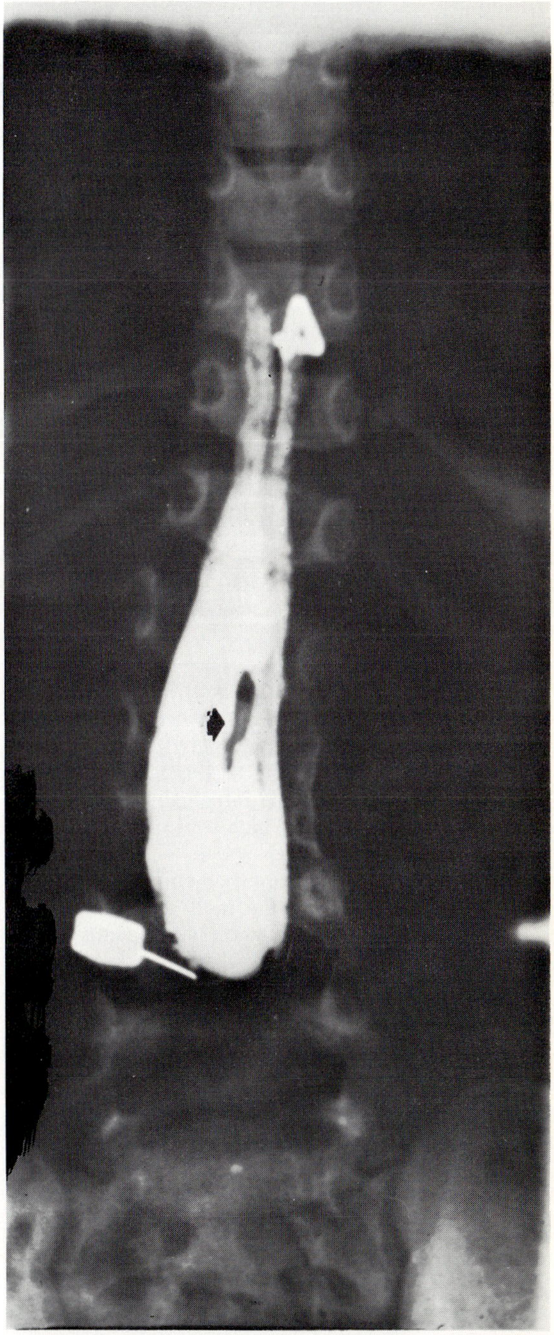

Fig. 21. Diastematomyelia. Myelogram (same child as in Figure 20) demonstrating level of spicule and splitting of cord.

even more justified. This has recently been demonstrated in a series of children by Sharrard et al. Such return of neurologic function is probably due to the prevention of stretching of the neural plate by underlying accumulation of fluid or pus, or by the biochemical alterations associated with drying of the

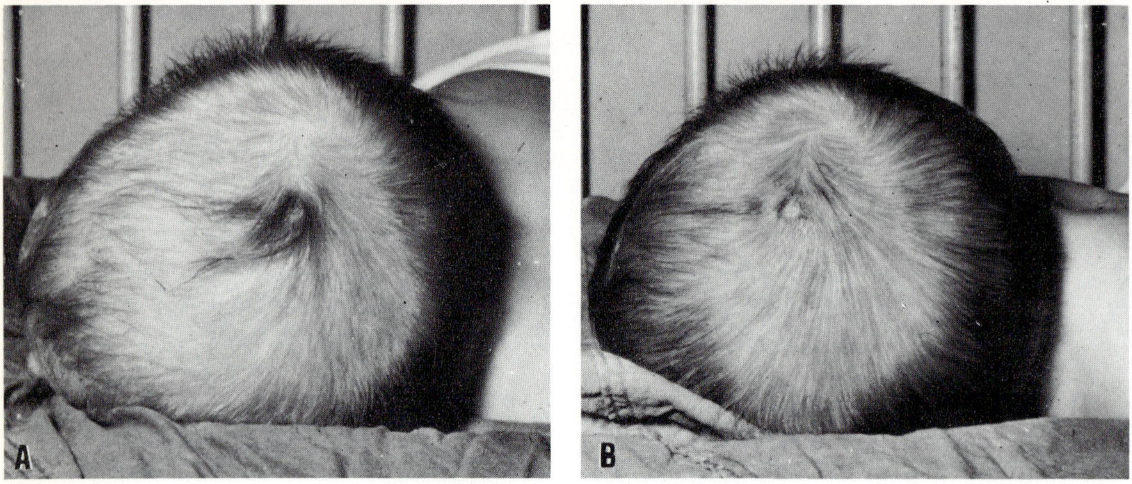

Fig. 22. Occipital dermal sinus. Child with recurrent meningitis. *A*. Head unshaven, sinus not readily apparent. *B*. Same child. Head shaven and sinus readily apparent.

neural plate. It may also be due, however, to a return of function residual in the neural plate, which has been lost upon birth because of trauma to the plate during delivery. In addition, early resolute surgical therapy seems justified in view of the natural history of children with meningomyelocele, which indicates that if the infant survives to 3 months of age, he has a 35 percent chance of living to the age of 12 years. Such children, if untreated, may well survive with neurologic loss which could have been prevented.

The paralysis secondary to meningomyelocele is part of the basic disease; the most serious complication of the disease is hydrocephalus. This occurs because of malformations within the brain, most commonly the Arnold-Chiari hindbrain malformation, and because of obliteration of the subarachnoid pathways by ascending infection secondary to an open cerebrospinal fluid fistula at the site of the meningomyelocele. Since better methods of treating the hydrocephalus are now available, many more normal children are being salvaged, and more rigorous therapy can be applied to the back defect.

It is the author's current philosophy, therefore, for the reasons stated above, that all meningomyeloceles be repaired as soon after birth as possible, regardless of the neurologic function of the child or the clinical indication of the hydrocephalus at this time, unless the child be afflicted with other congenital malformations which will limit life. Kidney and bladder function are evaluated radiographically, the legs placed in casts, if needed, and early ventriculography performed. Hydrocephalus is treated with a ventriculojugular shunt during the initial hospitalization. Patients are sent home on sulfisoxazole therapy and followed monthly by the neurosurgeon, orthopedist, urologist, and rehabilitation specialist at a birth defects center. The long-term rehabilitation potential of such children is shown in Table 2. With such a program, 80 percent of the children reach 3 years of age, and the developmental quotient is normal in 60 percent of the survivors.

DIASTEMATOMYELIA. In this condition, the spinal cord is divided into two halves, each of which may undergo modification of structure. It is most common in the lumbar and midthoracic areas. The two cords are separated by a fibrous or bony spicule, which can often be seen on x-ray (Fig. 20). Each half of the divided cord has its own pial investment, but the arachnoid and dura may be shared. Neurologic symptoms are produced in children because of the different rates of elongation of the spinal cord and vertebral column, with increasing pressure of the spur upon the ascending spinal cord with growth. Symptoms progressively develop, usually at about the age of 4 years or later. Therefore, diagnosis of diastematomyelia in the low thoracic or lumbar area is an indication for prophylactic surgery in a young child, to prevent the development of neurologic symptoms. Operations in older children with lesions at a higher level, where the ascent of the cord is not so great, are more questionable, unless progressive neurologic symptoms develop. Myelography (Fig. 21) is indicated prior to surgery. The operative results are generally good; and if there is a question, exploratory laminectomy is warranted, because of the low risk of harming the patient with careful surgery.

DERMAL SINUS. Dermal sinus tracts may occur at any place along the spinal axis but are most common in the lumbosacral area. They result developmentally from a failure of the neural ectoderm to separate from the skin ectoderm with a sinus tract covered by epithelial tissue, leading down to or through the dura. There may or may not be a spina bifida occulta on radiographs of the spine. Sinuses should be looked for in all children with recurrent, unexplained meningitis. If a sinus tract is found, it should be excised with preparations made for laminectomy and intradural exploration, if necessary. When possible, sinus tracts should be excised prior to infection, for once infection has taken place, the scarring around the intradural contents of the sinus is extreme and enhances the difficulty of the surgery.

In addition to spinal dermal sinuses, cranial dermal sinuses may occur at any place in the midline of the skull and scalp but are most common in the occipital region. The tracts, which appear as defects in the midline in the occipital bone, are directed obliquely and have hyperostosis around the bone edges (Fig. 22A and B). Prophylactic excision of such sinus tracts is indicated to prevent intracranial suppuration and abscess formation. It is advisable to study the child with pneumoencephalography prior to excision of the sac to determine whether there is intracranial extension, which should be surgically excised if it exists. A normal air study does not rule out intracranial extension, which can be explained by the fact that the brain and cyst are formed and developed over the same period of time, with the cerebral tissue not being displaced by the cyst, but merely failing to develop in the region.

REFERENCES

BRAIN

DeMyer, W. Technique of the Neurologic Examination: A Programmed Text. New York, McGraw-Hill Book Co., 1969.

Dodge, P., and Porter, P. Demonstration of intracranial pathology by transillumination. Arch. Neurol., 5:594, 1961.

Gorlin, R., and Pindborg, J. Syndromes of the Head and Neck. New York, McGraw-Hill Book Co., 1964.

Leiber, B., and Olbrich, G. Die Klinischen Syndrome. München/Berlin, Urban & Schwarzenberg, 1966.

Nellhaus, G. Head circumference from birth to eighteen years. Pediatrics, 41:106, 1968.

O'Neill, E. M. Normal head growth and the prediction of head size in infantile hydrocephalus. Arch. Dis. Child., 36:241, 1961.

——— Minimal rates of head growth in the first four months of life. Arch. Dis. Child., 37:415, 1962.

MICROCEPHALY

Book, J., Schut, J., and Reed, S. A clinical and genetical study of microcephaly. Amer. J. Ment. Defic., 57:637, 1952.

Bray, P., Shields, W., Wolcott, G., and Madsen, J. Occipitofrontal head circumference—an accurate measure of intracranial volume. J. Pediat., 75:303, 1969.

Davies, H., and Kirman, B. Microcephaly. Arch. Dis. Child., 37:623, 1962.

Greenfield, J. G., et al. Neuropathology. Baltimore, Williams & Wilkins Co., 1963.

Pryor, H., and Thelander, H. Abnormally small head size and intellect in children. J. Pediat., 73:593, 1968.

Winick, M., and Rosso, P. Head circumference and cellular growth of the brain in normal and marasmic children. J. Pediat., 74:774, 1969.

MEGALOCEPHALY AND MEGALENCEPHALY

Dennis, J., Rosenberg, H., and Alvord, E., Jr. Megalencephaly, internal hydrocephalus and other neurological aspects of achondroplasia. Brain, 84:427, 1961.

Ford, F. Diseases of the Nervous System in Infancy, Childhood and Adolescence, 5th ed. Springfield, Ill., Charles C Thomas Co., 1966.

Hook, E., and Reynolds, J. Cerebral gigantism: Endocrinological and clinical observations of six patients including a congenital giant, concordant monozygotic twins, and a child who achieved adult gigantic size. J. Pediat., 70:900, 1967.

Salmon, J., and Flanigan, S. Megalencephaly, a clinical study with chromosomal analysis. J. Neurosurg., 21: 409, 1964.

MEDIAN FACIAL DEFECTS AND HOLOPROSENCEPHALY (ARHINENCEPHALY)

Currarino, G., and Silverman, F. Orbital hypotelorism, arhinencephaly, and trigonocephaly. Radiology, 74: 206, 1960.

DeMyer, W., and White, P. EEG in holoprosencephaly (arhinencephaly). Arch. Neurol., 11:507, 1964.

——— Zeman, W., and Palmer, C. G. Familial alobar holoprosencephaly (arhinencephaly) with median cleft lip and palate. Report of a patient with 46 chromosomes. Neurology, 13:913, 1963.

——— Zeman, W., and Palmer, C. G. The face predicts the brain: diagnostic significance of median facial anomalies in holoprosencephaly (arhinencephaly). Pediatrics, 34:256, 1964.

Potter, E. Pathology of the Fetus and Newborn. Chicago, Year Book Publishers, 1952.

Yakovlev, P. Pathoarchitectonic studies of cerebral malformations. III. Arhinencephalies (holotelencephalies). J. Neuropath. Exp. Neurol., 18:22, 1959.

MEDIAN CLEFT FACE SYNDROME: HYPERTELORISM, MEDIAN CLEFT LIP, AND FRONTAL ENCEPHALOCELE

DeMyer, W. The median cleft face syndrome. Neurology, 17:961, 1967.

Waardenburg, P., Fanceschetti, A., and Klein, D. Genetics in Ophthalmology. Springfield, Ill., Charles C Thomas Publ., 1961, 1963, Vol. I, Vol. II.

HYDRANENCEPHALY

Farmer, T. W., ed. Pediatric Neurology. New York, Harper & Row, 1964.

Hamby, W. B., Krauss, R. F., and Beswick, W. F. Hydranencephaly: Clinical diagnosis. Presentation of seven cases. Pediatrics, 6:371, 1950.

Poser, C. M., Walsh, F. C., and Schneinberg, L. C. Hydranencephaly. Neurology, 5:284, 1955.

AGENESIS OF THE CORPUS CALLOSUM

Carpenter, M. B. Agenesis of the corpus callosum. A study of 18 cases diagnosed during life. Neurology, 4:200, 1954.

Koch, F., and Doyle, P. Agenesis of the corpus callosum. J. Pediat., 50:345, 1957.

Mountcastle, V., ed. Interhemispheric Relations and Cerebral Dominance. Baltimore, Johns Hopkins Press, 1962.

HYDROCEPHALUS

Adams, R. D., Fisher, C. M., Hakim, S., Ojemann, R. G., and Sweet, W. H. Symptomatic occult hydrocephalus with "normal" cerebrospinal fluid pressure. A treatable syndrome. New Eng. J. Med., 273:117, 1965.

Bering, E. A., Jr. Dynamics of cerebrospinal fluid. Clin. Neurosurg., 5:77, 1958.

——— Circulation of the cerebrospinal fluid, demonstration of the choroid plexuses as the generator of the force of flow of fluid and ventricular enlargement. J. Neurosurg., 19:405, 1962.

——— Hydrocephalus: changes in CSF in ventricles. J. Neurosurg., 20:1050, 1963.

Bouton, J. Primary melanoma of the leptomeninges. J. Clin. Path., 11:122, 1958.

Bowsher, D. A. A Possible Mechanism of Hydrocephalus. Ciba Foundation Symposium on the Cerebrospinal Fluid. Boston, Little, Brown and Co., 1958, p. 282.

Bruce, A. M., Lorber, J., Shedden, W. I. H., and Zachary, R. B. Persistent bacteraemia following ventriculo-caval shunt operations for hydrocephalus in infancy. Develop. Med. Child Neurol., 5:461, 1963.

Dandy, W. E., and Blackfan, K. D. Internal hydrocephalus, an experimental, clinical and pathological study. Amer. J. Dis. Child., 8:406, 1914.

Davson, H. Physiology of the Ocular and Cerebrospinal Fluids. Boston, Little, Brown and Co., 1956.

Farmer, T. W. Pediatric Neurology. New York, Paul B. Hoeber, Inc., 1964.

Fishman, R. A., and Greer, M. Experimental obstructive hydrocephalus. Arch. Neurol., 8:156, 1963.

Foltz, E. L., and Shurtleff, D. B. Five year comparative study of hydrocephalus in children with and without operation (113 cases). J. Neurosurg., 20:1064, 1963.

——— and Shurtleff, D. B. Conversion of communicating hydrocephalus to stenosis or occlusion of the aqueduct during ventricular shunt. J. Neurosurg., 24:520, 1966.

Friedman, S., Zita-Gozum, C., and Chatten, J. Pulmonary vascular changes complicating ventriculovascular shunting for hydrocephalus. J. Pediat., 64:305, 1964.

Gibson, J. B., Burnows, D., and Weir, W. P. Primary melanoma of the meninges. J. Path. Bact., 74:419, 1957.

Heisey, S. R., Held, D., and Pappenheimer, J. R. Bulk flow and diffusion in the cerebrospinal fluid system of the goat. Amer. J. Physiol., 203:775, 1962.

Hoffman, J. J., and Freeman, A. Primary malignant leptomeningeal melanoma in association with giant hairy nevi. Report of two cases. J. Neurosurg., Part I, 26:62, 1967.

Ingraham, F. D., and Matson, D. D. Neurosurgery of Infancy and Childhood. Springfield, Ill., Charles C Thomas, Publ., 1954.

Laurence, K. M. The natural history of hydrocephalus. Lancet, 2:1152, 1958.

Lin, J. P., Goodkin, R., Tong, E., Epstein, F. J., and Vinaguerra, E. Radioiodinated serum albumin (RISA) cisternography in the diagnosis of incisural block and occult hydrocephalus. Radiology, 90:36, 1968.

Matson, D. D. Clinical classification and evaluation of hydrocephalus. *In* Disorders of the Developing Nervous System. Springfield, Ill., Charles C Thomas, Publ., 1961.

——— Hydrocephalus. Clin. Neurosurg., 13:324, 1966.

——— Neurosurgery in Infancy and Childhood, 2nd ed. Springfield, Ill., Charles C Thomas, Publ., 1969.

Mathews, E. S., Sanchez, G., and Ransohoff, J. A preliminary report on a biological fluid transfer system for the treatment of hydrocephalus. Develop. Med. Child Neurol. (Suppl.), 13:103, 1967.

Ojemann, R. G., Fisher, C. M., Adams, R. D., Sweet, W. H., and New, P. F. J. Further experience with the syndrome of "normal" pressure hydrocephalus. J. Neurosurg., 31:279, 1969.

Pudenz, R. H., Russell, F. E., Hurd, A. H., and Shelden, C. H. Ventriculoauriculostomy: a technique for shunting cerebrospinal fluid into the right auricle. J. Neurosurg., 14:171, 1957.

Ransohoff, J. Ventriculopleural anastomosis. J. Neurosurg., 11:295, 1954.

——— and Hiatt, R. B. Ventriculo-peritoneal anastomosis in the treatment of hydrocephalus; utilization of the suprahepatic space. A preliminary report. Trans. Amer. Neurol. Ass., 77:147, 1952.

——— Shulman, K., and Fishman, R. A. Hydrocephalus, a review of etiology and treatment. J. Pediat., 56:399, 1960.

Rayport, M., Ransohoff, J., and Zimmerman, H. M., eds. Proceedings of the Rudolf Virchow Medical Society in the City of New York. Horn (Austria), Ferdinand Berger, 1967, p. 281.

Russell, D. S. Observations on the pathology of hydrocephalus. Medical Research Council, Special Report Series No. 265. London, Her Majesty's Stationery Office, 1949.

——— Rubinstein, L. J., and Lumsden, C. E. Pathology of Tumors of the Central Nervous System. Baltimore, Williams and Wilkins Co., 1963.

Scarff, J. E. Nonobstructive hydrocephalus treatment by endoscopic cauterization of the choroid plexus; long-term results. J. Neurosurg., 9:164, 1952.

——— Treatment of hydrocephalus: a historical and critical review of methods and results. J. Neurol. Neurosurg., Psychiat., 26:1, 1963.

Shick, R. W., and Matson, D. D. What is arrested hydrocephalus? J. Pediat., 58:791, 1961.

Selverstone, B. Studies of the Formation and Absorption of the Cerebrospinal Fluid Using Radioactive Isotopes. Ciba Foundation Symposium on the Cerebrospinal Fluid. Boston, Little, Brown and Co., 1958, p. 147.

Shulman, K., ed. Workshop in Hydrocephalus. Department of Neurosurgery, Univ. Pennsylvania School of Medicine and The Children's Hospital of Philadelphia, 1965, p. 157.

Strenger, L. Complications of ventriculovenous shunts. J. Neurosurg., 20:219, 1963.

Welch, K., and Friedman, V. The cerebrospinal fluid valves. Brain, 83:454, 1960.

Wislocki, J. B., and Ladman, A. J. The Fine Structure of the Mammalian Choroid Plexus. Ciba Foundation Symposium on the Cerebrospinal Fluid. Boston, Little, Brown and Co., 1958, p. 55.

Yashon, D. Prognosis in infantile hydrocephalus. J. Neurosurg., 20:105, 1963.

——— Jane, J. A., Cassell, S., Cameron, G., and Sugar, O. Cerebrospinal fluid diversion in infantile hydrocephalus. Arch. Neurol., 15:541, 1966.

DEFECTS OF THE CLOSURE OF THE NEURAL PLATE

Alter, M. Anencephalus, hydrocephalus, and spina bifida. Arch. Neurol., 7:411, 1962.

Badell Ribera, A., and Swinyard, C. A. Rehabilitation of children with spina bifida cystica. Excerpta Medica Int. Congress Series No. 76, September, 1964, p. 180.

Cameron, A. H. The spinal cord lesion in spina bifida cystica. Lancet, 2:171, 1956.

Doran, P. A., and Guthkelch, N. Studies in spina bifida cystica (General survey and reassessment of the problem). J. Neurol. Neurosurg. Psychiat., 24:331, 1961.

Laurence, K. M. *In* Norman, A. P., ed., Congenital Abnormalities in Infancy. Philadelphia, F. A. Davis Co., 1963, pp. 21-81.

Lorber, J. The prognosis of occipital encephaloceles. Develop. Med. Child Neurol. (Suppl.), 13:75, 1966.

——— Results of treatment of myelomeningocele. Develop. Med. Child Neurol., 13:279, 1971.

Mealey, J., Jr., Dzennis, A. J., and Hockey, A. A. The prognosis of encephaloceles. J. Neurosurg., 32:209, 1970.

Schwiddle, J. T. Spina bifida. Survey of two hundred twenty-five encephaloceles, meningoceles, and myelomeningoceles. Amer. J. Dis. Child., 84:35, 1952.

Sharrard, W. J. W., Zachary, R. B., Lorber, J., and Bruce, A. M. A controlled trial of immediate and delayed closure of spina bifida cystica. Arch. Dis. Child., 38:18, 1963.

Shulman, K., and Ames, M. Results of intensive treatment of fifty consecutive children born with myelomeningocele. New York J. Med., 68:2656, 1968.

Smith, E. The pathogenesis and management of spinal myelomeningocele. Med. J. Aust., II:801, 1960.

Sugar, M., and Kennedy, C. E. The use of electrodiagnostic techniques in the evaluation of the neurological deficit in infants with myelomeningocele. Neurology, 15:787, 1965.

Till, K. *In* Wilkinson, A. W., ed., Recent Advances in Pediatric Surgery. Boston, Little, Brown and Co., 1963, pp. 240-259.

Vogel, F. S., and McClenahan, J. L. Anomalies of major cerebral arteries associated with congenital malformations of the brain. Amer. J. Path., 28:701, 1952.

Chapter 3
THE STATIC ENCEPHALOPATHIES

SIDNEY CARTER and ARNOLD P. GOLD

Chronic and nonprogressive cerebral dysfunction results from varied causes and produces multiple clinical syndromes. The clinical picture is dependent on the site and extent of the lesion and the developmental age at time of occurrence. The developing nervous system is more susceptible to insults occurring during the first trimester than later in pregnancy.

Cerebral palsy results from involvement of motor areas of the brain. Mental retardation usually follows diffuse cerebral involvement; however, small lesions occurring early in gestation may interfere with normal cerebral maturation and have as a consequence intellectual deficit. Impairment of the special senses, vision and hearing, follows involvement of select areas of the brain and their pathways. Convulsions most commonly result from cortical lesions. Speech disturbances may be a reflection of diffuse cerebral involvement or a focal lesion involving the speech area. Behavioral disorders and learning disabilities have a less well-defined anatomic localization. These syndromes may occur as isolated clinical phenomena or in any combination. Spastic diplegia may be the only manifestation of cerebral palsy; however, mental deficit, seizures, impairment of vision and/or hearing, or behavioral disturbances may accompany this motor deficit.

These defects of cerebral function may be the result of well-recognized anatomic or biochemical lesions, but in many impaired children the cause is not always apparent, may be unrecognized, or is yet to be defined. Prenatal factors affecting the developing nervous system are both endogenous and exogenous. The fetus may be affected by faulty implantation of the ovum, chromosomal anomalies, infections, trauma, radiation, and toxic substances. Later in pregnancy, maternal toxemia and diabetes may produce damage to the nervous system. Anoxia and trauma are the most commonly encountered causative factors in the natal period. Postnatally, infections, inborn errors of metabolism, trauma, toxins, and vascular disease are often incriminated.

Children with chronic nonprogressive lesions of the brain are being recognized with increasing frequency. More prevalence studies are needed, but available figures illustrate the magnitude of this common pediatric problem. It is estimated that 1 out of 1,000 live births will be severely retarded, 3 per 1,000 moderately retarded, and 25 per 1,000 mildly retarded. In the United States, 5,500,000 individuals have some degree of retardation. Cerebral palsy affects approximately 400,000 children. Approximately 5 percent of all children will have one or more seizures. Incidence of organically induced behavioral disturbances and/or specific learning disabilities is not available, but these conditions greatly outnumber any of the other clinical syndromes.

The Syndrome of Minimal Cerebral Dysfunction

Varied terminology has been applied to children with deviant behavior, specific learning disabilities, or both. These terms include Strauss syndrome, choreiform syndrome, minimal cerebral palsy, minimal cerebral damage, minimal cerebral dysfunction, the hyperkinetic child, organic reaction syndrome, brain-injured child, nonmotor brain damage, and chronic brain syndrome; they have a common feature in suggesting organicity as a basis for the observed clinical manifestations. The term minimal cerebral dysfunction appears to be satisfactory, in that it implies impaired cerebral function without implicating specific areas of the brain. This diagnosis is then used in describing children with normal or near normal intellect who demonstrate abnormal behavioral patterns, specific learning disabilities, or both.

CLINICAL MANIFESTATIONS. The clinical syndrome is variable, and the manifestations may change with age. Deviant behavior, learning disabilities, speech disorders, and poor coordination are the most common presenting complaints.

Behavioral patterns most frequently encountered are those relating to hyperactivity, but underactivity or even normal behavior can be seen. Hyperkinetic behavior is often evident in infancy with restlessness, irritability, and poor sleep patterns. Overactive behavior in the older child is without direction, is purposeless, and shifts from moment to moment. The hyperkinesis fluctuates; it is most marked when the child is confronted with new or stressful situations and is often diminished in familiar settings. Overactivity tends to diminish spontaneously at about 12 years of age and in most instances is significantly modified by 15 years. Less frequently, the behavior may be manifested by hypoactivity, in which the child is placid and retiring.

Behavioral changes closely related to the hyperactivity include a short attention span, irritability, low frustration threshold, impulsivity, distractibility, and social immaturity. Short attention span is characterized by difficulty in focusing and maintaining prolonged attention on a given task, with an inability to eliminate the distraction produced by minimal or trivial auditory, visual, or tactile stimuli. Impulsivity and distractibility are contributing factors. Shortened attention is variable and may be replaced by perseveration. During these periods, there is rigidity of behavior with an abnormal preoccupation for a single object or detail, and a resistance to change with failure to respond appropriately to changing stimuli. Emotional lability may be prominent, and the affective response inappropriately changes from one moment to another. Frustration threshold is often low, and insignificant conditions can provoke uncontrollable rage, unintentional aggressive outbursts, and temper tantrums. Social function is at a level below the chronologic or mental age. This social immaturity results in play with children of a younger age.

Specific learning problems unrelated to intellectual potential or deviant behavior are an additional feature of the minimal brain dysfunction syndrome. Impaired perceptual performance, above all for spatial relationships, results in academic difficulties primarily involving reading and number concepts. Specific reading disability, dyslexia, implies that the inability to read is unrelated to mental retardation, sensory impairment, inadequate schooling, poor motivation, or developmental lag. Reading is either not present or below age level and may be complicated by mirror reading. Some children also have an inability to write or to spell. They will often demonstrate mirror writing or letter reversals, and may be unable to discriminate p from q, b from d, n from u, and w from m. In some, there is inadequate ability to calculate. Many of these children are ambidextrous, which, with dyslexia, is attributed to failure to develop cerebral dominance.

Difficulties in abstract thinking are a common feature of the syndrome and are more evident with increasing age. During the early school years, learning is at a relatively concrete level, with little demand on abstract ideation. This disability may further complicate the difficulties in learning encountered by many of these children or may be the initial educational problem in some who have been previously successful at a concrete level with the use of rote memory.

Language difficulties are common. Some children remain nonverbal, but more commonly there is delay in the development of speech patterns. Once established, there are problems in the formation of phrases and sentences and a prominent tendency to preserve more immature modes of expression. Speech may be characterized by a paucity, misuse, and poor articulation of words. Flow of expressive language may be either slow, hesitant, or explosive.

Coordination is frequently impaired, and the children are often clumsy and awkward. Poor fine muscle coordination is initially demonstrated by difficulties with buttoning, zippering, or tying shoelaces. Subsequent manifestations are noted in the manipulation of scissors, coloring within a figure, drawing a straight line, and eventually poor handwriting. More gross incoordination is evident in the delay in learning to hop, skip, ride a bicycle, and catch a ball.

Social incompetence and environmental rejection result in secondary emotional symptoms characterized by aggression, destruction, withdrawal, and fantasy life.

Neurologic examination characteristically reveals a paucity of gross abnormalities. However, minimal subtle signs are usually present. Gait may be lumbering and awkward. After 7 years of age, there may be impaired tandem walking and difficulty in hopping and skipping. Examination of the motor system reveals impairment of rapid alternating movements, choreiform activity of extended fingers, and occasional tightness of various muscle groups, including hamstrings, posterior tibials, and pronators. Not uncommonly, there is a right-left confusion and a failure to establish handedness. The deep tendon reflexes may be asymmetric, but the plantar responses are usually physiologic. Eye muscle imbalance of the convergent or divergent types is commonly observed; it tends to diminish with age. Poor speech patterns are often associated with drooling and inability to perform rapid lateral tongue movements.

LABORATORY FINDINGS. There are no specific laboratory studies to confirm the clinical diagnosis. Urine test for phenylketonuria should be performed. Electroencephalograms are not in themselves diagnostic; they may be normal or show abnormalities

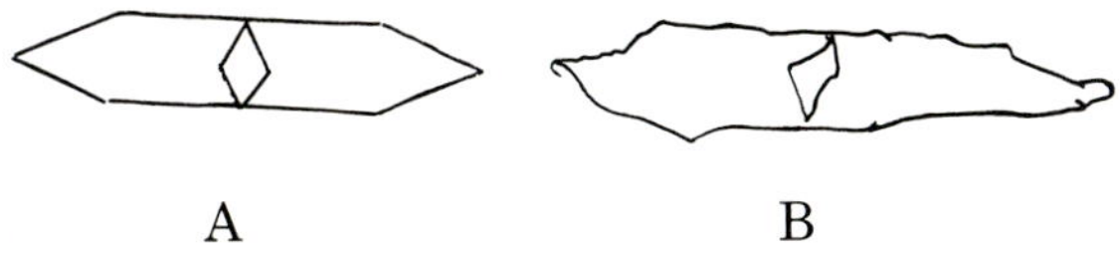

Fig. 23. Copying difficulties in a 9-year-old boy with brain damage. *A.* Sample. *B.* Copy.

of organization with voltage and frequency changes or even multispike and spike and wave activity. Plain radiographs of the skull are normal. Pneumoencephalography and cerebral arteriography are contraindicated.

Psychologic testing is the most helpful ancillary procedure in that it supplies further evidence to support the concept of impaired cerebral function and provides a guide of intellectual potential. Signs of organicity include discrepancies between a higher verbal and lower performance scale, which may be as great as 40 points, scatter on the subtests, and, above all, perceptual difficulties on the Bender Visual Motor Gestalt Test. Deviant perceptual performances (Fig. 23) are manifested by difficulty in copying forms and designs which are often correctly identified orally. There may be rotation or reorientation of the major axis of the figure. Difficulties with number concepts and abstract ideation may also be noted.

DIAGNOSIS. There is no isolated finding that is diagnostic of this clinical syndrome. Diagnosis can be accomplished only by combining the historical data with the results of the examinations. Differential diagnosis includes variants of the normal and psychiatric disturbances. Many normal children show hyperactivity which is more readily controlled and is unassociated with a short attention span, low frustration tolerance, or distractibility. Psychiatric disorders which may require differentiation include some neuroses, the character disorders, and certain psychoses. Not uncommonly, the child with minimal cerebral dysfunction may present with prominent emotional manifestations. These apparent functional phenomena usually result from frustrations produced by learning disabilities and the excessive demands made by the parents, peers, and school. Many physicians, including some psychiatrists, incorrectly interpret these secondary manifestations as primary emotional phenomena.

TREATMENT. A sound therapeutic program includes family counseling, a dynamic educational program, and medications to improve behavior.

Family counseling is of primary importance. Explanation of the physical nature of the disability not infrequently relieves parental anxiety and guilt. The family must be made to accept the handicap. Unnecessary pressures should be eliminated, realistic goals formulated, and a structured environment with consistent discipline and demands established. The family physician is often most effective in providing adequate parental guidance. A seriously disturbed parent-child relationship may require psychiatric assistance.

Educational planning depends on the nature of the disability and the intellectual endowment. Adequate school placement is difficult to obtain even in the most sophisticated community. All too often, the neurologically impaired class is a heterogenous group with children of varied learning problems and intellectual abilities. Ideally the class should be small in size, limited to children of similar intellectual endowment and learning problems, and directed by a teacher trained in remedial education. Efforts should be made to minimize distraction and competition. Emphasis should be placed on individual performance and the use of concrete teaching aids. In some instances, residential placement may be desirable for both the child and family.

Drug therapy is unpredictable, and a particular agent may lose its effectiveness with time. Four groups of compounds have been particularly effective: amphetamines, methylphenidates, phenothiazines, and diphenylmethane derivatives.

Amphetamines. Dextroamphetamine sulfate (Dexedrine) is the most effective amphetamine. The apparent paradoxic effect of this drug is most frequently observed in youngsters demonstrating barbiturate-induced hyperactivity. Dexedrine is administered in daily doses of from 5 to 30 mg given after breakfast and lunch. Initially 5 mg is given, and this is gradually increased on succeeding days until the desired clinical effect is observed or serious toxic reactions become prominent. Undesirable side effects that usually necessitate discontinuance of this compound are either increased hyperactivity with irritability and emotional lability or, more rarely, marked lethargy. Prior to prescribing the drug, the parents should be alerted to the difficulty with sleep for the first three or four nights and anorexia that generally improves spontaneously in a few weeks. These findings are usually not sufficient to warrant discontinuation of the compound.

Amphetamine sulfate (Benzedrine) has a dosage and pharmacologic activity similar to Dexedrine. Occasionally a child will show a poor response with one compound while the other will be effective.

Methylphenidates. Methylphenidate hydrochloride (Ritalin) is often effective in children with hyperactivity. Response is similar to that observed with the amphetamine group and in therapeutic doses is less likely to result in sedation, lethargy, anorexia, and insomnia. After an initial trial with 5 mg orally, the school-age child requires 5 mg three times daily; if necessary, this is further increased to a total daily dose of 60 mg. Side effects are similar to those of the amphetamines and when present are managed in similar fashion.

Phenothiazines. Thioridazine (Mellaril) is the most effective and least toxic of the phenothiazine group of agents in managing the hyperkinetic behavioral syndrome. A preschool child generally requires 10 mg three to four times a day and the older child 25 mg two to four times a day. Toxic reactions are rarely seen but include extrapyramidal disorders, leucopenia, and agranulocytosis. These side effects are indications for prompt discontinuation of the drug. The specific treatment of extrapyramidal complications is discussed under basal ganglia diseases (p. 71).

Chlorpromazine (Thorazine) is often effective in controlling the acutely agitated child but has limited value in the long-term management of the hyperkinetic youngster. Thorazine is usually given in dosages of 20 to 80 mg/day, but up to 300 mg/day may be necessary to achieve the desired results. Extrapyramidal reactions or jaundice as complications of therapy are rarely observed in children. Drowsiness, nasal congestion, dryness of the buccal mucosa, and postural hypotension are infrequent side effects, but their presence is not an indication for discontinuing the drug. Increased sensitivity to light may be so marked in some children that the drug cannot be tolerated.

Other phenothiazines have limited usefulness in the hyperkinetic child because of relatively low therapeutic value or high incidence of toxic side effects. Specifically, prochlorperazine (Compazine) should not be prescribed in the pediatric age group because of the relatively high frequency of extrapyramidal involvement with this drug.

Diphenylmethane Derivatives. Diphenhydramine hydrochloride (Benadryl) is occasionally effective, especially in anxious children with repetitive motor activities such as tics, head banging, and body rocking. The preschool child generally requires 10 mg three to four times a day, and after 6 years of age, 25 mg three times daily may be necessary. Lethargy is a frequent minor side effect with this compound and, if disturbing, can be controlled by the addition of 2.5 to 5 mg of Dexedrine to the therapeutic regimen.

PROGNOSIS. The eventual outcome is dependent on the nature of the disability, the intellectual potential, the establishment of realistic goals, and the avoidance of secondary emotional features by a well-structured and accepting family and a sound educational experience. With this program, it is hoped that the individual will develop social competence and independence. The relatively recent definition of this entity precludes any definitive statement concerning long-term prognosis.

Cerebral Palsy

NIELS L. LOW

Cerebral palsy is the name given to a group of diverse nonprogressive syndromes affecting the brain and manifesting themselves by impairment in motor function. This term is usually limited to conditions which presumably had their onset before birth, during the perinatal period, or in the first few years of life. Since the clinical manifestations as well as the causes are variable, cerebral palsy is not a specific medical diagnosis; it may include mental retardation, learning disabilities, and seizures in addition to the motor deficit.

ETIOLOGY. Either genetic or acquired factors may be responsible for these syndromes. The acquired causes usually result in damage to the fetal central nervous system during the early gestational period. They may be related to faulty implantation of the ovum or to diseases of the mother. Extreme nutritional deficiencies, infections, injuries, toxins, and radiation can interfere with the developing fetal brain, leading to permanent motor defects.

During the perinatal period a rapid succession of events occurs which may damage the brain and result in cerebral palsy. Prematurity is one of the most common associated conditions and predisposes the neonate to asphyxia and cerebral hemorrhage. In certain instances prematurity may result from preexisting abnormalities, and it may be difficult to determine whether the brain damage is the result or the cause of prematurity. Twenty to 25 percent of cerebral palsied children have birth weights less than 2,500 g. Pathologic studies indicate that the most common mechanism leading to brain injury is asphyxia. Multiple births are also frequently associated; these neonates are often of low birth weight and may have associated premature labor and expulsion. Asphyxia seems to be an important damaging factor, especially in the second-born twin. Another factor is the birth process, which can cause venous stasis. This primarily involves the deep-draining veins, with resultant hemorrhage from microscopic extravasation or actual rupture of these vessels. These vascular complications are often the result of asphyxia.

Kernicterus from neonatal hyperbilirubinemia has been recognized as one of the causes of the athetoid type of cerebral palsy. In such children nerve deafness, paresis of upward gaze, or mental retardation may occur.

In the postnatal period, there are many disease processes which are of etiologic significance. Infectious conditions, meningitis, or encephalitis may damage the brain. Marasmus and dehydration with subsequent venous thrombosis are occasional causative factors. Arterial occlusions occurring before or after birth which lead to infantile hemiplegia are not well understood.

PATHOLOGY. Gross malformations, regardless of basic origin, are found in about one-third of autopsied cerebral palsy children. In the other two-thirds the changes, often microscopic, may be primarily cortical or subcortical. The cortical lesions are characterized by laminar degeneration, fall-out of neurons, and cortical atrophy with narrowing of gyri and widening of sulci. The subcortical defects consist of atrophy of white matter, gliosis in the deep central structures, sometimes with cyst formation. Numerically, the cor-

TABLE 3. *Clinical Classification of Cerebral Palsy*

Spastic cerebral palsy
- Spastic hemiplegia
- Spastic tetraplegia
- Diplegia
  1. Spastic
  2. Atonic
- Spastic paraplegia
- Monoplegias and triplegias

Dyskinetic cerebral palsy
- Athetosis
- Other forms

Ataxic cerebral palsy

Mixed syndromes

tical changes are significantly more common in the postnatally acquired group, and the subcortical abnormalities are more frequently found in conjunction with perinatal complications. Athetosis, the aftereffect of kernicterus, show symmetric demyelination of the globus pallidus and the subthalamic nucleus.

CLINICAL CLASSIFICATION. The various syndromes are classified according to the predominant clinical manifestations. The classification given in Table 3 is descriptive and simple. The groups are defined as follows:

Spastic Cerebral Palsy. The spastic types of cerebral palsy are due to involvement of the upper motor neurons and are characterized by increased tone of the involved musculature, exaggeration of the deep tendon reflexes, clonus, abnormal reflexes (extensor plantar response), and a tendency to contractures (Fig. 24).

1. *Hemiplegia* implies that both extremities on the same side are involved; the upper extremity is usually more severely affected than the lower. In addition to increased deep tendon and periosteal reflexes in the involved arm and leg, there usually is some weakness of the peripheral muscles, especially dorsiflexors at the wrist and the ankle, and the forearm supinators. Because of this weakness and the tendency to contracture, the upper extremity tends to be kept flexed at the elbow, wrist, and fingers. In mildly affected children, the handicap may not be apparent while the patient rests in a sitting or standing position, but walking and especially running accentuate the abnormal position. In the mildest cases, the following maneuver is useful in eliciting spasticity: on supination of the previously outstretched pronated arm, there will be flexion of the elbow on the involved side.

The child with spastic hemiplegia characteristically walks more on the toes than on the heel, with a resultant circumduction of the affected leg in order to compensate for the apparent lengthening. Mildly affected children appear to have a normal gait; they walk well on tiptoes but are unable to walk on the affected heel with the toes elevated. This functional asymmetry may be enhanced by running. Further evidence of a mild hemiplegia may be obtained from an examination of the child's shoes. The unaffected side shows normal heel wear, while the involved side demonstrates a scuffed toe and a relatively unworn heel. The signs of upper motor neuron involvement are often elicited in the paretic extremities. Characteristically, there is increased tone with tightness of the adductors of the thigh, the hamstrings, and the posterior calf muscles. This results in an inability to abduct fully the thigh, extend the leg at the knee, and dorsiflex the foot. The involved extremities, especially the upper, may be shorter in length and have a reduced muscle volume.

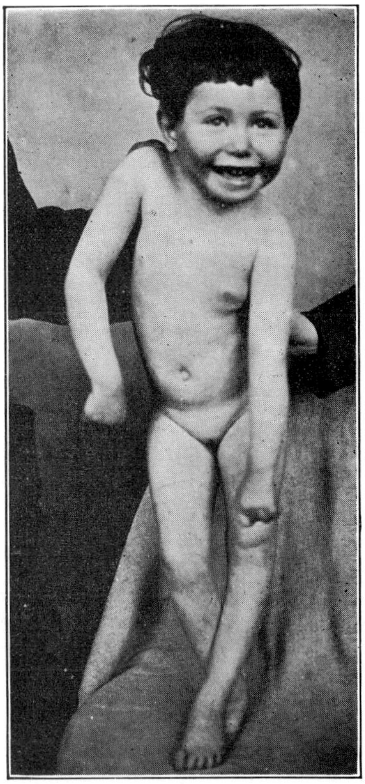

Fig. 24. Child with spastic type of cerebral palsy.

In addition to the weakness, the involved hand may show cortical sensory impairment with inability to discriminate objects (astereognosis). This is best demonstrated by having the child without the aid of vision identify familiar small objects placed in his hand. Useful function can rarely be attained in the presence of such a deficit.

There may be evidence of a central facial weakness and a homonymous hemianopsia.

2. The designation *tetraplegia* or *quadriplegia* is used when spasticity involves all four extremities to approximately the same degree. The clinical manifestations described above are present symmetrically, or nearly so, on both sides. Tightness of the hip

adductors and the hamstring muscles (knee flexors) is usually more marked in this condition than in hemiplegia. A few children with spasticity in all extremities have more involvement of the arms than the legs. Some clinics use the term "double hemiplegia" in these instances.

Such children with equal involvement of all four extremities usually manifest pseudobulbar palsy. Speech is unintelligible or dysarthric, swallowing is impaired, and lingual protrusion and palatal movement are restricted, but the gag reflex is usually present. These clinical manifestations are the result of bilateral involvement of the corticobulbar fibers and are considered an upper motor neuron lesion involving brainstem function.

3. *Spastic diplegia* is characterized by greater involvement of the lower than the upper limbs. The demarcation between tetraplegia and diplegia is not always clear and depends frequently on individual judgment regarding degree of involvement of the upper and lower extremities. The incidence of these two conditions in the literature varies because some clinics do not differentiate children with tetraplegia from those with diplegia. The child with typical spastic diplegia is frequently the result of a premature birth and is recognized by the clinical signs of spasticity in lower extremities while the abnormal findings in the upper limbs are relatively mild. In the young child the arms and hands may appear free of involvement, and only careful reexaminations may later demonstrate slight findings, such as weakness of dorsiflexors of the wrist or abnormal posturing when running.

Atonic diplegia is an unexplained variant of this form of cerebral palsy. It is characterized by marked delay in all motor milestones, decreased tone of the musculature of the lower extremities with increased range of passive movement, normal or increased deep tendon reflexes, and mental retardation. The presence of deep tendon reflexes differentiates atonic diplegia from anterior horn cell and peripheral nerve disease. A characteristic sign is flexion of the hips when the child is suspended upright under the arms (Foerster's sign). Atonic diplegia is a stage in the development of the affected child. As these children become older, hypertonicity usually supervenes and the hyperextensibility disappears. Because of this developmental change, this diagnosis usually can be made only in children between 6 months and 4 years of age.

4. *Spastic paraplegia* refers to the involvement of both legs with complete sparing of the upper extremities. Paraplegia is most often due to spinal cord pathology and only rarely results from brain disease. The differentiation between diplegia and paraplegia may be difficult, since hand involvement in diplegia may not be readily evident. Paraplegia, like spastic diplegia, is characterized by adduction spasm of thighs leading to a scissoring gait, tendency to flexion-contracture at the knees, and tightening of the heel cords (Achilles tendons) with resulting toe gait.

5. *Monoplegias* and *triplegias* are rare conditions. The terms are self-explanatory; they refer to involvement of only one or of three extremities. In triplegia, one arm is usually the limb that is spared.

Dyskinetic Cerebral Palsies. Dyskinesia implies an impairment of volitional activity by uncontrolled and purposeless movements which disappear during sleep. These movement disorders are often related to lesions of the basal ganglia. The most common type is athetosis, which is characterized by relatively slow, wormlike, writhing movements involving usually all four extremities, but also the face, the neck, and, to a lesser degree, the trunk. A child may display a similar pattern for years, but the clinical picture may vary somewhat with age. When the movements have a jerky component, they resemble chorea, and the term choreoathetosis is used. The abnormal movements are less apparent when the patient is relaxed, but increase under stress or tension. During various periods of the natural life cycle of this form of cerebral palsy, abnormal movements, rigidity, and dystonia may be seen. These variations do not justify a separate classification with arbitrary definitions and separations.

Athetosis is most commonly quite symmetric, but some degree of asymmetry may occur. Athetosis involving only one extremity or part of one is exceedingly rare. Because of the continuous movements of extremities and trunk, hypertrophy of some muscles is common, especially around the neck and in the paravertebral area. The athetosis due to kernicterus often has associated nerve deafness and paresis of upward gaze.

Lesch-Nyhan syndrome results from an inborn error of purine metabolism in which there is a deficiency of hypoxanthine-guanine phosphoribosyltransferase. The condition is characterized by choreoathetosis, mental retardation, self mutilation, and hyperuricemia.

Ataxic Cerebral Palsy. The ataxic variety of cerebral palsy is characterized by ataxic phenomena from early childhood and a lack of progression of the disease. It is related to a static lesion of the cerebellum or its pathways. Involved children have a wide-based gait, have difficulty in turning rapidly, perform fast repetitive movements poorly, and show decomposition on the finger-to-finger and finger-to-nose pointing test. Any evidence of progression, foot deformity, abnormal sensory findings, or familial history of ataxia would exclude the diagnosis of this form of cerebral palsy. The ataxic type has the best prognosis for functional improvement.

Mixed Forms. The clinical manifestations of more than one type of cerebral palsy may be present in some children. The combination of spasticity and athetosis is seen most frequently; ataxia and athetosis may be found. Although it may be difficult to separate the features of multiple involvement, the clinical phenomena in a child with a mixed form are characteristically the summation of the findings of both types involved.

ASSOCIATED CONDITIONS. Children who have motor disabilities which fall within the definition of cerebral palsy may have additional syndromes. The most common of these are seizure disorders and mental retardation.

The frequency of convulsions in children with cerebral palsy is difficult to assess, but approximately 25 to 35 percent of all cerebral palsied children have epilepsy. Seizures are more common in the postnatally acquired forms of cerebral palsy. They are present in over 40 percent of the children with hemiplegia and are less common in the other spastic varieties. Dyskinetic children have less than a 1 in 10 chance of developing convulsions, and ataxic patients less than 1 in 20.

Seizures may be evident in early infancy, but are more frequent in the 2 to 6 year age group. In some, the onset may be delayed until the second decade. The seizure type may in part be related to age of onset. Varied seizure patterns are seen. These include infantile spasms, grand mal, focal, multifocal, and psychomotor.

The prevalence of mental retardation is variously reported as being from 25 to 75 percent, but this figure is meaningless unless correlated with the type of cerebral palsy. The incidence is highest in the mixed group, less in the spastic type, still lower in athetosis, and least frequent in ataxia. Among the spastic children, retardation is found in decreasing frequency in the following types: severe tetraplegia, diplegia, paraplegia, hemiplegia, and monoplegia. Intelligence is statistically lower in cerebral palsy patients with seizures compared to those without epilepsy.

Aside from speech delay in mental retardation, cerebral palsy may be associated with a variety of speech disorders, including different degrees and expressions of aphasia, articulatory disturbances, apraxias, and abnormalities of rhythm.

Attention to visual handicaps is particularly important because of the high incidence of strabismus, refractive errors, and visual field defects. Visual-perceptual problems are commonly encountered in cerebral palsied children.

Deafness is uncommon except in children with athetosis due to kernicterus. Peripheral hearing loss (hypacusis) has to be differentiated from lack of response to speech and other auditory stimuli in children who are not deaf (central hearing loss or dysacusis).

INCIDENCE OF CEREBRAL PALSY. The difference among the various reported series is so great that no definitive frequency can be given. Most reports from the United States give a higher birth incidence than is found in the European literature. The most extensive survey throughout an entire country was made by Hansen in Denmark. He found a mean birth incidence (i.e., the number of cerebral palsied children per 1,000 births) of 1.3. This study also revealed that the birth incidence and the frequency of cerebral palsy in Denmark are on the increase.

Of all children with cerebral palsy, approximately 70 percent are spastic, 15 percent athetotic, 5 percent ataxic, and the remaining 10 percent have more than one type, usually spasticity with athetosis. In the Cerebral Palsy Clinic of the Columbia-Presbyterian Medical Center, the incidence of athetosis and ataxia has been decreasing over the last 10 years. Most spastics have either hemiplegia (40 to 45 percent) or diplegia (35 percent). Monoplegia and triplegia are rare forms.

LABORATORY DATA. The common laboratory tests, such as urinalysis, blood count, and sedimentation rate, are not contributory in the diagnosis and differential analysis of the cerebral palsies.

Plain roentgenograms of the skull are usually normal. Asymmetries may be seen in hemiplegic children, and relative microcephaly is not uncommon. Films of the skull should be a routine part of the work-up of cerebral palsied children.

Electroencephalography cannot be used as a diagnostic tool to differentiate cerebral palsy from other neuropathologic conditions, but clearly abnormal EEG's are common in all types of cerebral palsy, whether seizures are manifestly present or not. The most common EEG abnormality is spike seizure discharges. Asymmetries may occur with or without seizure discharges.

COURSE AND PROGNOSIS. By definition, cerebral palsy is the result of a static lesion of the brain which cannot be cured and does not progress; however, the clinical picture can change with time. Children with spasticity manifest a tendency to contracture, and without proper management the handicap may increase. Untreated spastics, who had walked earlier with or without aids, may become chairbound or bedridden. Frequent seizures may disable some children, and the associated repeated asphyxia may further reduce their intelligence. Apparent improvement may be seen in some nonretarded children with the athetotic or ataxic varieties of cerebral palsy.

While decreasing mortality among prematures and in children with meningitis increases the occurrence of cerebral palsy, the wide use of antibiotics and other improvements in medical care and socioeconomic conditions increases the life-span of these patients. The number of cerebral palsied adults is therefore likely to increase.

TREATMENT. The management of children with cerebral palsy varies with the child's age, the type and severity of involvement, presence or absence of seizures, and the degree of intellect. It is important that none of these aspects be regarded as isolated factors requiring treatment, but that the whole child and his family be properly cared for, including social and educational factors.

The motor aspects can be modified to a certain degree. Spastic children develop contractures, and this tendency can be counteracted by surgical and nonsurgical means. Tendons that are tight can be stretched by passive and active exercises. Stretching exercises can be made more effective with certain mechanical devices. Examples of such devices are short leg braces with an adjustable "stop" to prevent footdrop or toe-walking. This type of brace is sometimes used at night only to keep the foot dorsiflexed during sleeping hours. The Benesh Brace Boot (by Markell) prevents the patient's heel from slipping up within the shoe. Stretching of tight adductors of the thighs can be accomplished at night by a so-called "A" frame which separates the legs during resting hours. Various splints can be used to prevent contracture of wrist flexors, finger flexors, and thumb adductors. A variety of orthopedic procedures have been devised for the correction of contractures that do not respond to medical measures.

Athetosis and other forms of dyskinesia are affected only slightly, if at all, by exercises and appliances. In general, braces are contraindicated in athetosis.

Medications have been universally unsuccessful in reducing spasticity or influencing the abnormal movements of cerebral palsy. The management of seizures requires the daily use of anticonvulsants.

Significant mental retardation makes treatment a more difficult problem. Given two children with very similar physical handicap, one can expect better results in the child with normal or near-normal intelligence than in a retarded child. The best results can be obtained when parents and the child can actively cooperate in treatment.

Other ancillary methods of treatment can reduce the individual child's handicap. These include speech therapy for children with difficulties in verbal communication and early correction of visual handicaps. Psychotherapy may be of some value in occasional children; it is of more benefit in helping the family adjust to the handicapped child.

School placement has to be individualized just as are other forms of management. If the child is not retarded, and the physical handicap not severe, regular school placement is indicated. Special classes should be recommended only if the child is unable to perform adequately in a normal setting. Where available, classes for physically handicapped children of normal intellect or for the retarded should be recommended.

Institutional care may become advisable for severely retarded children who cannot be managed at home or who prove to be a significant social or emotional handicap to their siblings and parents.

REFERENCES

THE SYNDROME OF MINIMAL CEREBRAL DYSFUNCTION

Association for the Aid of Crippled Children. The Child with Brain Damage. New York, 1959.

Bax, M., and MacKeith, R. Minimal cerebral dysfunction. Little Club Clinics and Developmental Medicine No. 10. National Spastics Society. London, Medical Education and Information Unit, 1963.

Birch, H. G., ed. Brain Damage in Children: The Biological and Social Aspects. Baltimore, Williams and Wilkins Co., 1964.

Bortner, M. Evaluation and Education of Children with Brain Damage. Springfield, Ill., Charles C Thomas, Publ., 1968.

Chalfant, J. C., and Scheffelin, M. A. Central processings dysfunctions in children. NINDS Monograph No. 9, Public Health Service Publication. Bethesda, Md., 1969.

Clements, S. D. Minimal brain dysfunction in children. NINDB Monograph No. 3, Public Health Serv. Pub. No. 1415. Washington, D.C., 1964.

Cruickshank, W. M. The brain-injured child in home, school, and community. Syracuse, Syracuse Univ. Press, 1967.

Eisenberg, L. The management of the hyperkinetic child. Develop. Med. Child Neurol., 8:593, 1966.

Graham, F. M., and Berman, P. W. Current states of behavior tests for brain damage in infants and preschool children. Amer. J. Orthopsychiat., 31:713, 1961.

Haring, N. G. Minimal brain dysfunction in children. Public Health Service Publication No. 2015. Washington, D.C., 1969.

Kebanoff, S. G., Singer, J. L., and Wilensky, H. Psychological consequence of brain lesions and ablations. Psychol. Bull., 51:1, 1954.

Laufer, N. W., and Denhoff, E. Hyperkinetic behavior syndrome in children. J. Pediat., 50:463, 1957.

Mallison, R. Education as therapy. Seattle, Special Child Publications, 1968.

Money, J., ed. Reading Disability: Progress and Research Needs in Dyslexia. Baltimore, The Johns Hopkins Press, 1962.

Paine, R. S. Minimal chronic brain syndromes in children. Develop. Med. Child. Neurol., 4:21, 1962.

Passamanick, B., and Knobloch, H. Syndrome of minimal cerebral damage in infancy. J.A.M.A., 170:1384, 1959.

Siegel, E. Helping the Brain Injured Child. New York, Association for Brain-Injured Children, 1961.

Strauss, A. A., and Lehtinen, L. Psychopathology and Education of the Brain-Injured Child. New York, Grune and Stratton, Inc., 1947.

Tarnopal, L. Learning Disabilities. Springfield, Ill., Charles C Thomas, Publ., 1969.

Towbin, A. Organic causes of minimal brain dysfunction. J.A.M.A., 217:1207, 1971.

CEREBRAL PALSY

Andersen, B. Infantile Cerebral Palsy. Oslo, Oslo Univ. Press, 1957.

Christensen, E., and Melchior, J. Cerebral palsy—A clinical and neuropathological study. Clinics in Developmental Medicine No. 25. London, National Spastics Society, 1967.

Churchill, J. A. The relationship of Little's disease to premature birth. Amer. J. Dis. Child., 96:32, 1958.

Ellis, E. The physical management of developmental disorders. Clinics in Developmental Medicine No. 26. London, National Spastics Society, 1967.

Frost, P., Weinstein, G. D., and Nyhan, W. L. Diagnosis of Lesch-Nyhan syndrome by direct study of skin specimens. J.A.M.A., 212:316, 1970.

Gold, A. P., and Carter, S. Treatment of Cerebral Palsy. *In* Conn, H. F., ed., Current Therapy. Philadelphia, W. B. Saunders Co., 1969.

Hansen, E. Cerebral palsy in Denmark. Acta Neurol. Scand., 35:(Suppl.)146, 1960.
Heimer, C. B., Cutler, R., and Freedman, A. M. Neurological sequelae of premature birth. Amer. J. Dis. Child., 108:122, 1964.
Kurland, L. T. Definitions of cerebral palsy and their role in epidemiologic research. Neurology, 7:641, 1957.
Lesch, M., and Nyhan, W. L. A familial disorder of uric acid metabolism and central nervous system function. Amer. J. Med., 36:561, 1964.
Malamud, N., Itabashi, H. H., Castor, J., and Messinger, H. B. An etiologic and diagnostic study of cerebral palsy. J. Pediat., 65:270, 1964.
Perlstein, M. A., Gibbs, E. L., and Gibbs, F. A. The electroencephalogram in infantile cerebral palsy. Amer. J. Phys. Med., 34:477, 1955.
——— and Hood, P. N. Infantile spastic hemiplegia. I. Incidence. Pediatrics, 14:436, 1954.
——— and Hood, P. N. Infantile spastic hemiplegia. III. Intelligence. Pediatrics, 15:676, 1955.
——— and Hood, P. N. Infantile spastic hemiplegia. Amer. J. Phys. Med., 34:391, 1955.
——— and Hood, P. N. Etiology of postnatally acquired cerebral palsy. J.A.M.A., 188:126, 1964.
Schachat, W. S., Wallace, H. M., Palmer, M., and Slater, B. Ophthalmologic findings in children with cerebral palsy. Pediatrics, 19:623, 1957.
Towbin, A. The Pathology of Cerebral Palsy. Springfield, Ill., Charles C Thomas, Publ., 1960.

Mental Retardation

LAWRENCE T. TAFT and HERBERT J. COHEN

Mental retardation is one of the most significant problems facing our society. The effects of this condition are often profound and devastating to both the child and his family.

DEFINITION AND DESCRIPTION. Mental retardation is a symptom associated with many syndromes and diseases. An individual is labeled as being mentally retarded if he performs two standard deviations below the mean on a standardized psychologic test. However, different psychologic tests measure different aspects of cognitive functioning and the tests are not "culture free." A low intelligence quotient may not always be a reliable "symptom" of intellectual incompetency. IQ scores, in certain cases, can be profoundly changed by a modification of the environment, test preparation, test familiarity, and improved motivation.

The primary concern for the individual who performs poorly on standard IQ tests is whether he is able to adapt and successfully compete in society. IQ tests that measure cognitive abilities do have some predictive value in determining future adaptation to society's demands. However, these demands are quite variable. A child with a low IQ may be considered handicapped in some settings and not in others. The child with a mild intellectual deficit may be unrecognized until he starts school, since at that time his behavior must accord to stricter standards and his

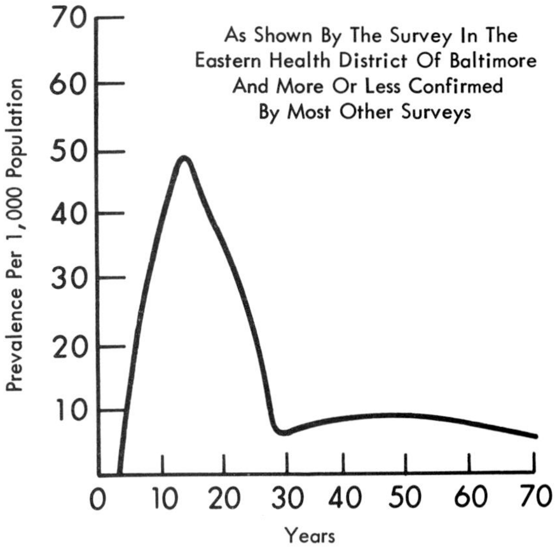

Fig. 25. Shape of curve for prevalence of mental deficiency.

intellectual competence in selected areas is first challenged. The same youngster, at the completion of school, may, once again, fade into the general population. He may then appear to function more competitively with his peers. Figure 25 illustrates the reported relative frequencies of mental retardation apparent at various ages. There is a decided drop in the frequency of identified cases after adolescence.

Adaptive difficulties can exist in individuals who function at any level on certain standardized psychologic tests. A child with an IQ score in the superior range may still have a reading disability and experience educational failure. It is unwise and incorrect to assume that the IQ tests used to delineate a specific population of "retardates" automatically absolve individuals who score slightly above this level from being functionally handicapped.

CLASSIFICATION AND ETIOLOGY. Degrees of mental retardation are defined by the terms mild, moderate, and severe. Mild retardation is equated with an IQ of 50 to 75, and indicates that the individual is both "educable and trainable." In general, most children in this category can reach a third to fifth grade level of academic achievement, and should be independent in activities of daily living. Prognostically, the majority of this group, especially those with an IQ greater than 65 and no severe emotional problems, can be expected to achieve an independent existence as an adult. They should be able to work as unskilled or semiskilled laborers, and be able to assume family responsibilities. Moderate mental retardation (IQ 25 to 50) implies that the individual will have no significant academic achievements but will be "trainable" and can go to school, primarily for training in self-care activities. The trainable individual may learn to read and write at a primer or

TABLE 4. *Pathophysiologic Classification of Mental Retardation*

Prenatally Determined

Chromosomal (autosomal)
- A. Down's syndrome (trisomy 21; translocation 15/21, 21/22, 21/21; mosaicism)
- B. Trisomy 13
- C. Trisomy 18
- D. Partial deletion of long arm of 18
- E. Partial deletion of chromosome 4-5 (cri du chat syndrome)

Chromosomal (sex)
- Klinefelter's syndrome (XXY, XXXY, XXXXY)

Metabolic*
- Abnormalities of amino acid metabolism
  - a. Hyperglycinemia
  - b. Hyperlipemia
  - c. Homocystinuria
  - d. Oasthouse urine disease
  - e. Congenital tryptophanuria
  - f. Hydroxyprolinuria
  - g. Cystathioninuria
  - h. Hartnup disease
  - i. Joseph's syndrome
  - j. Lowe's syndrome (oculo-cerebro-renal dystrophy)
  - k. Hypersarcosinuria
  - l. Phenylketonuria
  - m. Histidinemia
  - n. Hyper-beta-alaninemia
  - o. Hyperammonemia—type 2
  - p. Albinism—oculocutaneous form
  - q. Hypervalinemia
  - r. Congenital lysine intolerance
  - s. Methionine malabsorption
  - t. Maple syrup urine disease
  - u. Hydroxykynureninuria
  - v. Hyperprolanemia
  - w. Citrullinemia
  - x. Arginosuccinic-aciduria
  - y. Kwashiorkor
  - z. Wilson's disease (hepato-lenticular degeneration)
- Abnormalities of lipid metabolism
  - a. A-beta-lipoproteinemia
  - b. Alexander's disease
  - c. Cerebromacular degenerations (Bielchowski, Batten-Spielmeyer-Vogt, Kufs)
  - d. Cerebroside lipidosis (infantile and childhood)
  - e. Familial sudanophilic leucodystrophy
  - f. Ganglioside lipidosis (Tay-Sachs)
  - g. Globoid cell leucodystrophy (Krabbe)
  - h. Isovaleric acidemia
  - i. Kinky hair disease (Menke's disease)
  - j. Lipogranulomatosis (Farber's)
  - k. Pelizaeus-Merzbacher leucodystrophy
  - l. Neurovisceral lipidosis
  - m. Refsum's disease (heredopathia atactica polyneuritiformis)
  - n. Sphingomyelin lipidosis (Niemann-Pick)
  - o. Sulfatide lipidosis (metachromatic leucodystrophy)
  - p. Sweaty socks syndrome
- Abnormalities of carbohydrate metabolism
  - a. Galactosemia
  - b. Mucopolysaccharidoses
    - Hurler's Type
    - Hunter's Type
    - Sanfilippo's Type
    - Morquio-Ullrich
- Abnormalities of purine metabolism
  - a. Hyperuricemia
  - b. Hereditary orotic aciduria

TABLE 4. (continued)

Abnormalities of mineral metabolism
- a. Idiopathic hypercalcemia
- b. Pseudohypoparathyroidism
- c. Pseudo-pseudohypoparathyroidism

Syndromes† (classified as to prominent clinical findings)

Skin abnormalities
- a. Linear sebaceous nevi—convulsions
- b. Congenital icthyosis with spastic paralysis (Sjögren-Larsson syndrome)
- c. Adenoma sebaceum (tuberous sclerosis)
- d. Café-au-lait spots (neurofibromatosis)
- e. Telangiectasia (ataxia-telangiectasia)
- f. Incontinentia pigmenti
- g. Facial port-wine nevus (Sturge-Weber-Dimitri)

Cataracts
- Marinesco-Sjögren syndrome

Emaciation
- Leprechaunism

Obesity
- a. Laurence-Moon-Biedl
- b. Prader-Willi syndrome

Cleft lip and cleft palate
- a. Oral-facial-digital syndrome
- b. Oto-palato-digital syndrome

Facial anomalies prominent
- a. Cebocephalus
- b. Cerebro-hepato-renal syndrome
- c. de Lange's syndrome
- d. Dyscephalia mandibulo-oculo-facialis (Hallerman-Streiff syndrome)
- e. Leprechaunism
- f. Oculo-auriculo-vertebral dysplasia
- g. Rubinstein-Taybi syndrome (broad thumb and broad toe)
- h. Smith-Lemli-Opitz syndrome

Digit abnormalities
- a. Rubinstein-Taybi syndrome
- b. Oral-facial-digital syndrome
- c. Oto-palato-digital syndrome
- d. Smith-Lemli-Opitz syndrome

Tall stature
- Cerebral gigantism

Dwarfism prominent
- a. Bird-headed dwarf (Virchow-Seckel dwarf)
- b. Silver's syndrome

Cranial abnormalities
- a. Apert's (acrocephalosyndactyly)
- b. Craniofacial dysostosis (Crouzon's disease)
- c. Happy puppet syndrome
- d. Hydrancephaly
- e. Hydrocephalus
- f. Cloverleaf skull (Kleebattschadel syndrome)
- g. Familial microcephaly
- h. Kinky hair disease (Menke's syndrome)

Muscle weakness
- a. Myotonic dystrophy
- b. Pseudohypertrophic muscular dystrophy

Fetal Teratogens

Chemical
- a. Dietary inadequacies
- b. Vitamin deficiencies
- c. Drugs

Physical
- a. Irradiation
- b. Trauma

TABLE 4. (continued)

- Infectious agents
  - a. Cytomegalic inclusion disease
  - b. Influenza
  - c. Rubella
  - d. Toxoplasmosis
  - e. Syphilis
- Metabolic
  - a. Toxemia
  - b. Placental dysfunction
  - c. Diabetes mellitus

Perinatally Determined

- Birth anoxia
- Kernicterus
- Prematurity
- Birth trauma

Postnatally Determined

- Head trauma
- Poisonings
  - Lead
  - Carbon monoxide
  - Arsenic
- Infectious
  - Meningitis
  - Encephalitis
- Cerebrovascular accidents
  - Aneurysm
  - Arteriovenous malformation
  - Thrombosis
- Metabolic
  - Hyponatremia
  - Hypernatremia
  - Hypoglycemia
- Postimmunization encephalopathies
  - Rabies
  - Pertussis
  - Smallpox
- Cultural–familial
- Psychogenic

*The metabolic abnormalities are listed as being prenatally determined since they are genetic disorders. Some may not become manifest until a later age.

†These are not listed as being prenatally determined since they all appear to be due to abnormalities in morphogenesis.

first grade level. Vocational placement is usually limited to employment in a sheltered workshop, and supervised care is necessary. Severe retardates (IQ less than 25) acquire no academic skills; they are usually not trainable and require custodial care.

It is also useful to classify individuals with an intellectual handicap in two subgroups, defined as: (1) true mental defects (biologic); and (2) functional mental retardation. Retardation in those with true mental defects may be due to either structural or metabolic brain defects. Such individuals are not able to perform within the normal range on formal psychologic testing even when they are functioning at their highest level. In contrast, functional retardation implies that the affected individuals have the capacity to perform within the normal range but are unable to do so because of such factors as emotional disturbance, deprivation, cultural disadvantage, discrimination, or educational handicaps.

Anatomic and etiologic classifications for mental retardation are often inadequate since the pathogenesis and neuropathology have usually not been correlated with clinical manifestations. In addition, brain damage or maldevelopment (e.g., absence of the corpus callosum), may not be asociated with mental retardation. The classification in Table 4 lists most known determinants and/or diseases that have been associated with mental retardation. Many are described in detail elsewhere. In the vast majority of mild retardates, no single etiologic factor can be identified. A comprehensive evaluation, including physical and neurologic examinations, and biochemi-

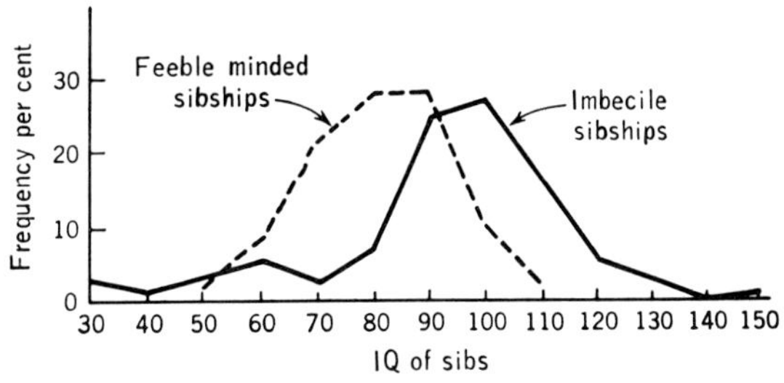

Fig. 26. Frequency distributions of the IQ's of sibs of feeble-minded and imbeciles with an IQ range of 30 to 68. (After Roberts. *Eugen. Rev.,* 44:71, 1952.)

cal and cytogenetic studies, usually fails to prove the presence of clear-cut cerebral pathology.

INCIDENCE AND DISTRIBUTION. Based on the psychologic criteria noted above, mental retardation is found in approximately 3 percent of the population. Seventy-five percent of retardates are in the mild category, 20 percent in the moderate group, and only 5 percent are classified as severely retarded. However, there are marked variations in this distribution, associated with chronologic, cultural, and socioeconomic factors.

The prevalence of mild retardation is highest in low socioeconomic classes. In contrast, moderate and severe retardates are distributed more evenly from among all of the social classes. This finding has created considerable controversy as to whether biologic factors or social (experiential) factors play the major role in causing mild mental retardation. Severe deprivation, protein malnutrition, and environmental factors have all been demonstrated to cause a diminished rate and level of learning, and subsequent subnormal mental functioning. The high frequency of retardation in the lower classes has suggested that polygenic or multifactorial hereditary patterns are paramount. As shown in Figure 26, Roberts has demonstrated that mild retardates have siblings with lower IQ's than siblings of more severe retardates. Twin studies have generally supported the notion that heredity is of primary importance in determining eventual IQ results. However, the phenotypic expression of any genotype does depend to some extent on environmental factors. It is probable that there are certain biologic determinants of behavior and that external stimuli modify their expressivity and vary the degree or type of responsiveness. Many factors may operate in a relatively covert manner. The absence of clearly demonstrable CNS pathology in the mild retardate may simply reflect the lack of refinement of our clinical diagnostic tools, and many subtle abnormalities in function may go undetected.

PRESENTING SYMPTOMS. Suspicion of mental retardation may be aroused either by the recognition of a specific syndrome with its overt anomalies or by a developmental lag. Down's syndrome is a classic example of the former and is usually recognized at birth, as are most cases where multiple anomalies are present. Retarded children with delayed development only are diagnosed at a later age. Severe mental retardation is manifested in the first year of life by marked lags in motor and adaptive behavior. However, the diagnosis of mental retardation in a child with only motor retardation must be made with cau-

TABLE 5. *High-Risk Factors Predisposing to Mental Retardation**

Family history

1. Deafness, blindness, neurologic diseases, cerebral palsy, epilepsy
2. Congenital malformations (including congenital dislocation of the hip)
3. Mental disorder
4. Elderly or very young mother

Prenatal

1. Rubella (certainly) and other virus infections (possibly) contracted in early pregnancy
2. Toxoplasmosis
3. Hyperemesis
4. Threatened abortion
5. Severe illnesses in the early months necessitating chemotherapy or major surgery
6. Exposure to radioactive substances during pregnancy
7. Blood group incompatibilities
8. Maternal diabetes mellitus
9. Maternal thyrotoxicosis and toxemia
10. Uterine hemorrhage
11. Hydramnios
12. Multiple pregnancy

Perinatal

1. Premature birth (39 weeks and earlier)
2. Low weight at birth in relation to gestational age
3. Postmature birth (42 weeks and later)
4. Abnormal presentation
5. Prolonged, precipitate, or instrumental labor
6. Birth asphyxia
7. Neonatal jaundice
8. Presence of any congenital abnormality
9. Induction of labor

Postnatal

1. Difficulties in sucking and swallowing
2. Convulsions
3. Cerebral palsy
4. Meningitis or encephalitis
5. Any serious illness or infection in first few months of life

Symptomatic group

1. Mother's suspicion that the child is blind, deaf, retarded, or otherwise abnormal
2. Inattention to sound or to visual stimuli
3. Delayed motor development
4. Delayed development of vocalization and speech

*From Sheridan. *Monthly Bull. Minist. Health (London),* 21:238, 1962.

TABLE 6. *Reasons for Early Diagnosis of Mental Retardation*

Early identification of treatable conditions
1. Metabolic (e.g., PKU, cretinism, galactosemia)
2. Surgical (e.g., subdural hematoma, hydrocephalus)

Genetic counseling for hereditable conditions
e.g.—Tuberous Sclerosis

Prevent complications by:
1. Parent counseling
2. Appropriate schooling
3. Behavioral management
4. Recommendations regarding recreation

tion since such children may have cerebral palsy and normal intelligence. Moderate retardates are usually delayed in motor and adaptive behavior in early infancy but are not sufficiently deviant from the norms to arouse suspicion unless their speech development is significantly delayed. Mild retardates are often unrecognized until they are subjected to the more exacting demands of a school curriculum and are in direct competition with youngsters of normal mental capacity.

The mild retardate may be identified by developmental screening examinations. The presence of any "high-risk" factors (Table 5) should alert the physician that certain infants and children deserve a more careful developmental evaluation. Developmental tests such as the Denver Developmental Screening Examination, the Gesell Test, or modified versions of the latter, are useful in this regard. Although these tests cannot define a child's exact future IQ, they do have reasonable predictive value in identifying mental subnormality. For a preschool and kindergarten age child (aged 5 to 6 years), the Meeting Street School Test may be of value in identifying children at risk of educational failure.

ROLE OF THE PHYSICIAN. The physician's primary responsibility, in the case of the retarded child, is to examine the patient and identify any specific etiologic and pathologic entities that are known to cause mental subnormality. A complete diagnostic evaluation should be performed on a child with symptoms of maldevelopment as soon as the problem is recognized. Though remediable conditions are not common, there are a few treatable conditions in which early institution of therapy can produce favorable results. Table 6 lists the important reasons for early diagnosis and early intervention.

PHYSICAL FINDINGS. The presence of congenital stigmata enumerated in Table 7 may provide a clue that fetal maldevelopment has occurred. These findings may be due to chromosomal defects or to first trimester teratogenic influences on the fetus. A search for skin lesions such as adenoma sebaceum, vitiligo, and café-au-lait spots is important to help exclude a familial degenerative disease such as tuberous sclerosis. The presence of organomegaly should lead to the suspicion of a lipid or carbohydrate storage disease. Careful eyeground examination can rule out optic atrophy, macular abnormalities, or pigmentary degeneration found in degenerative CNS diseases and chorioretinitis associated with congenital toxoplasmosis, cytomegalic inclusion disease, or rubella. Metabolic disorders, such as a cretinism or mucopolysaccharidosis, may be suspected if the child has coarse facial features. An unusual body or urinary odor may suggest an amino-aciduria. Constipation is a common finding in cretinism. Short stature is a frequent finding in both institutionalized and noninstitutionalized retardates. Not infrequently, complete investigations into known causes of short stature prove unrevealing. In these patients "brain damage" is assumed to be etiologically related to the dwarf stature, but the pathophysiologic mechanism is unknown. In nonbrain-damaged individuals short stature has been reported to be a consequence of emotional deprivation.

It is important to measure the head size at regular intervals. Appropriate graphs of normal values are available for premature as well as full-term infants and older children. A head circumference of three standard deviations or more from the mean should always be investigated. Head circumferences two standard deviations from the mean should be regarded with suspicion, especially if the circumference is out of proportion as compared with the child's percentiles for height and weight. In most cases of malnutrition, especially when this occurs after 1 year of age, the head size will grow at a relatively normal rate and will appear relatively large in comparison to body size. Microcephaly at birth suggests the possibility of: (1) prenatal rubella; (2) toxoplasmosis; (3) cytomegalic inclusion disease (CID); (4) Paine's sex-linked recessive microcephaly with amino-aciduria; (5) chromosomal aberration; or (6) fetal maldevelopment of unknown origin.

A head circumference that is normal at birth but subsequently has a slow rate of growth should arouse suspicion of: (1) perinatal brain damage; (2) a metabolic disorder (e.g., PKU); (3) a degenerative brain disease; or (4) rubella, CID, and toxoplasmosis acquired in utero.

LABORATORY STUDIES. Investigations include screening test for amino-aciduria, serum electrophoresis to measure IgM, since it is occasionally elevated in the perinatal period in congenital infections, and confirmatory serologic tests for toxoplasmosis, CID, and rubella. Skull x-rays should be performed on microcephalic or retarded children, since identification of cerebral calcifications, though uncommon, may assist in detecting previously undiagnosed cases of CID, toxoplasmosis, or tuberous sclerosis. In most cases of mental retardation, an EEG is usually of little specific diagnostic help. However, abnormalities associated with subdural hematomas, infantile spasms, and petit mal status have occasionally been found, and

TABLE 7. *Physical Stigmata Often Associated with Mental Retardation*

Head

Dolicocephaly
Brachycephaly
Scaphocephaly
Asymmetry
Acrocephaly
Macrocephaly
Microcephaly
Frontal bossing
Flat or prominent occiput

Facial Appearance

Birdlike
Elfinlike
Expressionless
Coarse features
Odd shape
Odd general appearance

Hair

Low hairline anterior or posterior
Hirsutism
Alopecia
Kinkiness
Abnormal texture
Eyebrow hair meets in midline
White forelock
Short and blond
Abnormal pigmentation

Nose

Beaked
Broad or broad bridge
Flat
Clefted
Saddle-shaped
Thin
Upturned

Mouth

Micrognathia
Cleft lip
Cleft palate
Thin, thickened, or fissured lips
Thick alveolus or mandible
Hypoplastic mandible
Prominent maxilla
Open mouth
High arched palate
Prognathia
Large protruding tongue
Fissured or lobulated tongue
Cleft uvula

Chest

Shield-like
Deformed
Narrow
Pectus excavatum
Pigeon breast
Wide-spaced nipples

Abdomen

Protuberant
Large umbilical hernia

Skin

Pigmentary changes
Simian creases
Abnormal dermatoglyphics
Nevi
Hemangiomata
Acrocyanosis
Adenoma sebaceum
Depigmented
Petechiae
Blotching
Café-au-lait spots
Dryness
Increased elasticity
Fistulae
Nevus flammeus

Eyes

Abnormal shape
Slant—mongoloid or antimongoloid
Blue sclera
Coloboma
Brushfield spots
Epicanthal folds
Hypo- or hypertelorism
Cataracts
Corneal clouding
Long curly eyelashes
Heterochromia
Glaucoma
Abnormal corneal slope or size
Nystagmus
Ptosis

Philtrum

Short
Long

Teeth

Abnormal crown formation
Absent
Supernumerary
Enamel hypoplasia or aplasia
Enamel hypomaturation and hypocalcification
Intrinsic staining
Malposition
Delayed eruption

Neck

Short
Webbed

Genitalia

Enlarged
Small
Ambiguous
Hypospadias
Cryptorchidism
Bifid or small scrotum

Back

Gibbus
Marked kyphosis or lordosis

TABLE 7. (continued)

Hands	Arms
Short metacarpals	Wide carrying angle
Broad	Enlarged wrists
Large or short	
Clawlike	**Feet**
Spadelike	Edema
Polydactyly	Short metatarsals
Clinodactyly	Rocker-bottom
Aplasia of digits	Talipes equinovarus or valgus
Broad distal digits (thumbs)	Syndactyly
Overlapping fingers	Dysplasia of toenail
Syndactyly	Overlapping toes
Proximally placed thumbs	Short toes
Simian creases	Broad big toe
	Increased distance between 1st and 2nd toe

these conditions require early and specific treatment. The deaf child may present with the clinical picture of pseudoretardation, and appropriate hearing tests should be made to exclude this possibility.

Routine cytogenetic studies are rarely abnormal in the great majority of retardates. Karyotypes should be selectively performed when there are physical stigmata or a family history to suggest a chromosomal disorder. Such studies can confirm the clinical diagnosis and prove of value for future family planning.

PSYCHOLOGIC TESTING AND SOCIAL BEHAVIORAL EVALUATION. A comprehensive assessment of a suspected retarded child should always include a clinical psychologic evaluation. It is common practice to use patterns of functioning on standard psychologic tests to help differentiate the environmentally deprived, genetically determined, and organically impaired patient. Psychometric testing, performed in a one-to-one setting by an experienced psychologist, can be helpful in determining the extent to which emotional factors, sensory impairments, or perceptual problems are impairing learning capacity. This aids in defining the patterns of disability which will assist the clinician in prescribing appropriate remediation and treatment.

The results of psychologic tests are influenced by the child's attitude towards testing, familiarity with test situations, levels of anxiety in a strange and demanding situation, and the general environment in which he has developed.

Though the psychologist can competently evaluate some of these factors, a psychiatrist and social worker can be of great assistance in this regard. In the presence of suspected behavioral aberrations that may depress intellectual function, a psychiatric evaluation should be performed. Children with infantile autism or childhood psychosis may appear retarded but actually may have better intellectual potential. The child who is hallucinating and whose thinking is heavily involved with fantasy may not perform up to his intellectual potential. The same is true of the overanxious or inhibited child with subpar performance. A psychiatric examination is useful in determining the importance of emotional factors and their influence on intellectual functioning.

Evaluation of the family by a social worker is extremely helpful in clarifying the family's attitude towards the retarded or handicapped child. A study of family dynamics, siblings and extended family relationships, and the family's economic situation, are essential in assisting the physician in formulating appropriate recommendations. The family may confide important information to the social worker that they will not tell to the physician. In these situations, the social worker can communicate with the family more effectively than can the physician. Social service counseling for the families of retarded children is most useful after the completion of the diagnostic evaluation. The social worker may also be helpful to the family in establishing contacts between the family and appropriate community resources.

In many areas of the country, centers have been established to evaluate children with suspected mental retardation. These diagnostic centers are interdisciplinary and usually consist of a pediatrician or pediatric neurologist, psychiatrist, psychologist, social worker, educational consultant, and a nurse. Speech, occupational, and physical therapists are often included. The team approach is often useful in delineating all the factors affecting the function of the referred patient. This is especially helpful in cases that present complex diagnostic problems. However, the full-team approach appears unnecessary in the more straightforward cases where the diagnosis, treatment, and prognosis are more obvious. In such cases a physician with knowledge of community resources for retardates may well be able to handle the problem effectively, without referral to a major diagnostic and treatment center.

TREATMENT. ***General Comments.*** Since the causes of mental retardation are complex and multifactorial, there is no single therapeutic approach which is universally applicable to all individuals with this condition.

Cases of mental retardation due to apparently treatable metabolic disorders, e.g., PKU, are rare and are among the few currently known disorders where a relatively uncomplicated procedure, such as dietary changes, may produce a major change in the course of the disease. Conditions such as hydrocephalus that can cause mental retardation can be corrected by neurosurgical procedures. With early treatment, the results are generally favorable.

The need to identify curable conditions accurately and promptly is of obvious importance. But it is essential to stress that any therapeutic recommendations in the more complex multifactorial cases of mental subnormality must be based on a thorough understanding of the relative importance of the organic, psychologic, genetic, and social (environment) components in producing the intellectual deficiency. The child's parents must be given a practical and meaningful interpretation of the child's problems and behavior, along with an understanding of the anticipated changes in function and behavior that occur with maturation. Physicians dealing with parents of retarded children must be forthright in indicating when the prognosis is poor and, at the same time, admit when the prognosis is uncertain. The need for periodic reevaluation, in order to assess a child's progress, must be stressed. If the physician is candid with the family and conveys, with compassion and sympathy, his genuine concerns about the child to the family, then shopping for "other opinions" will be minimized.

Educational Programs. The major burden in the treatment of mental retardation usually falls on the shoulders of the educator. Many clinics that care for retarded and handicapped children include a psychoeducational consultant in the diagnostic team. Consultants of this type have been developing and applying increasingly sophisticated diagnostic techniques which go beyond the simple determination of IQ level. Tests such as the Illinois Test of Psycholinguistic Abilities (ITPA) have been increasingly applied in order to separate the various sensory modalities and integrative components from the conceptual and memory functions involved in learning. Use of Frostig tests have assisted in pinpointing perceptual problems, and the recent work of Birch and Lefford has demonstrated the significance of visual, kinesthetic, and haptic integrative defects in brain-damaged children. In addition, Birch and Belmont have devised a test of visual-auditory integration, a function which appears to be defective in some individuals with language disturbances and learning disabilities.

The above diagnostic procedures, by pinpointing areas of weakness and strength, can be useful in developing an educational prescription for the mildly retarded child with learning difficulties. It must be stressed that, whatever the remedial techniques that are applied, the success in a particular child is usually dependent on the child's basic abilities or disabilities plus: (1) the interest, attitude, and enthusiasm of the instructor; (2) the motivation and cooperation of the child; (3) the amount of time allotted for instruction, which may be related to class size; and (4) the degree of structuring in the program. The difficulty in accurately determining the relative importance of all of these variables has complicated the task of assessing the true worth of many of the special educational techniques that are currently being applied.

Types of classes or educational programs for the retarded vary in each community. Despite the division of retarded children into educable and trainable categories, the educational methods for teaching the two groups do tend to overlap. Higher- and lower-track classes in each category, if available, may provide a useful means of selecting children with better or improved functioning and using available resources more efficiently and effectively. The higher-track educable child should achieve a fourth to fifth grade level in reading and math, but have limited ability to reason abstractly. The lower-track educable child will struggle to acquire third grade skills. The higher-track trainable child may be "trained" in activities of daily living and learn first and second grade math, reading, writing, and spelling. The lower-track trainable usually acquires no formal academic skills.

Social and Recreational Needs. Of all areas of treatment for the retarded child, this is the most sensitive area to deal with appropriately. The retarded child is generally rejected by his chronologic peers, by society in general, and often by his siblings and even his family. Yet, like any other child, he has social and recreational needs. These are usually unmet. In school he is usually isolated with other children who show similar problems. Meaningful social relationship with healthy models are few and far between. Retarded children and adolescents desperately need after-school social and recreational programs and these are usually unavailable.

Behavioral Modification. *Operant conditioning.* Experimental techniques to modify retarded children's behavior by training or conditioning via a system of rewards and/or punishments, using positive and negative reinforcement, are currently being more widely applied. These methods, commonly called "operant conditioning," have produced some dramatic improvement in gross functioning, and in achieving independence in activities of daily living, in moderate to severely retarded and emotionally disturbed children. Similar techniques applied to more mildly retarded children appear to have produced some successful results in improving learning and behavior under experimental and controlled conditions. The suitability of these techniques, and the advisability of the application of these procedures on a more widespread basis, is rather uncertain.

Drugs. Drug treatment in mentally retarded children has essentially been confined to the application of appropriate medications to treat specific symptoms in selected patients. No specific medications have as yet been demonstrated to improve overall mental functioning in retarded children.

Certain drugs have been useful in treating mentally retarded children with concomitant medical problems. Retarded children with epilepsy should be given appropriate anticonvulsant medications. An occasional child with petit mal status may appear retarded and/or autistic. When this is diagnosed by EEG and effectively treated, it may result in a dramatic improvement in mental functioning. The same dramatic results have been reported in a few individuals with psychomotor seizures. A substantial number of children with "minimal brain damage" are very hyperactive and have a short attention span, and appear to function as mildly retarded children. In many of these patients, the hyperkinesis diminishes when they are placed on Dexedrine or Ritalin, which often has a paradoxical effect on brain-damaged children. In such cases, an improved attention span may result in better academic performance and, on retesting, improvement in IQ scores.

The retarded child with significant emotional problems may also benefit from drug treatment. A high anxiety level, stemming from feelings of frustration, recurrent failure, and a sense of rejection, all may have adverse effects on the academic performance of the brain-damaged child, whether or not he functions in the retarded range. A child of this type benefits from tranquilizers such as the phenothiazines, though the effective dosage level may be quite variable. With a decrease in the level of anxiety, concomitant improvement in intellectual functioning may occur. However, it should be pointed out that drug therapy in brain-damaged, hyperactive, anxious, or emotionally disturbed children merely permits the expression of the underlying intellectual potential and has no direct effect in improving intelligence per se.

Vocational training. The majority of mild retardates appear to fade into the general employed population. Academic failure does increase the probability of unemployment, but factors other than IQ level may have a significant determining role in this regard. In an increasingly complex technologic society, the labor market for unskilled workers is shrinking, and job openings for mildly mentally retarded individuals are becoming more scarce. Thus, vocational training of mild retardates for semiskilled or repetitive jobs, in which some retarded individuals show greater perseverance than nonretardates, is essential. Individuals must be selected who are emotionally stable, and they must be placed in situations where they are supervised and not required to make significant decisions involving abstract reasoning.

For the mild retardate, success as an adult in the community is more dependent on good social and emotional adjustments than on academic achievement. The mild retardate is more likely to be ostracized when he has a: (1) personality disorder; (2) speech defect; (3) motor problem; or (4) cosmetic defect. Motivational factors are also paramount in determining a young retardate's ultimate success. Failures experienced in early childhood often lead to loss of initiative and a fear of competing. Zigler has shown how important motivational reinforcement may be in helping a retardate achieve at a higher level.

It is difficult to provide employment for the moderate to severely disabled and retarded. Sheltered workshops, "half-way houses" (part-time residencies and part-time outside employment), and closely supervised restricted employment programs provide only a few of the answers to this complex and challenging problem.

Institutionalization. One of the most difficult problems facing the physician who cares for a retarded child is the role of institutional placement. Surveys of institutions that care for retarded children indicate that the majority of the resident children fall into the moderate to severely retarded range. In general, the most severely defective, and in particular, the more deformed or stigmatized the infant or child, the earlier the referral for residential care will be initiated.

When dealing with parents of a young infant with multiple deformities or Down's syndrome, where the prognosis is relatively clear, the pediatrician's or family physician's role as a counselor to the family is often compromised by what the obstetrician may already have told the parents. If the pediatrician is the first to inform the parents of the diagnosis, his approach may be more flexible. A complete exposition of diagnosis and all the prognostic implications during the first interview is usually too overwhelming for most young parents. The details of the problem are best elaborated in a series of visits and discussions with, if possible, *both* parents, so that genetic as well as prognostic implications can be explored. Social service and psychiatric assistance may be necessary to deal with feelings of guilt or severe depression in some of the cases.

The question of institutional placement almost always arises early in infants with Down's syndrome or with stigmata that are usually associated with mental retardation. Immediate residential placement is usually difficult to arrange even if the parents decide they wish to institutionalize the child rather than take the baby home with them from the hospital. The physician's responsibility in such cases is to inform the families of the facts and prognosis, and describe, without bias, the realities and/or rewards that result from living with and rearing a retarded and stigmatized child. The physician may offer advice in these matters, particularly if he is well acquainted with the family's social dynamics and finances. However, he should not make the final decision about institutional placement. The family is on firmest ground when the decision is made by them, and the physician acts only as an advisor.

The above principles generally apply to children who are diagnosed as being retarded at any age. In order for the parents to make an intelligent decision concerning home care versus institutional placement, the family must be aware of the child's diagnosis and prognosis, the available nonresidential educational, social, and community facilities for the child, as well as the nature of the residential facilities for the community. Visits to these residential centers and state schools should be encouraged prior to a submission of an application for admission. When the parents come to the physician for advice concerning this matter, he, too, should be aware of the nature of the facilities in his community. Parents' groups such as the National Association for the Help of Retarded Children or Association for the Aid of Crippled Children are often useful in supplying this information to the physician and the family. Finally, when the physician does advise the family on the question of residential placement, he should consider the total effect of the retarded child on this particular family. He should also provide the family with some needed insight and, as far as is possible, be supportive.

Institutionalization is considered most often when the affected children are at the chronologic extremes of the pediatrician's practice. The parent of the severely retarded or stigmatized infant has good reason for considering early placement. The parent of the mild to moderately retarded child usually maintains that child at home with the help of community programs. However, as adolescence approaches, behavior problems increase and become unmanageable. Vocational and recreational opportunities seem unavailable. There is fear of sexual abuse to naive female retardates or unwarranted concern about sexual aggressivity in male retardates. As a result, parents of retarded children reconsider or first consider the idea of residential placement. This is particularly true if the parents are advanced in age and concerned about "who will care for the child after they are gone."

There has been considerable controversy and discussion concerning the faults of most state institutions for the retarded in the United States and elsewhere. Archaic philosophies and limited allocation of funds have created many large overcrowded institutions with poorly trained staffs and limited therapeutic programs. However, it can be firmly stated that the tide is now turning. The problems of institutional care are being debated, new programs being created, and new funds being provided. No longer will children be "put away" in institutions but, for those who are able, they will be sent there for rehabilitation and training.

Chromosomal (Autosomal) Disorders Associated with Mental Retardation

TRISOMY 21 (DOWN'S SYNDROME). This disease entity was first described by Langdon Down in 1866. It has more recently been demonstrated to be associated with a consistent cytologic anomaly, the presence of an excess of chromosomal material derived from all or part of chromosome number 21. Karyotypic analysis reveals that the majority of patients with Down's syndrome have 47 chromosomes with a trisomy of chromosome number 21 (Fig. 27). The underlying genetic mechanism for this event is nondisjunction.

A small percentage of individuals with Down's syndrome have a structural chromosomal abnormality called a translocation with a total chromosome number of 46. Translocations occur because of centric fusion of two chromosomes and most commonly involve chromosomes number 21 and 15. However, translocations involving chromosomes 21 and 25 have been reported.

There are individuals who have been found to be mildly or moderately affected whose cells karyotypically are mixtures of normal cells and cells trisomic for chromosome number 21. This condition is called mosaicism and results either from nondisjunction in early cell division of normal zygote or from the loss of a chromosome in a developing trisomic zygote.

There is a correlation with maternal age (Fig. 28). The trisomy 21 anomaly is encountered with increasing frequency with older mothers; while the rarer translocation anomaly is seen in younger mothers. However, the birth of a child with trisomy 21 may occur at any maternal age.

The etiology of the cytogenetic disturbance associated with Down's syndrome remains unknown. In addition to maternal age, autoantibodies (thyroid) and maternal radiation have both been implicated as possible etiologic factors.

Clinical Findings. Patients with Down's syndrome are usually recognized at birth and become more recognizable with advancing age (Fig. 29). No one symptom or combination of symptoms is diagnostic. Trisomy and translocation patients are clinically indistinguishable. However, mosaics have atypical signs, and normal intellect has been reported in some cases. The clinical features are listed in Table 8. The findings printed in italics are the most frequent ones reported.

Pathology. Extensive neuropathologic changes have been observed, but both the gross and microscopic abnormalities are variable and are not specific of Down's syndrome. Macro- and microgyria, delayed myelination of white matter, immature differentiation of ganglion cells, and abnormal embryonic cell piles are all fairly common findings. Thyroid, pituitary, adrenal, and thymus have been reported to show signs of maldevelopment and malfunction.

Intelligence. The intelligence of patients with Down's syndrome is variable and follows a bell-shaped curve, with a median IQ of 40 to 50 in home-reared children, and an overall range of 20 to 70. It has been reported that the rate of intellectual growth declines with passing years. This may

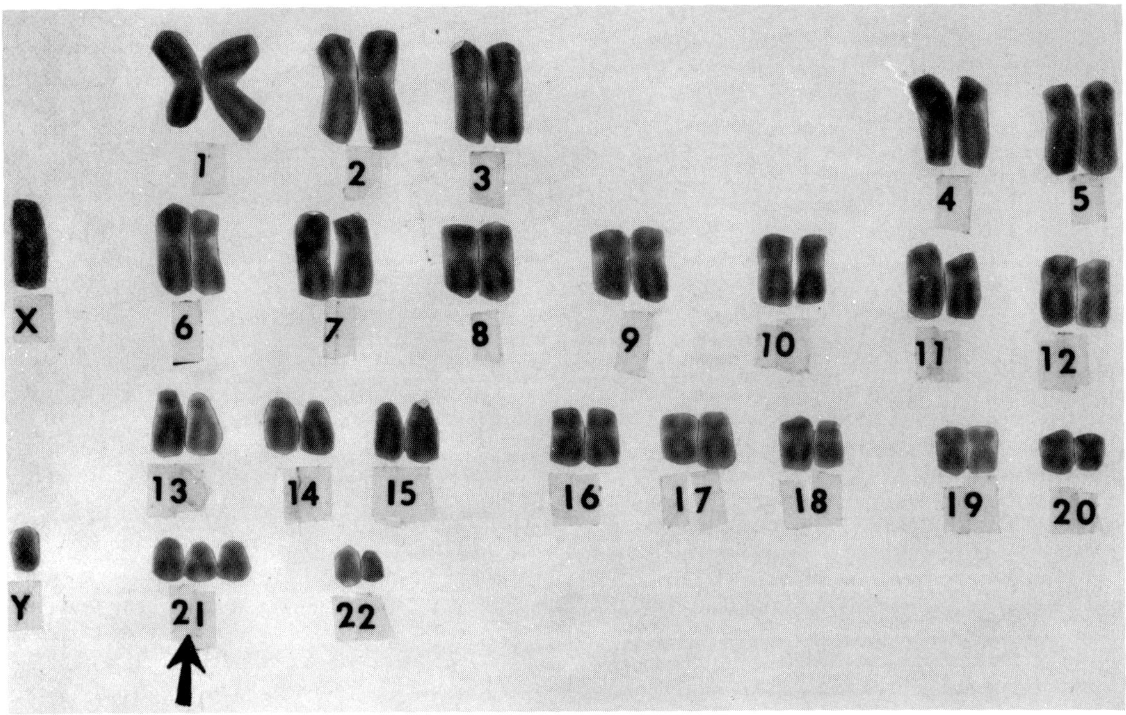

Fig. 27. Karyotype of child with Down's syndrome showing trisomy at chromosome 21 (arrow). (Courtesy of Drs. O. J. Miller and D. Warburton.)

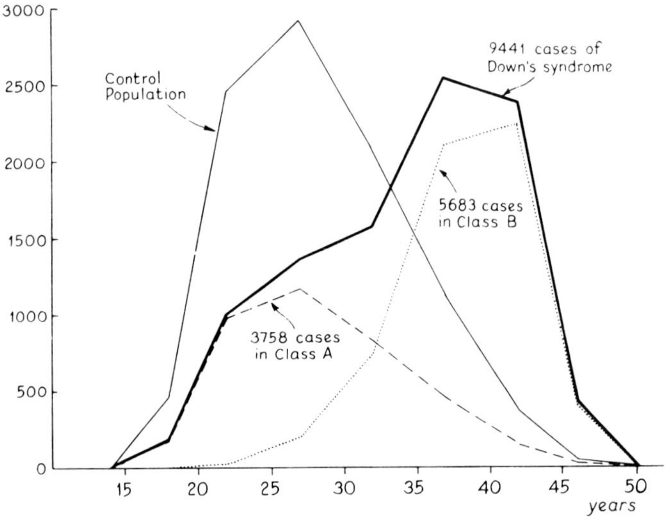

Fig. 28. Maternal age distribution of 9,441 cases of Down's syndrome with control population. (From Penrose and Smith. *Down's Anomaly*. Courtesy of J. & A. Churchill Ltd.)

reflect the possibility of CNS degeneration related to premature aging, or a possible arrest in psychologic and social capacities. It may be that since the tests have been standardized on normal individuals, they may not reflect "normal" maturation of children with Down's syndrome who have defective brains.

Development. Almost all uncomplicated Down's individuals ambulate by 3 to 4 years of age and over 90 percent develop simple language by 5 years of age. The aging process is more rapid. Cataracts

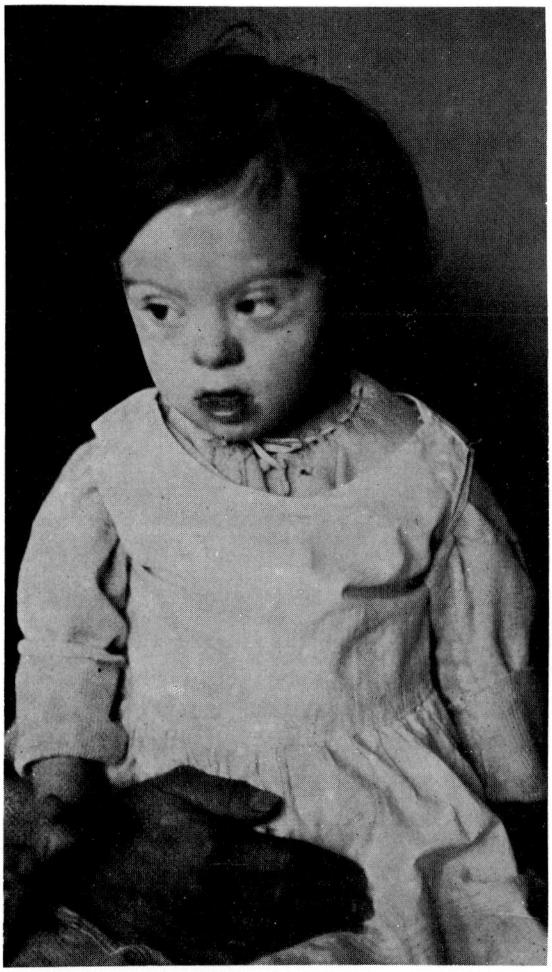

Fig. 29. Girl 4 years of age with Down's syndrome showing characteristic facies.

and arteriosclerosis are frequent complications in early adult life. A rapid metabolic turnover has been implicated as a possible cause for this phenomenon. For example, the life-span of polymorphonuclear leucocytes is shortened. This is illustrated by a decreased lobe count per cell.

Laboratory Findings. Laboratory investigations have yielded inconsistent findings, including the following reported abnormalities: serum serotonin is decreased; acid and alkaline phosphase of white blood cells are increased; and glucose-6-phosphate dehydrogenase of red blood cells is increased. Some variation and differences in these findings have been reported between the translocation and trisomic types.

Treatment. There is no specific medical treatment for this condition. Though many drugs have been tried in an attempt to improve this condition, treatments with vitamins, special diets, and thyroid medication have proved unsuccessful.

Prognosis. Individuals with Down's syndrome functioning within the mild to high moderate range of mental retardation can be educated to early grade level accomplishments. Many of these can find employment in a sheltered workshop. Very few, if any, become independent in the community. Their cosmetic defect adds to their problem in being accepted, even if their IQ permits them to compete vocationally.

The average life-span of patients is shortened and one half die by the end of the third year, mostly as a result of respiratory infections and congenital heart disease. Most of the remaining patients succumb by 40 to 50 years of age for reasons believed to be related to rapid aging processes. Leukemia occurs three times more frequently than in normal children.

Genetic Counseling. If the mother is under 35 years of age, karyotypically normal, and has a trisomic

TABLE 8. *Clinical Features in Down's Syndrome* *

Head	Microcephaly; *flat occiput*; brachycephaly
Eyes	*Inner and outer epicanthal folds slanted upwards and outwards;* bilateral speckling of iris (Brushfield's spots) around limbic area; strabismus; refractive error; cataracts in early adulthood
Ears	*Simple or aberrant helix formation;* low set
Nose	Usually small with flattened bridge
Mouth	Tongue large and fissured; *nasopharynx small* (causes mouth breathing); abnormal morphology and frequent absence of teeth
Neck	Short; occasional webbing
Hands	*Stubby, distal triradius; radial loop on digit IV and ulnar loops of all other digits;* digital loop between digits IV and V; *incurved short 5th fingers (clinodactyly) with single crease; single four finger breadth midpalmar crease (Simian line)* (usually bilateral)
Feet	Short and stubby; widespread 1st and 2nd toes; deep crease leading distally from angle of 1st and 2nd toes; distinctive dermatoglyphics
Abdomen	*Protruberant; umbilical hernia;* duodenal atresia; megacolon; microcolon
Skin	Dry; decreased elasticity
Heart	*Septal defects;* pulmonary stenosis; aortic stenosis
Genitalia	Male—testes undescended; small penis Female—labia minora underdeveloped; menopause early
Pelvis	Iliac wings large and flared; *iliac index measured on x-ray is decreased*
Neurologic	*Hypotonia*, normoreflexia; poor fine and gross coordination
Speech	Voice is usually low-pitched and "raucous"; speech has infantile omissions and substitutions

*The more common clinical features are italicized.

TABLE 9. *Comparison of the Findings in Trisomy D and Trisomy E*

	Trisomy D (13/15)	Trisomy E (16/18)
Incidence	0.45 per 1,000 live births	0.23 per 1,000 live births
Sex ratio	F > M	F > M
Maternal age	30.8 years	34.4 years (control 28.5)
Birth weight	Average or low	Small for gestational age
Rate of growth	Normal	Slow
Mental retardation	Severe	Severe
Seizures	Minor motor; apneic episodes	Occasional
Tone	Hypertonic or normal	Hypertonic
Hearing	Impaired	Normal
Head	Microcephaly; sloping forehead; abnormal calcification	Prominent occiput
Eyes	Microophthalmus; coloboma of iris; corneal opacities	Ptosis or lid abnormalities
Ears	Low set; abnormal helix	Low set
Mouth	Cleft palate; cleft lip	Small
Skin	Capillary hemangiomata Necrotic ulcers of scalp	Mottled; lanugolike hair
Hands	Polydactyly; flexed fingers, hyperconvex and narrow fingernails; retroflexible thumbs	Clenched fingers, index over third; syndactyly
Feet	Posterior prominence of heels, polydactyly	Big toe short and in hammer position; rocker-bottom feet
Heart	Dextrocardia; ventricular septal defect	Ventricular septal defect; patent ductus arteriosus
Kidney	Obstructive hydronephrosis	Double ureter
Hernia	Umbilical	Umbilical and inguinal
Genitalia	Abnormal scrotum; cryptorchidism; bicornuate uterus	—
Skeletal	—	Short sternum, small pelvis, small mandible; delayed ossification
Other	Accessory spleen; enlarged gallbladder (stenosis of bile duct); incomplete rotation of colon	Eventration of diaphragm
Dermatoglyphics	Distal axial triradius; Simian crease; arch fibular pattern in the hallucal area of foot	Simple area pattern for nearly ali digits; single flexion crease 5th finger; occasional Simian crease
Death	Early childhood	Early infancy

offspring, the risk of recurrence is low. In contrast, a mother over 35 years of age would have a six times greater risk of a recurrence.

If the propositus is found to have mosaicism or a translocation anomaly, chromosome studies should be performed on both parents, and on any siblings. A phenotypically normal individual may be a carrier of the translocation. Appropriate genetic counseling on recurrence risks can then be offered by the physician.

13/15 TRISOMY (D) (PATAU SYNDROME). The main clinical findings are listed in Table 9. These babies

A

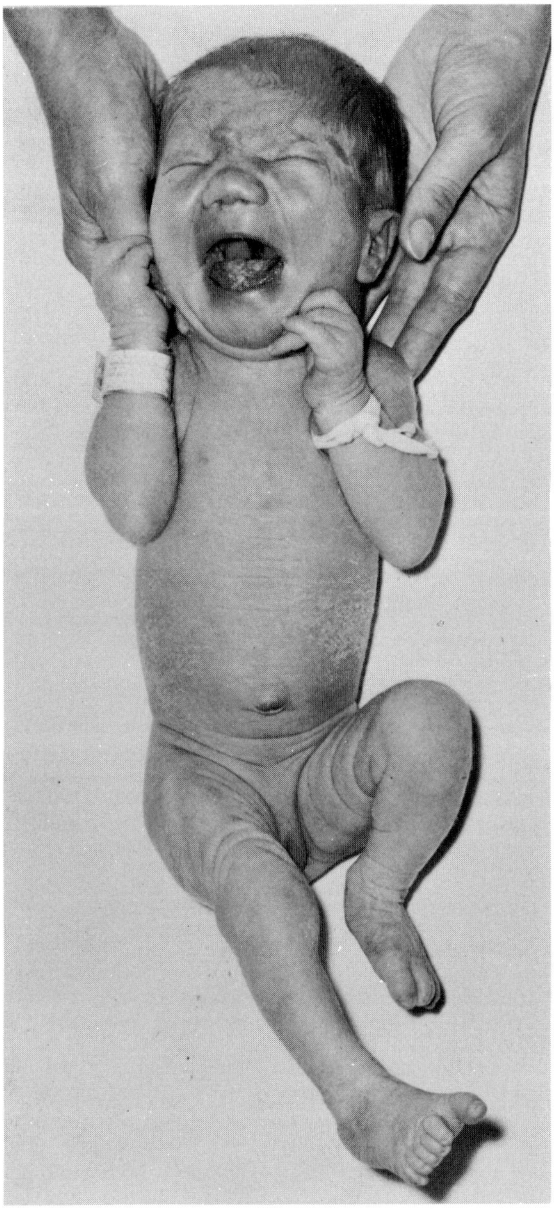

B

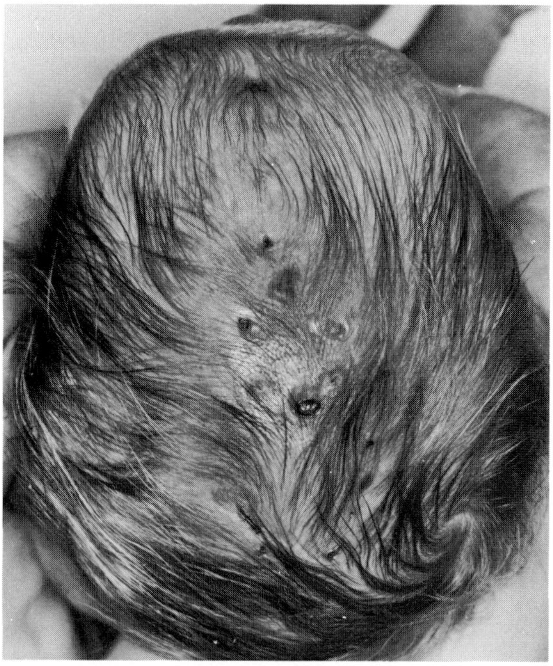

Fig. 30. Trisomy 13/15 (D) showing characteristic clinical features. *A.* (*Left*) Some of the anomalies associated with Trisomy 13: microphthalmia, cleft palate, and polydactyly. *B.* (*Above*) Typical necrotic ulcers seen in Trisomy 13. (Courtesy of Drs. J. Lindsten and P. Zetterquist.)

are usually easily recognized at birth since their deformities are quite vivid and distinctive (Fig. 30A and B). The majority have a cleft palate and lip, low-set malformed ears, microphthalmia, capillary hemangioma, polydactyly, and congenital heart disease. Familial D/D translocation has been described.

A shortened life expectancy is the rule, with death usually occurring in the first year of life.

TRISOMY E (18). The addition of an extra chromosome in the E group causes a distinct clinical syndrome (Fig. 31A, B, C, and D). Children with this chromosomal defect are of low birth weight and have numerous stigmata including a prominent occiput, micrognathia, low-set ears, overlapping of the second and third digits, multiple contractures (arthrogryposis), and rocker-bottom feet (Table 9). These infants fail to thrive, and usually die within the first few months of life. Congenital heart and renal anomalies are common postmortem findings. The few children who survive beyond the first few months of life have severe developmental retardation.

CRI DU CHAT SYNDROME (PARTIAL DELETION OF SHORT ARM OF CHROMOSOME 4 OR 5). Lejeune and his co-workers described this syndrome which is named after a characteristic cry of the infants so affected. Most observers have described the cry as resembling the mewing of a cat.

The clinical features (Fig. 32) are listed in Table 10. Findings such as an antimongoloid slant of the eyes, a moon facies, brachycephaly, epicanthi, and hypertelorism may suggest Down's syndrome. However, in this syndrome, increased maternal age is not common. Some familial translocations have been reported. Mental retardation is usually severe in cases of Cri du Chat, but despite this, the child's life-span is usually not significantly shortened.

MONOSOMY G (22/22 MONOSOMY, ANTIMONGOLISM). These patients are clinically almost the antithesis of the trisomy 21. Findings include antimongoloid slants of the eyes, hypertonia, and severe mental retardation. Only rare cases of monosomy G have been reported.

A B

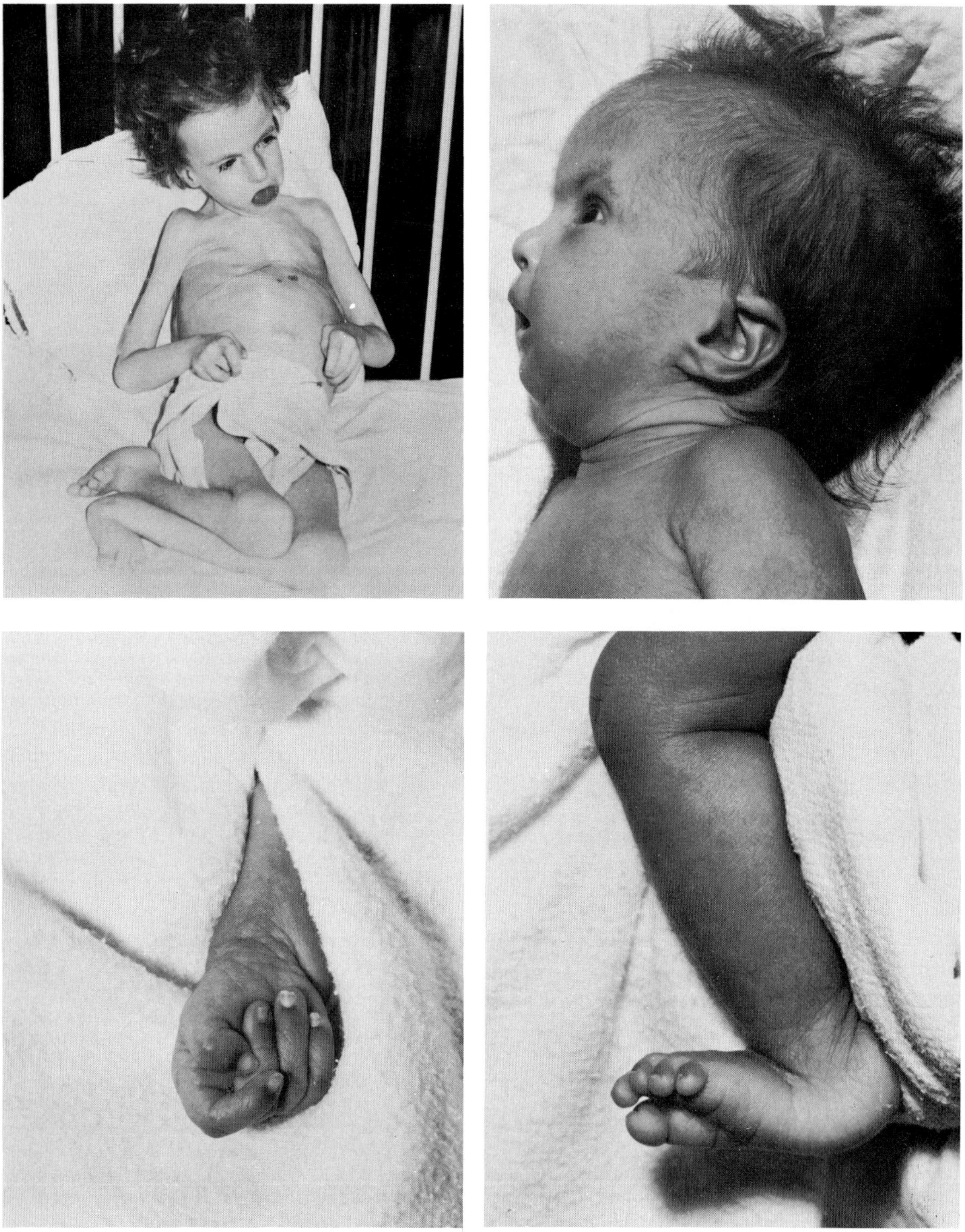

C D

Fig. 31. Trisomy 18 (E) showing characteristic clinical features. *A.* Note emaciation, flexion contractures of extremities, abnormal positioning of fingers, and "rocker-bottom" feet. *B.* Profile of face demonstrating micrognathia and low-set ears. C. Abnormal positioning of index finger with deviation to ulnar side, crossing backward over the middle finger. *D.* "Rocker-bottom" foot with short big toe. (Courtesy of Drs. W. W. Weber, P. Mamunes, R. Day, and Phebe Miller.)

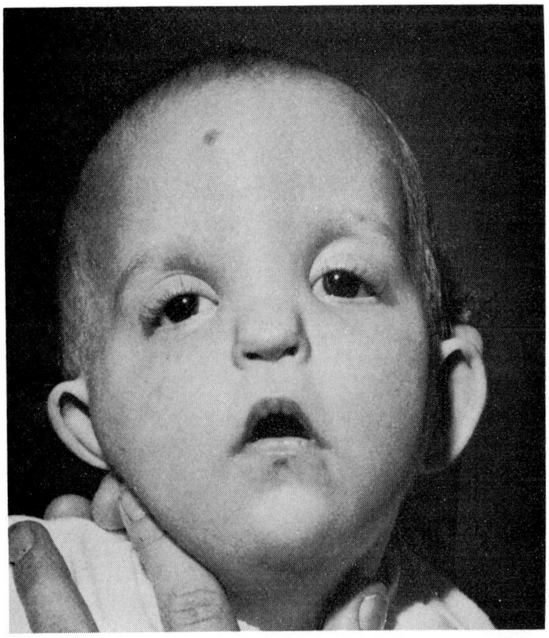

Fig. 32. Characteristic facies of Cat Cry syndrome (Cri du Chat). Note round moon face, hypertelorism, oblique palpebral fissures and low-set ears. (Courtesy of Drs. O. J. Miller and D. Warburton.)

RING CHROMOSOMES (A, 5, C, D, E, 16, 17, 18, AND X). Mental retardation is the one universal finding in the different ring chromosomal abnormalities. The clinical picture is variable. The findings are rarely distinctive enough to be identified as a single syndrome.

Sex Chromosome Abnormalities

KLINEFELTER'S SYNDROME (XXY). The extra X chromosome causes a eunochoid appearance. On examination, arm span is noted to be greater than height, facial and body hair is sparse, and the patient's voice is high-pitched. Gynecomastia is usually present. Testes are small but the penis is of normal size. Compared with the general population there is an increase in the prevalence of asthma and diabetes mellitus. Many, but not all, are mildly retarded. Psychotic illness appears also to be more common and usually is diagnosed as a "severe anxiety neurosis."

Laboratory findings include an increased output of urinary pituitary gonadotropins. A decreased uptake of ^{131}I by the thyroid gland is occasionally noted. Klinefelter patients are usually infertile. Testicular biopsy reveals clumping of the Leydig cells and abnormalities of the seminiferous tubules. Life-span is not usually shortened.

TURNER'S SYNDROME (XO). Mild mental retardation is infrequently a feature of the syndrome.

TABLE 10. *Clinical Findings in Cri Du Chat Syndrome (Partial Deletion of Short Arm of Chromosome 4 or 5)*

Always present

- Abnormal cry
- Severe mental retardation
- Microcephaly
- Hypertelorism
- Epicanthus
- Abnormal dermatoglyphics

Frequently present

- Failure to thrive
- Brachycephaly
- Moon face
- Antimongoloid slant
- Low-set ears
- Micrognathia
- Hypotonia
- Strabismus

Occasionally Present

- Short neck
- Optic atrophy
- Congenital heart disease

"SUPERFEMALE" SYNDROME (XXX and XXXX). In the XXXX syndrome all have been retarded, while normal intelligence may occur with the XXX syndrome. Short stature is a common characteristic in these patients.

"DOUBLE MALE" SYNDROME (YY, XYY, XXYY, and XXXYY). XYY individuals have been reported to have a tendency toward aggressive, psychopathic, and antisocial behavior. Mild mental retardation is occasionally associated with these findings. It is uncertain to what extent the mental defect or the chromosomal anomaly influences or determines the behavioral traits observed in this syndrome.

Combined or Multiple Cytogenetic Abnormalities

Down's syndrome has been noted in association with Klinefelter's syndrome. XXY trisomy has been reported in 6.25 percent of males with Down's syndrome in a survey done soon after birth, and in only 0.35 percent of older males with Down's syndrome. The reported difference in relative frequencies may mean that the combination increases the patient's risk for a shortened life-span. Down's syndrome has also been reported in association with XXX, Turner's syndrome, and trisomy D. Of particular interest are the reports of Down's syndrome in patients with sibs who have another type of trisomy (XXY, trisomy E, XXX). This association may reflect a familial predisposition towards chromosomal errors, although they may be purely chance happenings.

REFERENCES

Birch, H. G., and Lefford, A. Intersensory development in children. Monogr. Soc. Res. Child Develop., 28: Serial No. 89, 1, 1963.

——— and Lefford, A. Two strategies for studying perception in "brain-damaged" children. *In* Birch, H. G., ed., Brain Damage in Children: The Biological and Social Aspects. Baltimore, Williams and Wilkins Co., 1963.

——— and Belmont, L. Auditory-visual integration, intelligence and reading ability in school children. Percept. Motor Skills, 20:295, 1965.

——— Richardson, S. A., Baird, D., Horokin, G., and Illsley, R. Mental Subnormality in the Community. Baltimore, The Williams and Wilkins Co., 1970.

Chase, H. P., and Martin, H. P. Undernutrition and child development. New Eng. J. Med., 282:933, 1970.

Collman, R. D., and Stoller, A. A. Survey of mongolism and congenital anomalies of the central nervous system in Victoria, New Zealand. New Zeal. Med. J., 61:24, 1962.

Conen, P. E. The "D" syndrome. Amer. J. Dis. Child., 111:236, 1966.

Cravioto, J., DeLicardie, E. R., and Birch, H. G. Nutrition, growth and neurointegrative development: an experimental and ecologic study. Pediatrics, 38: (Suppl.)2:331, 1966.

D'Amato, G. Residential Treatment For Child Mental Health. Springfield, Ill., Charles C Thomas, Publ., 1969.

Denhoff, E., Siqueland, M., Komich, P., and Hainsworth, P. K. Developmental and predictive characteristics of items from the Meeting Street School Screening Test. Develop. Med. Child Neurol., 10:220, 1968.

Eisenberg, L. Behavioral manifestations of cerebral damage in children. *In* Birch, H. G., ed., Brain Damage in Children: The Biological and Social Aspects. Baltimore, Williams and Wilkins Co., 1963.

Frankenburg, W. K., and Dodds, J. B. The Denver Developmental Screening Test. J. Pediat., 71:181, 1967.

French, J. H., Graziani, L. J., and Scheinberg, L. C. Treatment of metabolic and endocrine causes of mental retardation. Mod. Treatm., 4:987, 1967.

Frostig, M., Lefever, D. A., and Whittlesey, R. B. A development test of visual perception for evaluating normal and neurologically handicapped children. Percept. Motor Skills, 12:383, 1961.

Gellis, S. S., and Feingold, M. Atlas of Mental Retardation Syndromes. Washington, D.C., U.S. Dept. of Health, Education and Welfare, 1968.

Gruenberg, E. M. Some epidemiological aspects of congenital brain damage. *In* Birch, H. G., ed., Brain Damage in Children: The Biological and Social Aspects. Baltimore, Williams and Wilkins Co., 1964.

Haeussermann, E. Estimating developmental potential for preschool children with brain lesions. Amer. J. Ment. Defic., 61:170, 1956.

Haggard, E. W. Social status and intelligence: an experimental study of certain cultural determinants of measured intelligence. Genet. Psychol. Monogr., 49:141, 1954.

Helm, A. W., and Wallace, T. G. The effects of repeatedly retesting the same group on the same intelligence tests: II. high grade mental defectives. Quart. J. Exp. Psychiat., 2:19, 1950.

Hsia, D. Y. Human Developmental Genetics. Chicago, Year Book Medical Publishers, 1968.

Illingworth, R. S. The predictive value of development tests in the first year with special reference to the diagnosis of mental subnormality. J. Child Psychol. Psychiat., 2:210, 1961.

Kirk, S. Early Education of the Mentally Retarded. Urbana, Univ. of Illinois Press, 1958.

——— and McCarthy, J. J. The Illinois Test of Psycholinguistic Abilities—an approach to differential diagnosis. Amer. J. Ment. Defic., 66:399, 1961.

Knobloch, H., and Pasamanick, B. An evaluation of the consistency and predictive value of the 40 week Gesell developmental schedules. Psychiat. Res. Rep., 13:10, 1960.

——— and Pasamanick, B. Predicting intellectual potential in infancy: some variables affecting the validity of developmental diagnosis. Amer. J. Dis. Child., 106:43, 1963.

Laufer, M. W., and Denhoff, E. Hyperkinetic behavior syndrome in children. J. Pediat., 50:463, 1957.

Lilienfeld, A. M., and Pasamanick, B. The association of maternal and fetal factors with the development of mental deficiency. Amer. J. Ment. Defic., 60:557, 1956.

Masland, R. L., Sarason, B., and Gladwin, T. Mental Subnormality. New York, Basic Books, Inc., Publ., 1958.

McCracken, J. S., and Gordon, R. R. Cri du Chat syndrome—a new clinical and cytogenetic entity. Lancet, 1:23, 1965.

Motulsky, A. G. Population genetics of mental retardation. *In* Jervis, G. A., ed., Expanding Concepts in Mental Retardation. Springfield, Ill., Charles C Thomas, Publ., 1968.

Parker, C. E. Mavalwala, J., Weise, P., Koch, R., Hatashita, A., and Cibilich, S. The 47, XYY syndrome in a boy with behavior problems and mental retardation. Amer. J. Ment. Defic., 74:660, 1970.

Penrose, L. S. A clinical and genetic study of 1280 cases of mental defect. Special Report Series No. 229, Medical Research Council, London, His Majesty's Stationery Office, 1938.

——— and Smith, G. F. Down's Anomaly. London, J. and A. Churchill Ltd., 1966.

Polani, P. E. Cytogenetics of Down's syndrome. *In* Jervis, G. A., ed., Expanding Concepts in Mental Retardation. Springfield, Ill., Charles C Thomas, Publ., 1968, Ch. 4.

Sheridan, M. D. Infants at risk of handicapping conditions. Monthly Bull. Minist. Health (London), 21: 238, 1962.

Sievers, D. J. Development and standardization of a test of psycholinguistic growth in preschool children. Unpublished Ph.D. Thesis, Univ. of Illinois, 1955.

Smith, D. W. The 18 trisomy and D trisomy syndromes. Pediat. Clin. of N. Amer., 10:389, 1963.

Stein, Z. A., and Susser, M. W. The social distribution of mental retardation. Amer. J. Ment. Defic., 67:811, 1963.

Taylor, A. I. Patau's, Edward's and Cri du chat syndrome. A tabulated summary of current findings. Develop. Med. Child Neurol., 9:78, 1967.

Telfer, M. A., Baker, D., Clark, G. R., and Richardson, C. E. Incidence of gross chromosomal errors among tall criminal American males. Science, 159:1249, 1968.

Tizard, J., and O'Connor, N. The employability of high

grade mental defectives: I. Amer. J. Ment. Defic., 54:563, 1950.

——— Psychological development of handicapped children. Brit. Med. J., 1:1041, 1960.

Uchide, I. A., and Soltan, H. C. Evaluation of dermatoglyphics in medical genetics. Pediat. Clin. N. Amer., 10:409, 1962.

Wertelecki, W., Schindler, A. M., and Gerald, P. S. Partial deletion of chromosome 18. Lancet, 2:641, 1960.

Chapter 4
THE DEGENERATIVE AND DEMYELINATING DISEASES OF THE NERVOUS SYSTEM

ARTHUR L. DREW, JR.

The progressive, degenerative, and demyelinating diseases of the nervous system present themselves clinically with a wide diversity of symptoms according to primary anatomic sites involved (Table 11). They have a number of features in common. They are essentially hereditable and thus can be presumed to be the result of transmissible enzymatic defects most of which, at the present time, are not clearly defined. The basic mode of inheritance is that of a single autosomal recessive gene, although examples of sex linkage and dominant Mendelian patterns are known. Recent transmission of Kuru and Creutzfeldt-Jakob disease from man to animal raises the possibility that some of the obscure degenerative diseases of infancy and childhood, for instance the spongiform encephalopathies, may be due to transmissible infective agents, "slow" or "temperate" viruses. Further, studies of subacute sclerosing panencephalitis reveal the presence of measles virus and suggest an atypical immune response as yet another pathogenic mechanism of progressive degenerative diseases of the nervous system.

Except for a few rare forms in which the degenerative processes are present at birth, this group of diseases is characterized by the insidious onset of progressive central nervous system degeneration in a previously normally functioning child. Thus, the history of developmental regression is of extreme diagnostic importance. Such a history should always be sought. There tends to be rather marked variability from case to case even within a given family. Numerous atypical, abortive, and transitional forms are encountered and described.

In none of this group of diseases is therapy satisfactory, although in the more chronic forms considerable symptomatic and supportive treatment can and should be offered. Genetic counseling is of great importance.

Although the genetic origin of many of these diseases is well established, details of pathogenesis are not clear. Nevertheless, it is possible to classify some general types. There is the group in which the evidence for the presence of an inborn error of metabolism has been established or strongly suspected. In this group, various amino-acidurias, hepatolenticular degeneration, cerebromacular degeneration, galactosemia, the mucopolysaccharidoses, and metachromatic leucodystrophy may be included. Another group consists of the diffuse cerebral scleroses and disseminated scleroses, in which the fundamental pathologic processes are primary demyelination. There are also a number of progressive degenerative syndromes involving the basal ganglia, spinal cord, cerebellum, and peripheral nerves to which the term "abiotrophy" has been applied. In these there is a slow, genetically predetermined, and systematic decay of neural elements. Disorders in which there are degenerative changes in the nervous system associated with skin lesions are classified as neurocutaneous or neuroectodermal syndromes.

The diagnosis of degenerative disease can be difficult, and the exact delineation of these progressive disorders presents a challenge to even the most sophisticated. They must be differentiated from the static nonprogressive entities such as cerebral palsy which often present with similar clinical manifestations. The importance of establishing a correct diagnosis has both prognostic and genetic significance.

Definition and classification has, in the past, been largely dependent, as indicated in Table 11, upon localization of the major site of the pathologic process. Involvement of the gray matter is suggested by the early appearance of seizures, especially the myoclonic variety, and progressive dementia. In white matter disease, the early manifestation may be a progressive spastic paralysis. Rapid advances in neuropathology and biochemistry are leading to a more precise definition of this group of diseases. More precise diagnostic methods are becoming available to the clinician. In an increasing number of cases, correct antemortem diagnosis is now possible. An awareness of the clinical features and the natural history of the disease, and the utilization of appropriate laboratory procedures all contribute towards establishing the correct diagnosis. The age of onset and rate of progression, ethnic origin, changes in head size, systemic and ophthalmologic abnormalities, and specific alterations in urine, blood, and spinal fluid, together with electroencephalographic, electromyographic, and nerve conduction studies, will provide invaluable clues in diagnosis. Good family histories and careful examinations of parents and sibs are mandatory in many of this large group of diseases. Cerebral biopsy, less frequently rectal biopsy, in carefully selected cases and where competent neuropathologic, histochemical, and electron microscopic studies are available, has proved to be of great value in the diagnosis and wider understanding of the degenerative diseases. Cerebral biopsies should not be done for the sole reason that a definitive diagnosis has not been made. They are justified when clinical and laboratory studies point to a

TABLE 11. *Classification of Degenerative Diseases of the Nervous System*

Diseases of Cerebral Gray Matter

Cerebral Storage Diseases	
Cerebromacular degeneration—Amaurotic familial idiocy (AFI)	
	Accumulated Material
Norman-Wood congenital AFI	GD_3 gangliosidosis
Tay-Sachs infantile AFI	GM_2 gangliosidosis
Tay-Sachs with visceral involvement	GM_2 gangliosidosis
Neurovisceral gangliosidosis	GM_1 gangliosidosis
Jansky-Bielchowsky late infantile AFI	
Batten-Mayou-Spielmeyer-Vogt juvenile AFI	lipofuscin
Kufs adult AFI	
Niemann-Pick disease	ceramide-P-choline
Progressive familial myoclonic epilepsy (Unverricht's disease)	Lafore bodies (mucopolysaccharides)
Gaucher's disease	ceramide-glucose
Fabry's disease	ceramide di- and trihexosidosis
Farber's disease	ceramide and gangliosidosis
Cerebral cholesterolosis	cholesterol
Heller's disease	
Mucopolysaccharidoses Types I-III	mucopolysaccharides
Krabbe's disease	ceramide-galactose
Glycogen storage disease Type VIII	glycogen

Nonstorage Cerebral Diseases
- Progressive degeneration of cerebral gray matter
- Alper's disease
- Necrotizing encephalopathy (Leigh's Disease)

Diseases of Cerebral White Matter

Leucodystrophies
- Pelizaeus-Merzbacher's disease
- Metachromatic leucodystrophy
- Globoid-cell leucodystrophy (Krabbe's disease)
- Spongy sclerosis (Canavan's disease)
- Sudanophilic (neutral fat, orthochromic) familial leucodystrophy
- Alexander's disease

Demyelinating Scleroses
- Acute disseminated encephalomyelitides
- Acute necrotizing hemorrhagic leucoencephalitis (Hurst)
- Multiple or disseminated sclerosis
- Neuromyelitis optica (Devic's disease)
- Balo's concentric sclerosis
- Schilder's disease (encephalitis periaxialis diffusa)

Degenerations of the Basal Ganglia
(The Extrapyramidal Syndromes)

- Juvenile parkinsonism
- Huntington's chorea
- Dystonia musculorum deformans
- Hallervorden-Spatz disease
- Hepatolenticular degeneration (Wilson's disease)
- Status demyelinisatus
- Dyssynergia cerebellaris myoclonica

Polymorphous Neuroabiotrophies

Cerebellar Degeneration
- Spinocerebellar degenerations
  - Friedreich's ataxia
  - Roussy-Levy syndrome
  - Marinesco-Sjögren and Garland-Moorhouse syndrome
  - Bassen-Kornzweig syndrome
  - Ataxia-telangiectasia

TABLE 11. (continued)

Polymorphous Neuroabiotrophies (continued)

Brainstem and Spinal Cord Degenerations
- Progressive infantile spinal atrophy (Werdnig-Hoffman disease)
- Familial juvenile amyotrophic lateral sclerosis
- Fazio-Londes disease
- Familial amyotrophic dystonic paraplegia

Cranial and Peripheral Nerve Degenerations
- Leber's optic atrophy
- Peroneal muscular atrophy (neuromuscular atrophy, Charcot-Marie-Tooth disease)
- Hypertrophic interstitial neuritis (Dejerine-Sottas disease)
- Heredofamilial mononeuritis multiplex with brachial predilection
- Congenital indifference to pain
- Refsum's syndrome
- Hereditary sensory neuropathy associated with spinal cord disease
- Primary amyloidosis
- Alport's syndrome

Neurocutaneous Syndromes

Tuberous sclerosis
Neurofibromatosis
Encephalotrigeminal angiomatosis (Sturge-Weber-Dimitri syndrome)
Von Hippel-Lindau's disease
Neurocutaneous melanoses
Disseminated hemangiomatosis
Ataxia-telangiectasia
Hemangiectatic hypertrophy of a limb
Rud's syndrome
Sjögren-Larsson's syndrome
Darier's disease
Incontinentia pigmenti
Linear nevus sebaceus
Basal cell nevus syndrome

specific but unconfirmed diagnosis and where specific therapy or genetic counseling are demanding considerations. Some of these processes become evident in early infancy, while others appear in later childhood or early adolescence. Tables 12 A, B, and C outline the more common and better understood entities to be discussed in the sections dealing with degenerative diseases of cerebral gray and white matter.

Diseases of Cerebral Gray Matter

Cerebral Storage Disease

Progressive and excessive accumulation of cerebral lipids within the body of the nerve cell with variable degrees of secondary demyelination is the common pathology of this group. Accumulation is usually the result of defects in enzymatic degradation of lipid components (Table 13).

The major class of cerebral lipids involved in these diseases is the *sphingolipids*. These are fatty acid esters of N-acyl-sphingosine (ceramide) to which phosphoryl choline, hexose, hexoside, and sulfate are joined to form sphingomyelin, cerebroside, ganglioside, glycolipid, and sulfatide.

N-acyl-sphingosine—fatty acid ⟶ ceramide
Ceramide—galactose—sulfate ⟶ sulfatide
Ceramide—glucose ⟶ glucocerebroside
Ceramide—galactose ⟶ galactocerebroside
Ceramide—P-choline ⟶ sphingomyelin
Ceramide—hexoside (S) ⟶ ganglioside

N-acetyl-neuraminic acid (sialic acid)

Svennerhold has proposed what appears to be the best available nomenclature for the complex gangliosides:

G — ganglioside
M — monosialic acid
D — disialic acid
T — trisialic acid
1 — tetrahexoside
2 — trihexoside
3 — dihexoside

GM_2-ganglioside, the Tay-Sachs ganglioside, is thus a monosialicganglioside trihexoside.

The second major grouping of cerebral lipids consists of the *glycerophosphatides*. This complex group includes a variety of phosphatide compounds formerly denoted as cephalins and lecithins.

TABLE 12A. *Differential Diagnosis of the Cerebral Degenerative Disorders of Infancy—Gray Matter*

	Tay-Sachs	Niemann-Pick	Gaucher's	Alper's	Subacute Necrotizing Encephalopathy
Age of onset	4-6 months	Under 6 months	Under 6 months	Under 1 year	Under 1 year, rarely late childhood
Rate of progression	Rapid Death 2-3 years	Rapid Death before 3 years	Very rapid Death before 2 years	Rapid Death before 3 years	Usually rapid Death before 3 years
Ethnic group	Almost all Jewish	50% Jewish	65% Jewish		
Genetic	Recessive	Recessive	Recessive Rarely, dominant		Recessive
Head size	Enlarges late	Normal	Normal	Reduces late	Normal
Skin and/or systemic	Normal	Hepatospleno-megaly Xanthoma of skin, rare	Hepatospleno-megaly	Normal	Normal
Eye	Cherry-red macula Optic atrophy	Cherry-red macula Optic atrophy	Normal	Normal	Optic atrophy
Seizures	Frequent, but late	Rare	Rare	Onset with seizures Myoclonus and other types	Seizures late and rare
Neurologic signs	Early: flaccid paresis Late: spastic paresis Dementia: early Hyperacusis	Spastic paresis Early: dementia	Early: retroflexion of head Strabismus Bulbar palsy Spastic paralysis Early: dementia	Spastic paresis Dementia Cortical blind-ness and deafness	Bulbar palsy Weak, infrequent cry Flaccid paresis with immobility
Blood	Absent fructose-1-P-aldolase ↑ SGOT ↑ Vacuolated lymphocytes	Vacuolated lymphocytes ↑ Serum lipids ↑ SGOT	↑ Acid phosphatase	Normal	Normal
Urine	Normal	Normal	Normal	Normal	Normal
CSF	Normal	Normal		Normal	Normal
Biopsy	+Rectal	"Foam cells"—bone marrow	Gaucher cells—bone marrow		
X-ray		Diffuse pulmonary infiltrates Demineralization of bone			
Electroretino-gram	Normal				

The final major category of cerebral lipids is the *sterol group*, represented by cholesterol, which comprises about 20 percent of the lipid content of the cerebral white matter in unesterified form. The breakdown of myelin results in an increase in esterified fraction. The triglycerides, normally not present in the central nervous system, accumulate with the myelin breakdown and have been reported as elevated in plasma of patients with Heller's disease.

The specific enzymatic defects have not as yet been determined in all of the cerebral storage diseases (Table 13). The substrate, or storage material, has been fairly well documented in a number of the cerebral lipidoses. Infantile amaurotic idiocy (Tay-Sachs disease) Type I GM_2-gangliosidosis is the result of a deficiency in hexosaminidase A. Type II GM_2-gangliosidosis is a deficiency in hexosaminidase A and B and a juvenile Type III GM_2-gangliosidosis

TABLE 12B. *Differential Diagnosis of the Cerebral Degenerative Disorders of Infancy—White Matter*

	Krabbe's	Metachromatic Leucodystrophy	Spongy Sclerosis (Canavan)	Palizaeus-Merzbacher	Maple Syrup
Age of onset	3-6 months	1-2 years, rarely late childhood	0-4 months	6-24 months	1-2 weeks
Rate of progression	Rapid Death by 2 years	Slow Death by 3-5 years	Rapid Death by 3 years	Slow May survive to adult life	Rapid Death weeks to month
Sex or ethnic group			Most Jewish	Predominantly males	
Genetic	Recessive	Recessive	Recessive	Sex-linked recessive	Recessive (?)
Head size	Normal	Enlarges late	Enlarges early	Normal	Enlarges early
Skin or systemic	Normal	Normal	Normal	Normal	Normal
Eye	Late: optic atrophy	Late: optic atrophy	Optic atrophy blindness	Slow optic atrophy	Optic atrophy
Seizures		Rare	Uncommon	Late	Early, uncommon
Neurologic signs	Spastic paresis Nystagmus Head retraction Bulbar palsy Dementia	Changes in gait Ataxia Combined upper and lower motor neuron signs Bulbar palsy, Blindness, Deafness, Dementia } late	Hypotonia ↓ Spastic diplegia ↓ Decerebrate rigidity	Pendular nystagmus Titubation of head ↓ Cerebellar signs in early childhood ↓ Spastic diplegia late childhood Slow dementia	Rigidity ↓ Decerebrate rigidity Opisthotonus
Miscellaneous		Reduced nerve conduction			+Paper chromatography
Blood	Normal	Normal	Normal	Normal	Hypoglycemia
Urine	Normal	Metachromatic bodies	Normal	Normal	Maple syrup odor +Dinitrophenyl-hydrazine
CSF	↑ Protein (150-300 mg%)	Normal or ↑ protein up to 200 mg%	↑ Pressure Protein normal or up to 200 mg%	Normal	
Biopsy	Brain	Sural nerve	Brain		
X-ray		Nonfilling of gallbladder	Suture separation		

has been reported with a partial deficiency in hexosaminidase A. In Gaucher's disease, glucocerebroside is the accumulated substance. The enzyme defect is a glycolipid-β-glucosidase. The accumulated material in Niemann-Pick's disease is sphingomyelin (ceramide-P-choline). In Fabry's disease, both dihexoside and trihexoside ceramides are stored as a result of a deficiency in trihexoside-β-galactosidase. Farber's disease is the result of ceramide and ganglioside storage. The enzymatic defect is not certain. Cerebral cholesterosis and Hand-Schüller-Christian disease are both characterized by cholesterol deposits. In metachromatic leucodystrophy, ceramide-galactose-sulfate (sulfatide) accumulates as a result of defective degradation, due to a deficiency of cerebroside sulfate sulfatase. A deficiency in thermolabile beta-galactosidase is believed responsible for the accumulation of mucopolysaccharide in Hurler's disease.

CEREBROMACULAR DEGENERATIONS. The traditional classification of these disorders has been based on the association of progressive gray matter degeneration with intracellular lipid storage, secondary white matter demyelination, and macular-retinal degenerative changes. Age of onset, ethnic grouping, and duration have been basic considerations in their nosology.

TABLE 12C. *Differential Diagnosis of the Cerebral Degenerative Disorders of Childhood*

				Cerebromacular Degeneration		
	Schilder's	**Subacute Inclusion Body Encephalitis***	**Progressive Familial Myoclonus Epilepsy**	**Late Infantile**	**Juvenile**	**Adult**
Age of onset	5-10 years	5-20 years	5-15 years	3-4 years	5-10 years	15-25 years
Rate of progression	Onset abrupt Death in months to 3 years	Variable Death in months to years	Slow Death in 3-10 years	Slow Death in 5-10 years	Slow Death in 10-15 years	Very slow
Genetic			Recessive	Recessive	Recessive	Recessive
Site of pathology	White matter	Predominantly gray matter	Gray matter	Gray matter	Gray matter	Gray matter
Eye	Early: optic neuritis Late: optic atrophy	Rarely chorioretinitis Late: optic atrophy	Normal	Pigmentary degeneration of macula Optic atrophy	Pigmentary degeneration of retina	Normal
Seizures	Early or late	Early: akinetic ↓ myoclonus	Early: grand mal ↓ myoclonus	Early	Relatively early	Early: myoclonus
Neurologic signs	Early: spastic parasis ↓ dementia Late: cortical blindness and deafness aphasia pseudobulbar palsy	Initial: impaired intellect emotional lability Early: dementia abnormal involuntary movements, ataxia, loss of speech Late: decerebrate rigidity	Progressive dementia Ataxia	Ataxia Spastic paresis Dementia Blindness	Blindness Dementia Parkinsonian syndrome Pseudobulbar palsy ↓ Total dementia Spastic quadriparesis	Dementia Ataxia
Laboratory	CSF—normal or ↑ protein ↑ gamma globulin	CSF Marked ↑ gamma globulin		Azurphilic granules in PMN leucocytes	Azurphilic granules in PMN leucocytes	
Electroretinogram				Abnormal	Abnormal	
EEG		"metronomic"				

*Etiologically related to a slow virus infection but clinical course is that of a degenerative disease process.

1. Congenital Amaurotic Familial Idiocy (Norman-Wood)
2. Infantile AFI (Tay-Sachs)
3. Late Infantile AFI (Bielchowsky-Jansky)
4. Juvenile AFI (Batten-Mayou-Spielmeyer-Vogt)
5. Adolescent-Adult AFI (Kufs)

More recent neuropathologic and biochemical studies have led to more discrete biochemical characterization of this group of disorders. The following outline, based on recent work, begins to classify these lipid storage diseases at the molecular level as gangliosidoses.

THE GANGLIOSIDOSES.

1. Congenital form: GD_3-gangliosidosis
2. Classical Tay-Sachs disease: GM_2-gangliosidosis with absence of anodal component of hexosaminidase (isoenzyme A)
3. Tay-Sachs disease with visceral globoside storage: GM_2-gangliosidosis with the absence of both anodal and cathodal components of beta-D-N-hexosaminidase
4. Neurovisceral gangliosidosis (Tay-Sachs with visceral involvement) (generalized gangliosidosis): GM_1-gangliosidosis with both fractions of beta-galactosidase absent.

Type 1: early infantile form with visceromegaly and skeletal changes
Type 2: onset 7 to 14 months without visceromegaly or skeletal changes

TABLE 13. *Metabolic Defects in Lipid Storage Diseases**†

Constellation of metabolic diseases is characterized by inabilities to degrade sphingolipids

Disease	Major Sphingolipid Accumulated	Enzyme Defect
Gaucher	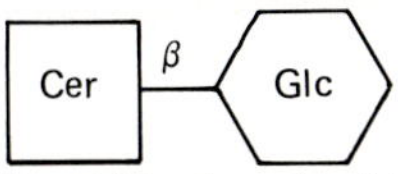 Ceramide glucoside (glucocerebroside)	β-Glucosidase
Metachromatic leucodystrophy	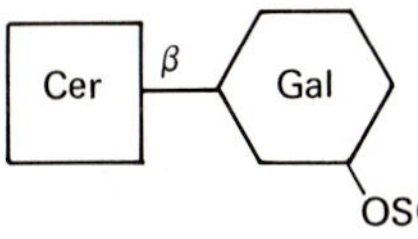 Ceramide galactose-3-sulfate (sulfatide)	Sulfatidase
Niemann-Pick	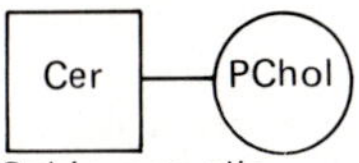 Sphingomyelin	Sphingomyelinase
Fabry	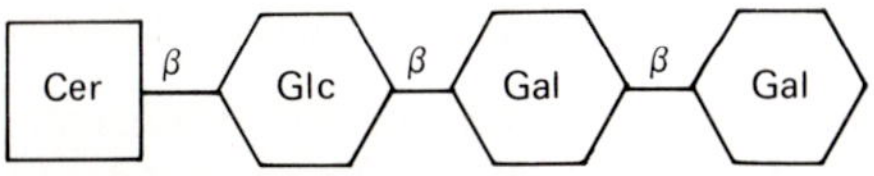 Ceramide trihexoside	β-Galactosidase
Tay-Sachs	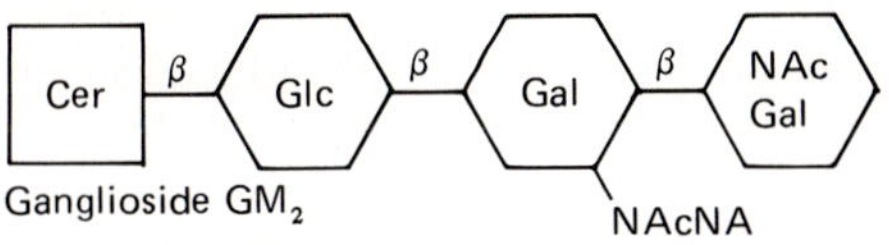 Ganglioside GM_2	Hexosaminidase
Generalized gangliosidosis	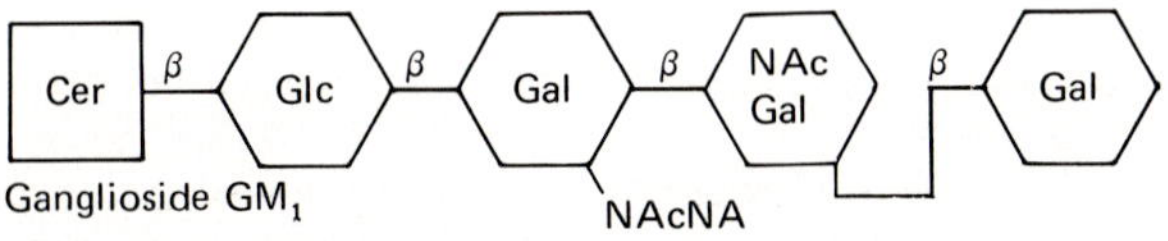 Ganglioside GM_1	β-Galactosidase

*From Brady. *Chemical Engineering News*, p. 61, Dec. 22, 1969.
†Cer = ceramide; Gal = galactose; Glc = glucose; PChol = phosphorylcholine; NacGal = N-acetylgalactosamine; NAcNA = N-acetylneuraminic acid.

A late infantile and juvenile form of GM_2-gangliosidosis has been described in which the anodal component of beta-galactosidase is absent.

OTHER SPHINGOLIPIDOSES.

1. Metachromatic leucodystrophy with the storage of ceramide-glucose-sulfate due to a defect in aryl-sulfatase
2. Nieman-Pick's disease—characterized by storage of sphingomyelin with a sphingomyelinase defect—several variants reported
3. Krabbe's disease—a defect in the metabolism of galactoceramide due to a deficiency in galactosyl ceramidase
4. Gaucher's disease—characterized by a defect in glycosyl ceramidase and the storage of glycosyl ceramide
5. Lactosyl ceramidosis—a partial defect in lactosyl ceramidase with the storage of galacto-glucose ceramide
6. Fabry's disease—a deficiency in hexosaminidase A and B with the storage of ceramide trihexoside

The presence or absence of vacuolated lymphocytes and azurophilic granules in the segmented white blood cells and the three architectural forms of storage material seen by electron microscopy are quite variable. The problem of determining the relation of genotype to phenotype in many of the gangliosidoses is as yet unsolved.

It has been demonstrated that, in a large percentage of the late infantile (Bielchowsky-Jansky) and juvenile (Batten-Mayou-Spielmeyer-Vogt) forms of amaurotic family idiocy, lipofuscin is the abnormally deposited or stored material. The term ceroid

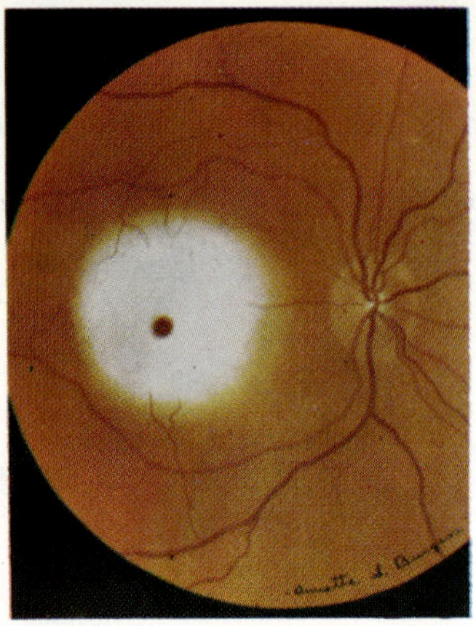

Fig. 33. Cherry-red spot in the fundus of a child with Tay-Sachs disease.

lipofuscinosis has been proposed, but as lipofuscin is an ubiquitous product of neuronal death it is far from certain that this finding represents the primary defect in the late forms of cerebromacular degenerations.

Despite the age of onset, all the cerebromacular degenerations share a progressive downhill course. Loss of vision, seizures of the myoclonic variety, dementia, ataxia, decerebration, and paralysis are the common clinical features. Abdominal distension, megalencephaly, hirsutism, thickening of facial features, and increased pigmentation of the skin are also noted in those surviving any length of time. Microcephaly is a feature of the Batten-Spielmeyer-Vogt form.

Infantile Amaurotic Familial Idiocy (Tay Sachs Disease). The symptoms of the infantile form are first noted at 4 to 6 monthes of age, when it is observed that the infant's development, previously normal, appears to slow and then stop. Initially, there are apathy, muscular hypotonia, loss of previously acquired functions, and failure of vision with inability to follow or fixate. After a few months there are abnormal sensitivity to sound (hyperacusis) and progressive regression with increasing spasticity, blindness, and dementia. Seizures, usually myoclonic in type, may occur, and ultimately the head may enlarge. Examination of the fundi demonstrates optic atrophy and the pathognomonic "cherry-red spot" (Fig. 33), in which the perimacular areas show a grayish dystrophic change and the capillary elements of the choroid are seen as a bright red spot at the fovea. In contrast to the late infantile and juvenile forms where true tapetoretinal degeneration occurs, the electroretinogram (ERG) in Tay-Sachs disease is normal. The course is as a rule no longer than 18 to 24 months, although expert nursing care may lead to survival for several years.

Pathologically the neuronal cell bodies and some dendrites are grossly distended by fine lipid granules and are often vacuolated. These changes occur in cortex, cerebellum, basal ganglion, spinal cord, brainstem, and sympathetic ganglion. In cases surviving longer, secondary demyelination of fiber tracts and cystic softening of the brain with prominent gliosis are also seen. The stored lipid is a ganglioside containing neuraminic acid which, by electron microscopy, is found within the neuronal body as a membranous inclusion.

The clinical diagnosis can be supported by the demonstration of increased serum glutamic oxalacetic transaminase and an increased number of vacuolated lymphocytes in peripheral blood. The absence of the enzyme fructose-1-phosphate aldolase in the peripheral blood confirms the clinical diagnosis. Rectal biopsy and histochemical study of the ganglion cells in the sympathetic plexuses and cerebral biopsy can also confirm the clinical diagnosis. Cerebral biopsy is the most definitive method of diagnosis during life. The demonstration of a deficiency of either anodal or cathodal components of beta-D-N-hexosaminidase in the patient and/or fibroblast tissue cultures will be the most elegant definitive method of diagnosis.

Neurovisceral lipidosis (GM_1-gangliosidosis) (generalized gangliosidosis), a recessive disease with abnormal storage of GM_1-ganglioside in cerebral gray matter, spleen, liver, and renal glomerular epithelium, is usually fatal in the first 2 years of life. Radiographic changes resembling Hurler's disease are present. Beta-galactosidase deficiency leads to faulty degradation of the GM_1-ganglioside. Two forms of GM_1-gangliosidosis are described: an early infantile "pseudo-Hurler" form and a late infantile form without visceromegaly or skeletal changes.

Classical Tay-Sachs disease is inherited as a simple autosomal recessive trait having a high degree of penetrance and little variability in expression. Despite the markedly increased frequency in those of Jewish background, the disease has been reported among every ethnic group. The frequency among Jews originating from eastern Europe is higher than among Jews from other regions.

No favorable specific therapy is available. Supportive measures and parental genetic counseling should always be carried out.

LATER FORMS OF CEREBROMACULAR DEGENERATION. The other forms of cerebromacular degeneration are less typical clinically. The onset is somewhat later in life, varying from 3 years of age to adolescence. Mental deterioration, seizures, and progressive visual involvement are the earlier signs. Increasing evidence of pyramidal tract disease, ataxia, the onset of myoclonic seizures, and optic atrophy with pigmentary degeneration of the retina should lead to the suspicion of the diagnosis of late cerebromacular degeneration. The pigmentary degeneration is more marked in the macular and perimacular areas. Unlike the infantile form, there is no predilection for Jews. The genetic expressivity and penetrance are more variable. Progressive deterioration and the retinal changes should lead to clinical suspicion. The presence of vacuolated lymphocytes or azurophilic granules in the granulocytes of patient and heterozygous parents will be of some diagnostic significance. More specific enzymatic techniques are desirable and perhaps will be available in the very near future. Further diagnosis will depend upon cerebral biopsy or autopsy. The specific sphingolipid involved is as yet undetermined. However, the electron microscopy picture in the Batten-Spielmeyer-Vogt variety of the disease is totally different from that in Tay-Sachs. Presumably they are distinct biochemical entities. Pathologic findings are quite similar to the infantile form, but perhaps due to the longer course, secondary demyelination and gliosis are more prominent. Therapy is unknown; supportive measures for both patient and parents are all that can be offered at the present time. Batten-Spielmeyer-Vogt, Bielchowsky, and Kufs diseases are autosomal recessive genetic diseases.

GENERALIZED LIPIDOSES. There are a number of other diseases in which lipids accumulate in the cell bodies of the cerebral gray matter. These include Gaucher's disease, Niemann-Pick disease, Farber's disease, Fabry's disease, Heller's disease, cerebral cholesterosis, and the Hand-Schüller-Christian syndrome, as well as eosinophilic granulomas. These last two are granulomatoses of the reticuloendothelial system in which the central nervous system may become involved secondarily as a result of pressure effects of dural and skull granulomas or less commonly by actual involvement of the brain.

Niemann-Pick Disease. This disease, in which ceramide-P-choline (sphingomyelin) is accumulated in foam cells, classically occurs in early infancy. The salient features are developmental arrest followed by progressive cerebral deterioration not unlike that seen in Tay-Sachs disease, hepatosplenomegaly, and blindness. Death usually occurs before the third year. The maculae show the "cherry-red" spot described in the infantile form of cerebromacular degeneration, although it is not reported in all cases. A few instances of later onset and more protracted course have been reported. In rare cases there is no evidence of cerebral involvement. Diagnosis can be established by demonstrating the characteristic "foam cells" in liver biopsy and bone marrow aspiration. Vacuolated lymphocytes in the peripheral blood have been reported. Pathologically there is ballooning of neuronal cells with secondary demyelination depending upon the duration of illness.

Gaucher's Disease. The infant with Gaucher's disease fails to thrive from birth. Enlargement of spleen and liver is found early. Strabismus, difficulty in swallowing, a feeble cry, and progressive decerebrate rigidity point to central nervous system involvement. Blindness and macular degeneration are not features of the cerebral forms of Gaucher's disease. Death usually occurs before the second year. Antemortem diagnosis can be made by bone marrow aspiration and demonstration of the characteristic Gaucher's cells. Acid phosphatase levels are elevated. The storage cells contain increased amounts of ceramide glucose (glucocerebroside). In the nervous system some neuronal cytoplasmic accumulation of cerebrosides occurs, particularly in the brainstem nuclei. There are Gaucher's cell infiltrates in the cortex. In the juvenile and rare adult forms of cerebral Gaucher's disease, more definite cerebral neuronal cerebroside accumulation is found, possibly because of the slightly longer course of the disease.

Progressive Familial Myoclonic Epilepsy (Unverricht's Disease). This disease is a distinct clinical entity with a recessive pattern of inheritance. The disease usually has its onset with seizures in the first decade of life, with a later development of almost constant myoclonus of the stimulus-sensitive type. Ataxia and progressive mental deterioration subsequently appear. Terminally Parkinsonian features are evident, with death in early adulthood. Pathologically Unverricht's disease is a specific entity exhibiting Lafora bodies as both intracellular and extracellular inclusions. These bodies have the histochemical reactions of an acid mucopolysaccharide and resemble amyloid.

Similar clinical pictures, when examined pathologically, may be found to be late forms of cerebral lipidosis (Batten-Spielmeyer-Vogt). Others have proved to be one of a number of other progressive degenerative conditions such as dyssynergia cerebellaris myoclonica (Ramsey-Hunt), subacute sclerosing panencephalitis, Friedreich's ataxia, and hepatolenticular degeneration in which the site of major pathologic involvement is in the brainstem, dentate and olivary nuclei, and cerebellar peduncles. All give clinical manifestations very similar to those of the progressive familial myoclonic epilepsy. In the Lafora type of progressive familial myoclonus, pathologic changes are more generally distributed than in the other degenerative diseases exhibiting myoclonic syndromes.

Farber's Disease. Also called disseminated lipogranulomatosis, this disease produces central nervous system changes with ballooned-out nerve cells similar to those found in Tay-Sachs disease. The disease is familial. Lipogranulomas of the viscera are widespread, and there is severe joint involvement suggesting the periarticular changes of rheumatoid arthritis. The lipid involved appears to be a ceramide, probably sphingomyelin.

Fabry's Disease. This disease is characterized by the selective storage of ceramide dihexoside and ceramide trihexoside in the nerve cells of the sympathetic nervous system, the myenteric plexuses, and subcortical nuclei of the central nervous system. Angiokeratoma corporis diffusum universalis, or Fabry's disease, has its onset in children as paroxysmal episodes of fever. Paresthesia and dysthesia of the extremities and proteinuria are early features. Skin lesions are highly characteristic of this disorder. At approximately 7 to 10 years of age, minute round bluish-red or black, blood-filled cavities are noted over the

TABLE 14. *The Mucopolysaccharidoses*

	Hurler	Hunter	Sanfilippo
Genetic	Autosomal recessive	Sex-linked recessive	Autosomal recessive
Clinical	Dwarf, visceromegaly, gargoyle facies, corneal clouding, severe mental retardation, marked skeletal involvement	Less marked than Hurler, deafness, no corneal clouding	Childhood onset of severe mental retardation; minimal facial, skeletal, and visceral involvement
Urine	Chondroitin sulfate Heparitin sulfate	Chondroitin sulfate Heparitin sulfate	Heparitin sulfate

lower portion of the body and scrotum. The disease progresses into adult life with mild diabetes insipidus, elevated blood pressure, anhidrosis, and progressive renal failure. Fabry's disease is considered to be an inborn error of metabolism and represents a rare form of the lipid storage diseases.

Cerebral Cholesterosis. This is a familial disease in which there is the marked accumulation of free cholesterol in the cerebellar and cerebral white matter. Extensive demyelination occurs. Clinically ataxia, mental deterioration, myoclonus, and bulbar paralysis occur. Xanthomas of the tendons are seen, and cataracts are frequent. In one variant form, accumulation of cholesterol is most marked in the basal ganglia and brainstem.

Heller's Disease. Normal development through the first 2 years of life followed by gradual loss of speech during the fourth or fifth year, together with increasing motor restlessness and progressive dementia, should lead to a suspicion of Heller's disease. Few, if any, neurologic findings are seen in dementia infantilis. The abnormal EEG and early normal development aid in differentiating Heller's disease and childhood schizophrenia. Abnormal increases in plasma glycolipids and total lipids together with decrease in bound neuraminic acid in spinal fluid have been reported. Several biopsy reports link the condition with the cerebral lipidoses, although dementia infantilis may be a demyelinating disease. An important differential diagnostic consideration is subacute sclerosing panencephalitis (SSPE).

THE MUCOPOLYSACCHARIDOSES. Six syndromes resulting from the abnormal storage of mucopolysaccharides have been described. The differentiating features of the three discussed below are indicated in Table 14.

Hurler's Disease (Gargoylism) (Type I). This condition has been shown to be a mucopolysaccharide storage disease. Not only is the central nervous system involved, but the skin, kidney, spleen, liver, heart, and skeletal system also contain excessive amounts of mucopolysaccharide glycolipids. The parenchymal cells of these organs and the cells of the reticuloendothelial system are distended and vacuolated. The nerve cells of the cerebral cortex are distended by a glycolipid substance akin to, and possibly identical with, the gangliosides. Similar changes, though less marked, are seen in the nerve cells of the spinal cord. A marked deficiency of a specific thermolabile beta-galactosidase has been reported in the liver of patients with Hurler's disease. Large amounts of compounds containing chondroitin sulfate-B and heparitin sulfate are excreted in the urine and can be detected by a urinary screening test (Fig. 34).

Clinically the Hurler's patient has macrocephaly and thick coarsened features, with the eyebrows joining in midline (Fig. 35). The tongue is thickened, tonsillar and adenoidal tissue are enlarged, and speech is thick and heavy. Relative dwarfism, kyphoscoliosis, thickening of the joints with progressive loss of mobility, protruding abdomen, umbilical hernia, hepatosplenomegaly, deafness, and corneal opacities make a typical case of Hurler's disease easily diagnosed. Radiographically there is thickening of the temporomandibular joint surfaces, an enlarged navicular-shaped sella turcica, and a curious characteristic beak-shaped formation of the lower thoracic and lumbar vertebrae. There is broadening of the metacarpals, and flat, broad ribs are seen. Large metachromatic granules are found within the polymorphonuclear elements of the peripheral blood and in fibroblasts cultured from the skin.

Mental retardation and physical incapacitation are progressive. Death usually occurs by age 10 to 12 and may be due to hydrocephaly but more often is due to cardiac failure.

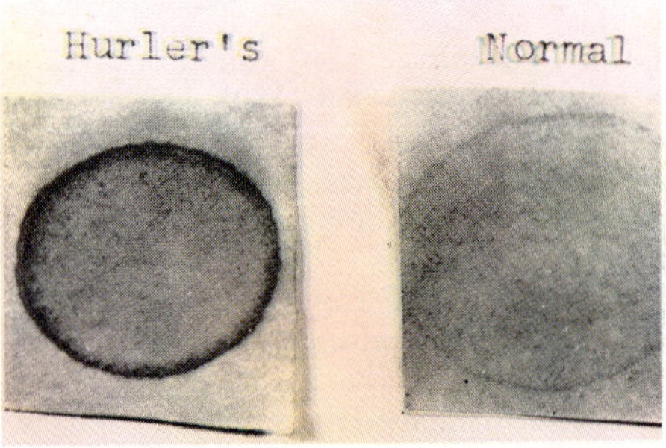

Fig. 34. Berry spot test for detection of mucopolysaccharidoses.

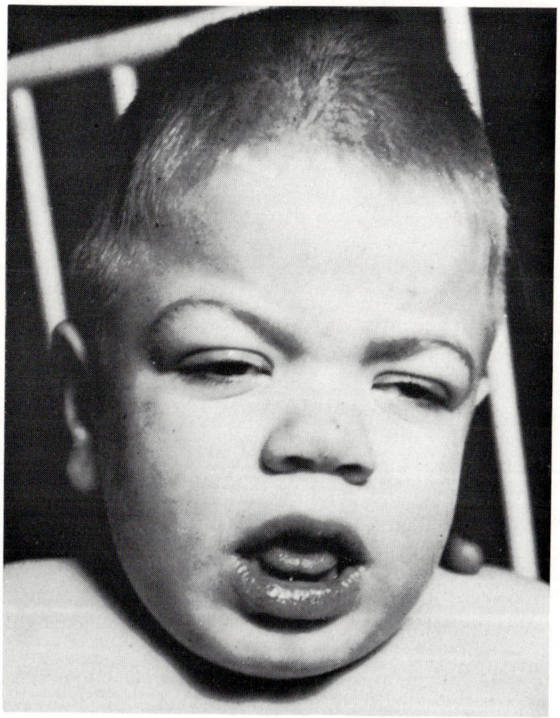

Fig. 35. Hurler's disease. Characteristic facies.

Hunter's Disease (Type II). This is the sex-linked recessive form and is less common than Hurler's disease. As a rule the clinical manifestations are less severe and more slowly progressive. Corneal clouding and deafness are not present. In both Hurler's and Hunter's diseases, true progressive megencephaly may lead to obstructive symptoms requiring a Holter valve or other shunting procedure. Fibroblast and leucocyte cultures from cases of both Hurler's and Hunter's continue to show abnormal accumulation of mucopolysaccharide as the result of inefficient degradation of the mucopolysaccharide. If fibroblast cultures of both Hunter's and Hurler's strains are mixed, the accumulation of mucopolysaccharide is corrected in about 10 days of mixed culture growth.

Sanfilippo's Disease (Type III). Only heparitin sulfate is excreted. Physical and radiographic manifestations are milder than in either type I or II, but mental retardation and severely disturbed behavior is progressive.

GLYCOGEN STORAGE DISEASES. ***Type VIII.*** This disease is characterized by slow speech and motor development with progressive spasticity and decerebration. Hepatomegaly is present early but disappears. Increased urinary catecholamines are found. Phosphorylase activity is reduced in the liver. This is inherited as a recessive trait.

Type II (Pompe's Disease). In this disorder an alpha-glucosidase deficiency results in generalized glycogen storage and may be associated with progressive and extensive neurologic involvement and progressive dementia.

Nonstorage Degeneration of Cerebral Gray Matter

The diseases of the cerebral gray matter which have been discussed can be grouped as "storage" diseases in which abnormal amounts of compounds are deposited within the neuronal cell body. There exist several other diseases involving the gray matter which cannot be strictly classified as "storage" diseases.

Progressive Degeneration of Cerebral Gray Matter (Poliodystrophy, Poliodysplasia). This condition is probably due to a variety of causes; it is not likely that the familial forms, the postencephalitic, postepileptic, and traumatic cases share a common etiology. The cases reported show a great diversity of signs and symptoms, and striking variability of duration and age of onset. Pathologically some cases show a diffuse degeneration of cerebral gray matter, and in others the pathologic findings are local or regional.

From the clinical point of view, progressive mental deterioration, seizures, myoclonic twitching followed by progressive spasticity, blindness, and often deafness should lead to the suspicion of progressive degeneration of the cerebral gray matter. Optic atrophy, abnormal involuntary movements, and ataxia occur. There are marked differences in clinical manifestations from case to case.

Alper's Disease. Diffuse cerebral degeneration in infancy has been reported as occurring in a familial distribution with quite uniform pathologic findings. There is an extensive neuronal loss and an increase in microglia, with gliosis of cerebral and cerebellar cortices, thalamus, and basal ganglia. The onset is with convulsions and myoclonus, followed by progressive mental and motor involvement, often associated with cortical blindness and deafness. The similarity of the clinical manifestations together with the uniform pathologic findings indicates that this form of poliodystrophy can be considered as a separate entity.

Necrotizing Encephalopathy (Leigh's Disease). This is characterized by the focal gray matter degeneration of the brainstem, basal ganglia, and subthalamic nuclei. There is extensive cranial nerve nuclear involvement. Pathologically the distinguishing features are spongy, necrotic areas of rarefaction with late cavitation. The onset usually occurs during the first year, often in the first or second month. The duration varies from several months to 2 or 3 years. Cases have been reported showing a later onset with survival from 10 to 12 years. Thus, it appears there is a chronic as well as a subacute form of infantile necrotizing encephalopathy.

Clinically the infant is quiet, cries infrequently, and has much difficulty in feeding due to bulbar cranial nerve palsy. Vocalization and speech deteriorate; spasticity and seizures occur later in the disease. Laboratory investigations are not rewarding. There is no therapy. Two adult forms of spongiform encephalopathy have now been shown to be "slow" virus diseases.

Diseases of the Cerebral White Matter

Recent advances in neurochemistry and electron microscopy have led to a number of classifications of white matter diseases. The term *dysmyelination* has been suggested for those diseases of white matter in which an inborn error of metabolism and enzymatic defect leads to faulty myelin formation, in contrast to the *demyelinating* or myelinoclastic group of diseases, in which there appears to be an abnormal myelin degeneration.

The myelinoclastic diseases are represented by multiple sclerosis, Devic's neuromyelitis optica, concentric sclerosis of Balo, and the diffuse sclerosis of Schilder. Acute necrotizing hemorrhagic leucoencephalitis and the acute disseminated encephalomyelitides secondary to infection and immunization procedures are also myelinoclastic diseases.

The second large grouping consists of the diseases of dysmyelination which are almost certain to be due to inborn errors of metabolism, with enzymatic defects which interfere with or prohibit the continuing normal processes of myelination. This group of diseases is made up of the leucodystrophies or diffuse scleroses. Demyelinating diseases are the result of exogenous agents, while the leucodystrophies are the result of endogenous defects.

Demyelinating diseases are of two general types. First, there are those in which are found multifocal perivenous lesions showing evidence of inflammation. Second, there are those with multifocal lesions but without evidence of inflammation. The first group is probably best thought of as an example of autoimmune disease; i.e., autosensitization to some component of myelin. The noninflammatory group is of even more uncertain cause and includes a number of conditions such as central pontine myelinolysis, progressive multifocal leucoencephalopathy, subacute combined degeneration, and the encephalopathies secondary to hypoxia and asphyxia.

Classification of the dysmyelinating leucodystrophies is subject to considerable debate. The principal source of confusion lies in the precise relationship of the leucodystrophies to the sphingolipidoses or cerebral storage diseases. One hypothesis is that the stored material in certain of the leucodystrophies represents the accumulation of myelin precursors or perhaps abnormal products of myelin formation which accumulate because of enzyme defects blocking normal myelin formation. The alternative is that the stored material represents products of myelin degeneration. As knowledge accrues, both hypotheses will probably be supported in one or more of the clinicopathologic entities to be discussed.

Krabbe's disease (globoid-cell leucodystrophy), metachromatic leucodystrophy, and Pelizaeus-Merzbacher's disease are the more common clinical types of true leucodystrophy. Krabbe's and metachromatic leucodystrophy can also be considered storage diseases.

Leucodystrophies

PELIZAEUS-MERZBACHER'S DISEASE. This is a rare, sex-linked, recessive genetic disorder present from infancy. An autosomal dominant form of late onset has been described. The distinguishing feature is the presence of an arrhythmic dancing type of nystagmus noted shortly after birth. Other cerebellar signs are noted early in life. Progression is slow with remission lasting several years. In later childhood, spasticity, optic atrophy, dysarthria, and ataxia are seen. Intellectual deterioration is slow. Duration is variable, and sometimes death occurs before puberty, although patients living well into adult life are known. Pathologically, hypoplasia of axons and lack of stainability of myelin are the main features. There is little evidence of myelin breakdown. Chemically there is no evidence of the storage of sphingolipids nor any increase in cholesterol esters, which clearly distinguishes this disease as a separate entity from either the sphingolipidoses or the demyelinating diseases. There appears to be a basic defect in the process of myelination.

The normal or only slightly elevated spinal fluid protein helps to distinguish this disease from some of the other leucodystrophies. No specific treatment is available.

METACHROMATIC LEUCODYSTROPHY (SULFATIDE LIPIDOSIS). This is an autosomal recessive disease due to a deficiency of the enzyme aryl sulfatase. The condition may become manifest anytime during childhood, most frequently about the age of 2 years. Late childhood and adult onset also occurs. Loss of ability to walk with hypotonia and areflexia are early manifestations and are subsequently replaced by spasticity and progressive paralysis. Optic atrophy, seizures, and myoclonus together with signs of progressive cerebellar involvement are noted. Atypical forms of this disorder have been described with isolated manifestations of abdominal distension, simulating intestinal obstruction, or progressive loss of speech. Decerebrate rigidity usually occurs within 2 or 3 years. A longer course may occur in those children with a later onset. An infantile form with onset at 1 to 2 years is distinguished from a juvenile form with onset age 4 to 10 years. The cerebrospinal fluid protein is characteristically elevated up to 200 mg percent. Nonfilling of the gallbladder is a common feature. Prolongation of peripheral nerve conduction time is usually found. Diagnosis may be made by sural or dental nerve biopsy with the demonstration of the accumulation of metachromatic-staining galactosphingosulfatides. Metachromatic sulfatides can be found in the urinary sediment or demonstrated chromatographically. The latter finding is highly suggestive but not pathognomonic. Urinary or leucocyte aryl sulfatase A deficiency is diagnostic of this disorder.

Pathologically there is widespread symmetric demyelination of the central nervous system and an accumulation of sulfatides and nonlipid hexosamine. Sulfatide deposits show marked metachromasis. Liver, kidney, and bile duct epithelia are also involved. Electron microscopy reveals the cerebroside sulfuric acid ester accumulations to be chiefly in the cytoplasm of the oligodendroglia, astrocytes, and large macroglial cells. By electron microscopy no inclusions are reported in the neuronal cells. By more conventional techniques intraneuronal deposits have been reported.

GLOBOID-CELL LEUCODYSTROPHY (KRABBE'S DISEASE). This is inherited as an autosomal recessive disease. At about 3 to 6 months of age, a previously normal infant develops stiffness of the lower extremities, spasms with head retraction, and extension of lower limbs. Flexion of the upper extremities occurs subsequently. Incessant crying is prominent. The disease finally terminates in decerebrate rigidity and death from bulbar paralysis. Rarely does the infant survive more than two years. The cerebrospinal fluid protein is usually elevated in the range of 150 to 300 mg percent, with a normal gamma globulin content and colloidal gold curve and a significant decrease in beta globulins. There is symmetric diffuse demyelination of the cerebral white matter. The characteristic globoid cells of mesodermal origin, possibly microglia or adventitial cells of vessels, are distended with a protein-bound glycolipid containing cerebrosides. These cells can be considered as large macrophages attempting to remove products of myelin catabolism. Defective synthesis of sulfatides and accumulation of ceramide-galactose due to an enzymatic defect in cerebroside sulfatransferase has been reported.

SPONGY SCLEROSIS (CANAVAN'S DISEASE, FAMILIAL SPONGY DEGENERATION OF THE NEURAXIS). This disease is probably an autosomal recessive trait with a higher frequency in those of Jewish ancestry. The onset is in the first months of life with arrest of psychomotor development, hypotonia, and seizures. The neck becomes flaccid, and a progressive spastic diplegia culminates in decerebrate rigidity. Optic atrophy ends in blindness. Macrocephaly occurs often with the separation of the sutures of the skull as a result of diffuse edema of both gray and white matter. Increased spinal fluid pressure may be observed, and the erroneous diagnosis of hydrocephalus may be considered. Protein content of the cerebrospinal fluid is usually normal. Death usually occurs prior to the second year of life. Widespread demyelination, cerebral edema, and a characteristic spongy vacuolation are noted pathologically. As in Pelizaeus-Merzbacher's disease, there is evidence of a defect in normal myelination and some suggestion of demyelination. The relationship of this condition to subacute spongiform encephalopathy of adults is unknown.

SUDANOPHILIC (NEUTRAL FAT, ORTHOCHROMIC) FAMILIAL LEUCODYSTROPHY. This disease is pathologically characterized by the symmetric loss of myelin in cerebral and cerebellar white matter. Lipid-distended phagocytes are noted around the areas of demyelination. Clinically the onset occurs in late childhood with signs of progressive pyramidal tract and cerebellar involvement. Aphasia may occur. The loss of myelin and the increase in esterified cholesterol place this form of leucodystrophy closer to the demyelinating diffuse scleroses. However, its familial occurrence with a sex-linked inheritance and the symmetric nature of the lesions serve to warrant its retention in the group of dysmyelinative leucodystrophies. Addison's disease, often initially asymptomatic, is frequently associated with this disorder and may be the cause of coma and sudden death.

ALEXANDER'S DISEASE. This extremely rare and recently reported disorder, also known as dysmyelinogenic leucodystrophy, has been classified as both a storage disease and a leucodystrophy. The onset is in infancy with death usually occurring by the second year. All cases have been male, except one reported juvenile case. Clinically there is progressive dementia with spastic quadriplegia and enlargement of the head. Seizures are a common feature. Pathologically, eosinophilic staining material is deposited at all the interfaces of brain, brainstem, and spinal cord. Few deposits are noted in the cerebellum. In addition, there is widespread demyelination of cerebrum and cerebellum, with more severe involvement of the frontal lobes and less severe destruction in the occipital lobes. The eosinophilic material has histochemical properties suggestive of neurokeratin and appears to be located in the astrocytic footplates. The original case was reported as a fibrinoid degeneration of astrocytes, and another case was reported as megalencephaly with hyaline panneuropathy.

Demyelinating Scleroses

In contrast to the leucodystrophies, this group of diseases is myelinoclastic and pathologically multifocal, perivenous, and inflammatory. The absence of a familial distribution of cases further tends to distinguish these diseases from the familial leucodystrophies. Etiology is obscure, and several concepts of pathogenesis have been offered. The destructive action of some enzyme present in blood or cerebrospinal fluid, viral infection, capillary thrombosis, and autosensitization to some component of myelin have all been proposed as etiologically significant. At the present time, the autoimmune concept appears to be most tenable. Demyelinating diseases can be further separated into the diffuse and disseminated forms. Schilder's disease represents the diffuse demyelinating scleroses. The disseminated demyelinating scleroses include acute and chronic multiple sclerosis, acute necrotizing hemorrhagic leucoencephalitis, and the acute disseminated encephalomyelitides which follow infection and immunization procedures. Neuromyelitis optica and the concentric sclerosis of Balo are probably subtypes of the disseminated form of acute multiple sclerosis.

ACUTE DISSEMINATED ENCEPHALOMYELITIDES. These diseases occur following rubella, rubeola, variola, varicella, and occasionally the ill-defined "influenza" syndrome. Immunization against variola, rabies treatment, and rarely pertussis immunization may be followed by an acute episode of disseminated encephalomyelitis. Signs of an acute encephalitis with evidence of multiple sites of central nervous system involvement are associated with an elevation of spinal fluid protein and a lymphocytic pleocytosis in the spinal fluid. Fever, convulsions, stupor, ocular palsies, dysarthria, paraplegias, and cerebellar ataxia, together with urinary and fecal incontinence, may occur in various combinations. Severe forms of the disorder will leave permanent neurologic deficits. About 15 percent of all cases are fatal. There is no specific therapy. Unlike other forms of disseminated sclerosis, recurrences are rare.

Acute Necrotizing Hemorrhagic Leucoencephalitis (Hurst Disease). This is a fulminating and usually fatal disease following some minor upper respiratory infection. Pathologically one or more large hemorrhagic and necrotic foci of demyelination are found in brain, spinal cord, and brainstem. Presenting signs and symptoms depend upon the site of the lesion or lesions. Headache, fever, and signs of meningitis are present. Cerebrospinal fluid protein is elevated, and up to several hundred leucocytes may be present. These cells are predominantly neutrophilic, in contrast to the lymphocytic pleocytosis of the acute disseminated encephalomyelitides described above. No specific form of therapy is available.

Multiple or Disseminated Sclerosis. This disease is relatively rare in children. Although it has been observed in the first decade, the diagnosis should be made with extreme circumspection. The diagnosis is based upon the occurrence of multiple attacks and evidence of multiple sites of neurologic involvement. Preferential sites of involvement are segmental portions of the brainstem, spinal cord, and cerebellum. Cerebral symptoms are uncommon. In order of frequency, one encounters motor weakness of the extremities, retrobulbar neuritis, paresthesias, diplopia, disturbance of balance, and bladder difficulties. No characteristic laboratory features are present other than an occasional mild pleocytosis with some increase in spinal fluid protein. Gamma globulin may be elevated, and a first-zone colloidal gold curve elevation is a frequent finding. These cerebrospinal fluid findings are not pathognomonic. The disease may be present in the absence of any abnormalities in the cerebrospinal fluid. Pathologically the findings consist of scattered areas of demyelination with little or no evidence of tissue reaction. The gray matter is usually spared. The disease occurs sporadically, and between attacks the symptoms may clear partially or even completely. Over a period of years, there is a tendency for slow, progressive neurologic disability.

Neuromyelitis Optica (Devic's Disease). Somewhat more common in children is neuromyelitis optica (Devic's disease). Although there are cogent neuropathologic reasons for believing that this is in every way identical with disseminated or multiple sclerosis, the clinical picture is sufficiently uniform to consider this as a special subclass of disseminated sclerosis. The disease is characterized by the association of a transverse myelitis and bilateral optic neuritis. These may develop simultaneously or one after the other. Visual loss is severe and is usually accompanied by ophthalmoscopic signs of inflammation of the nerve head itself. Involvement of the spinal cord, as a rule, produces a complete transverse myelitis. It may, however, be disseminated. On pathologic examination some cases presenting with this symptom complex show the classical lesions of multiple sclerosis. Others may show pathologic changes best classified as subacute or acute necrotizing hemorrhagic myelitis. In some cases of neuromyelitis optica, large confluent plaques of demyelination may occur within the cerebral hemispheres. In these cases there is invariably an elevation of cerebrospinal fluid protein and a mononuclear pleocytosis.

Recovery may be quite rapid and complete in several weeks. Some cases are associated with permanent residua, and those which fall in the classification of subacute necrotic myelopathy are usually fatal. No specific therapy is known, and management is entirely symptomatic.

Balo's Concentric Sclerosis. This condition has many of the histopathologic features of multiple sclerosis. However, in Balo's disease the lesions are primarily confined to the cerebral white matter. The distinguishing features are the occurrence of alternate concentric bands of destruction and preservation of myelin. Whether or not this form of the disease should be considered as a variant of diffuse cerebral sclerosis rather than disseminated sclerosis has not been determined.

SCHILDER'S DISEASE (ENCEPHALITIS PERIAXIALIS DIFFUSA). Schilder's disease shows an extensive demyelination of the cerebral white matter. The process is asymmetric and tends to originate occipitally, spreading forward to parietal, temporal, and frontal lobes. Histologically the lesions resemble those of disseminated or multiple sclerosis. The finding of increased esterified cholesterol and the decrease of myelin lipids further identifies Schilder's disease with the demyelinating diseases. The age of onset may be at any time past infancy, with a peak incidence between the ages of 5 and 10. The onset is acute, often with seizures, progressive visual loss, and gait disturbance. Progression is occasionally interrupted by short periods of quiescence. There is progressive dementia, frequent loss of hearing, aphasia, and paralysis. Spastic quadriplegia and decerebration are the final stages within a few months to several years after the onset. The frequent loss of vision is attributable to cerebral as well as optic nerve demyelination with a complex pleural picture of cortical blindness and optic neuritis. In contrast to the leucodystrophies, sensory and motor deficits tend to precede the dementia. Increased intracranial pressure may simulate brain tumor. Laboratory findings are nonspecific, although there may be some elevation of cerebrospinal fluid protein with an increased gamma globulin content and a first-zone colloidal gold curve. Prognosis is fatal and treatment is unknown. Antemortem diagnosis can be confirmed by cerebral biopsy.

SUBACUTE SCLEROSING PANENCEPHALITIS (SUBACUTE INCLUSION BODY ENCEPHALITIS [DAWSON], SUBACUTE SCLEROSING LEUCOENCEPHALITIS [VAN BOGAERT], AND PANENCEPHALITIS [PETTE AND DORING]) (SSLE;SSPE). Isolation of measles virus from brain biopsy material, the growth of measles virus from brain biopsy in tissue culture, and transfer of an unidentified encephalogenic agent from human brain biopsy to ferrets, strongly implicate the measles virus as the etiologic agent in SSPE. Clinically, intellectual deterioration and affective lability are often the early signs. This is followed by the appearance of myoclonic jerks and choreoathetosis. The age of onset is seldom before late childhood or adolescence, and the disease usually runs its course over months to years with eventual blindness, spastic quadriplegia, and virtual decortication. The electroencephalogram may be helpful in diagnosis when it exhibits slow high-voltage complexes appearing in a rhythmic metronomic fashion. This change is not pathognomonic. The presence of a markedly elevated gamma globulin or a strongly positive first-zone colloidal gold curve with increased immunoglobulin-G associated with M gradients serves to distinguish this condition from Schilder's disease and the other progressive degenerative cerebral disorders. Pathologically there is diffuse demyelination of hemispheric white matter and marked gliosis which is disproportionate to the myelin loss. Numerous eosinophilic-staining intranuclear bodies may be found in both nerve cells and the oligodendroglia. The entire central nervous system is involved, the changes being most pronounced in the cerebral hemispheres.

Degenerations of the Basal Ganglia
(The Extrapyramidal Syndromes)

A number of progressive degenerations involving the basal ganglia and its connections are seen in children. Clinically they are characterized by abnormal involuntary movements (hyperkinesia), paucity of spontaneous movement (bradykinesia), and rigidity. While athetosis, tremor, chorea, and dystonia may all be seen in other degenerative or acquired diseases of the central nervous system, those diseases in which these features are prominent are included in this group. The common pathologic features are degeneration and demyelination of the subcortical nuclear masses and their connections.

PARKINSONISM. A rare juvenile form of parkinsonism has been described as occurring either sporadically or occasionally in a familial distribution. The symptoms of resting tremor, paucity of spontaneous movement, and rigidity may become apparent in the early part of the second decade. The course is chronic, leading over a number of years to incapacity as a result of the rigidity and tremor. The pathology is essentially a progressive degeneration of the globus pallidus. Therapy is symptomatic and consists of the use of the belladonna group of alkaloids. Neurosurgical intervention probably has a place in the management of juvenile paralysis agitans. L-DOPA therapy may prove to be of therapeutic value as it has in adult parkinsonism.

HUNTINGTON'S CHOREA. Huntington's chorea has a mean age of onset of 44 years. There are confirmed reports of cases of Huntington's chorea which began at the age of 3 years; in less than 1 percent of patients with Huntington's chorea is the onset in the first decade. The disease is inherited as a dominant autosomal trait. The main pathologic lesions are found in the basal ganglia. Both caudate nucleus and putamen show a marked to complete loss of nerve cells. There is an astroglial reaction throughout these areas. Other extrapyramidal nuclei are invariably involved. The cerebral cortex is affected in all patients showing neuronal destruction and some glial hypertrophy. In some, a panatrophy of the cerebellar hemisphere is reported.

The clinical manifestations in childhood are rarely typical of those seen in the adult form of Huntington's chorea. The cases reported in childhood are essentially hypokinetic, in contrast to the characteristic choreatic movements seen in the adult forms. Bradykinesia, muscular rigidity, convulsive disorder, and progressive mental deterioration are the characteristic features in the childhood cases. However, the adult choreic clinical picture does occur in children and may lead to confusion with other hyperkinetic syndromes.

While it may be permissible on occasion to make a clinical diagnosis of Huntington's chorea in an adult in whom a family history is absent, it appears at the present time that because of the atypical features of the childhood form of the disease, the diagnosis should not be made in children unless there is a verified family pedigree of Huntington's chorea. No therapy is known. A variety of medications used for adult forms of extrapyramidal syndromes has been tried in a limited series of cases. No success can be reported. The disease is more

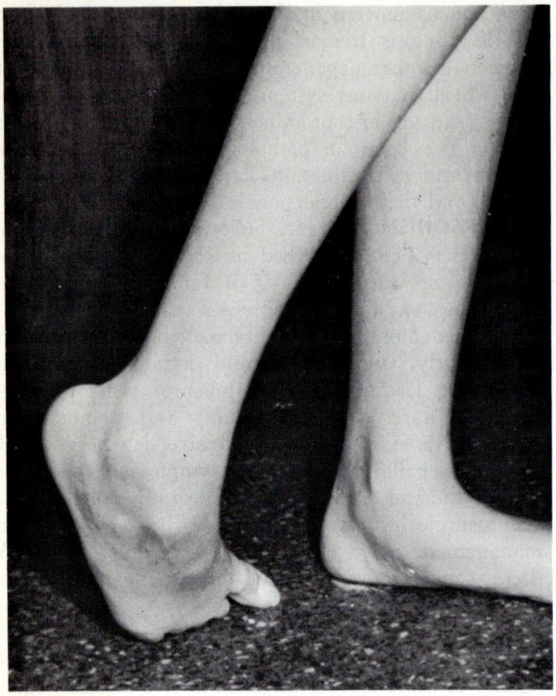

Fig. 36. Typical dystonic posturing of foot in early dystonia musculorum deformans.

rapidly fatal in children, lasting usually only three to five years after the first clinical manifestations. No specific metabolic error has been found in Huntington's chorea, although increases of dopamine have been reported in the urine.

DYSTONIA MUSCULORUM DEFORMANS. This disease has its onset about the fifth year with a slow, progressive course to complete incapacity in six to eight years. Some cases may show a less severe progression. The characteristic clinical manifestations of this inherited disease are slow, writhing dystonic movements involving neck, trunk, and extremities. The disease often has its onset with a bizarre gait disturbance that is frequently interpreted as a functional disorder (Fig. 36). Facial grimacing may also be present. In a typical case the eventual outcome is complete incapacity and the assumption of fixed dystonic postures. Pathologically, widespread but nonspecific degenerative changes are seen in the subcortical nuclear masses and cerebellum. Therapy has been entirely symptomatic. Some success in control of the movements may be achieved by thalamotomy. Since the disease is essentially a progressive one, unilateral thalamotomy may give relief for variable periods of time until the opposite side of the body becomes severely involved and a second operation may be indicated.

HALLERVORDEN-SPATZ DISEASE. This is a dominantly inherited, slowly progressive syndrome of dementia, spasticity, and a dyskinesia of the athetotic variety with some dystonic features. Emotional incontinence is common, and optic atrophy may be a late manifestation. Seizures and sensory impairment are not usually present. The disease usually has its onset in middle to late childhood, and death results within a period of 5 to 20 years. Pathologically, diffuse neuronal degeneration is found in cerebral and cerebellar white matter but particularly in the pallidum and the dentate nuclei. The cortical spinal tracts are severely degenerated. Neuroplasmic swellings in the gray matter are common. The characteristic pallidonigral hyperpigmentation is not always striking. The neuroplasmic swellings have led to the disease being described as a neuroaxonal dystrophy.

Increased iron is deposited in the globus pallidus and there is a delayed (about 10 days) "leakage" of radioactive iron into the area of the globus pallidus but no increased systemic uptake of iron. In one case in the author's experience, a significant increase of iron was found in the hair. Thus, there are a number of indications that this condition represents some type of abnormality of iron metabolism.

HEPATOLENTICULAR DEGENERATION (WILSON'S DISEASE). This is an autosomal, recessively inherited, progressive disease characterized by progressive degeneration of the basal ganglia and hepatic cirrhosis. The disease is now identified as an inborn error of metabolism, the primary defect being the failure of proper formation of the copper-containing protein ceruloplasmin. The biochemical findings consist of a decreased level of plasma ceruloplasmin, an increase in the plasma nonceruloplasmin copper, and an increased urinary copper excretion.

Pathologic changes are seen throughout the central nervous system but are most marked in the basal ganglia. Increased amounts of tissue copper are found in the affected areas. A nodular cirrhosis of the liver is found, and it has been shown that the characteristic Kayser-Fleischer ring is due to deposition of copper within Descemet's membrane (Fig. 37).

The onset of disease is usually in the second decade. However, with the increasingly accurate methods of diagnosis provided by ceruloplasmin determinations, the diagnosis can be established earlier, often by the fourth or fifth year. Early symptoms may be unsteadiness of gait and trembling of the hands. Signs of increasing hepatic insufficiency may precede, accompany, or follow the neurologic involvement. Similarly, intellectual dulling or psychiatric symptoms, emotional lability, and anxiety states may occur with, before, or after the development of the neurologic picture. Neurologically Wilson's disease may mimic other progressive degenerations of the basal ganglia. Both bradykinetic and hyperkinetic forms are seen. The characteristic tremor is a posture-holding "wing-beating" type, but an atypical cerebellar intention tremor or the tremor at rest as in parkinsonism may be seen. Dysarthria, facial grimacing, excessive salivation, and progressive rigidity are other features of the disease. Many patients exhibit the typical Kayser-Fleischer circumcorneal

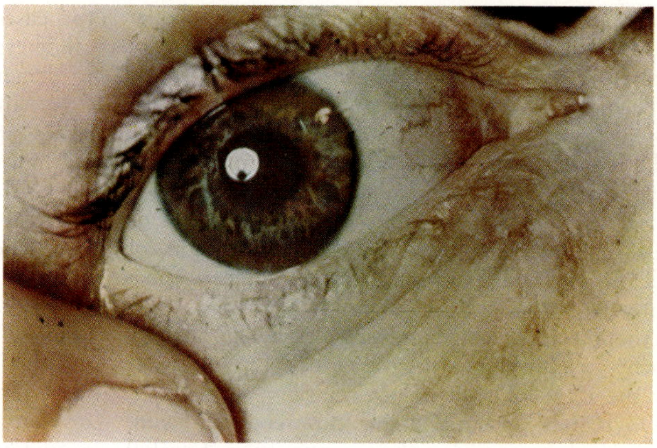

Fig. 37. Kayser-Fleischer ring. Note pigmentary change initially involves superior or inferior pole of Descemet's membrane.

greenish-yellow ring at the junction of cornea and sclera. At the present time, a diagnosis can be established by the demonstration of decreased ceruloplasmin content. However, some cases have been reported in which a normal ceruloplasmin is found.

Differential diagnosis includes all the progressive degenerations of the basal ganglia, and Wilson's disease must always be suspected in any child with juvenile cirrhosis.

Treatment is aimed at reducing dietary copper intake and removing copper from the tissues. The latter is accomplished by the use of dimercaprol or penicillamine. Without treatment, the disorder leads to death within five to six years. Therapy has been of considerable value in both adult and childhood cases.

ESSENTIAL OR FAMILIAL TREMOR. This condition is most apt to manifest itself in early adolescence but may appear in well developed form in childhood. There is a fine rhythmic tremor of the hands and fingers, accentuated by fatigue and emotional stress and little affected by movement or intention. It is best demonstrated with hands and arms extended and fingers spread. When benign tremor occurs as a sporadic case, Wilson's disease and other basal ganglia diseases must be ruled out. The condition most often appears as a dominant trait, and examination of other members of the family is most helpful. Considering the benign nature of the condition, treatment is rarely required. Rarely, thalamotomy may be effective in those severely involved.

STATUS DEMYELINISATUS. This disease has been described as a progressive degeneration of the lenticular nuclei. The onset is in infancy, and death occurs after variable periods of time up to the middle of the second decade. The condition has been reported as occurring on a familial basis. The symptoms are increasing rigidity, athetoid and dystonic movements, and progressive dementia.

DYSSYNERGIA CEREBELLARIS MYOCLONICA. Extremely rare, this disorder is familial. The exact mode of inheritance is uncertain, but in at least one case a dominant form of inheritance seemed most probable. The onset is with myoclonic muscular twitching involving the extremities as well as the face. Moderate to mild mental retardation is present. As the disease progresses, the myoclonic phenomenon tends to disappear, to be replaced by progressive cerebellar ataxia and severe intention tremor. Seizures may occur but are not as prominent a feature as they are in familial myoclonus epilepsy. Differential diagnosis from Wilson's disease should be made. The principal pathology appears to be in the dentate system. Familial paroxysmal choreoathetosis (Mount and Reback) may become of differential diagnostic interest in this and other diseases of the basal ganglia leading to hyperkinesia.

Polymorphous Neuroabiotrophies

A great variety of progressive degenerative disorders involving, in various combinations, cerebellum, brainstem, spinal cord, and peripheral nerves have been described in children. These diseases occur in familial distributions as recessive, dominant, and sex-linked traits. As syndromes they occur in many intermediate and transitional forms. Their exact interrelationships are unclear, and there are many pathologic similarities. One common feature is that cause is completely unknown, and therapy is unavailable. These disorders can best be classified in terms of the major clinical-pathologic symptomatology.

Cerebellar Degeneration

Pure, progressive degeneration of the cerebellum is rare in children. The more frequent age of onset is some time after 20 years. A familial history is present in a significant number of these cases. The first symptoms may be unsteady gait and dysarthria, followed by progressive cerebellar ataxia. Pathologically there is atrophy of the cerebellum with marked loss of Purkinje cells. Both pathologically and clinically these cases begin to merge with the spinocerebellar degenerations. There is often atrophy of the spinocerebellar tracts and the posterior columns, giving symptoms of position and vibratory sensory loss. Optic atrophy may occur, and other manifestations of brainstem and spinal cord involvement may be present.

Differential diagnosis from other forms of progressive cerebellar ataxias, cerebellar neoplasm, and in older cases multiple sclerosis must be made. One helpful diagnostic feature is the demonstration of significant cerebellar atrophy by pneumoencephalography.

Another form of progressive cerebellar atrophy occurring in children is that described by Louis-Bar under the term of ataxia-telangiectasia.

Olivocerebellar and olivopontocerebellar degenerations have been reported to occur on a familial basis. Rare cases are described in children, but for the most part, these are diseases affecting adults.

THE SPINOCEREBELLAR DEGENERATIONS. *Friedreich's ataxia* is the best known member of this group of disorders. It is genetically transmitted in both dominant and recessive modes. Sex distribution is equal. The age of onset is usually prior to 20 with the average being between 10 and 13 years. Cases have been reported earlier than this. Progression is steady, and ambulation becomes impossible within 5 to 8 years. The usual duration of disease is about 16 years, although considerably longer and shorter courses have been reported. The pathologic changes in the spinal cord consist primarily of degeneration in the dorsal columns and spinocerebellar and pyramidal tracts. However, peripheral nerves, medulla, pons, and cerebellum may also be involved. The spinal cord is usually smaller than normal, and the dorsal roots are atrophic.

Ataxia, dysarthria, nystagmus, posterior column sensory loss, reflex changes, and musculoskeletal deformities are the cardinal manifestations of this disorder. Ataxic gait is the earliest clinical sign. The ataxia begins in the lower extremities, but as the disease progresses, trunk, upper extremities, head, and neck become involved. Speech becomes dysarthric, and there may be impaired laughing, chewing, and breathing due to marked incoordination. A nodding head tremor is frequent, and nystagmus appears in over half the cases.

Sensory impairment characteristically involves the dorsal columns, with diminution of position and vibratory sensation.

Muscular weakness is a common feature of the disease, and prominent wasting as the result of disuse is seen late. However, in some families lower motor neuron atrophy is present early in the disease. The distribution of the atrophy is distal and similar to that seen in Charcot-Marie-Tooth disease.

Deep tendon reflexes are almost always absent in the lower extremities, and late in the disease those in the upper limbs may disappear. Abdominal reflexes are retained. A Babinski sign is almost a constant finding.

Optic atrophy is present in about 10 percent of the cases. Occasionally there may be involvement of other cranial nerves. Mental impairment progressing to dementia may be present in some cases.

Musculoskeletal deformities are common. Pes cavus and retraction and flexion of the toes with equinovarus tendency results in the typical "Friedreich's foot." Kyphoscoliosis is observed in the majority of children.

There are no distinctive laboratory features other than the frequent occurrence of electrocardiographic abnormalities suggesting progressive degeneration of the cardiac muscle. Terminal cardiac failure due to interstitial myocarditis is not infrequent. No treatment is available, and death usually occurs as a result of infection complicated by cardiac failure.

The Roussy-Levy syndrome, a variant of Friedreich's ataxia, is of principal importance because of its significantly better prognosis. This syndrome is either nonprogressive or excessively slow in its development. The salient features are pes cavus and areflexia of the lower extremities, often of the upper as well. The absence of ataxia, dysarthria, and nystagmus distinguishes it from the classical Friedreich's ataxia. Muscle wasting in the lower leg and hypothenar eminences occur in some families. A dominant genetic pattern is usual. Pathology is not well documented but is probably similar to that of Friedreich's ataxia with little or no spinocerebellar degeneration.

Other variants of spinocerebellar degeneration include cases of progressive ataxia occurring as hereditary syndromes associated with mental retardation, cataract, and pyramidal tract signs, together with poor growth and development. Another form of spinocerebellar degeneration is hereditary spastic ataxia with central retinal degeneration and vestibular impairment. In clinical practice, cases intermediate between Charcot-Marie-Tooth disease, familial spastic paraplegia, Roussy-Levy syndrome, progressive spinal atrophy, and the more typical form of Friedreich's ataxia are common.

Congenital spinocerebellar ataxia (Marinesco-Sjögren or Garland-Moorhouse) is recessively inherited and is associated with cataracts and mental retardation. Neurologically it is characterized by limb ataxia, dysarthria, areflexia, and pyramidal tract signs. Retarded somatic and mental maturation is a constant feature. Frequently, there is a dolichocephalic skull with epicanthic folds and strabismus.

Familial spastic paraplegia is a hereditary disorder characterized by the childhood onset of progressive spasticity of the lower extremities, with associated hypereflexia, and the Babinski sign. The course is slowly progressive. Muscle atrophy is not part of this syndrome, and ataxia is not seen. Pathologically the degeneration is limited to the pyramidal tracts in the spinal cord.

There are two well recognized metabolic disorders in which there may be primary cerebellar involvement. *Hartnup disease* is manifested by cerebellar ataxia, a pellagroid skin rash, and moderate mental retardation. The disease is believed to be an inborn error of tryptophan metabolism with an associated amino-aciduria. The skin lesions and the cerebellar ataxia are inconstant and apparently reversible by administration of nicotinic acid. Ataxia may appear acutely and may be associated with acute delirium and hallucinations.

The Bassen-Kornzweig's syndrome is a recessively inherited disorder associated with a deficiency of beta-lipoprotein. In early childhood there is a prominent steatorrhea. Characteristic features are cerebellar and dorsal column signs together with retinal degeneration and retinitis pigmentosa. The red blood cells have many thorny projections from their surfaces. This acanthocytosis is a highly characteristic diagnostic feature.

Brainstem and Spinal Cord Degenerations

The feature that distinguishes this group of progressive neuroabiotrophies from the spinocerebellar degenerations is the fact that the predominant pathologic changes occur in the spinal cord and specifically in the pyramidal tracts or anterior horn cells. Again there are a number of combinations and intermediate forms.

These progressive degenerations of the spinal cord are characterized by the wasting of muscles and motor weakness. The cause is entirely unknown, but the strong familial tendency points to the operation of genetic factors. At present no treatment is known other than symptomatic relief.

The principal lesions are in the cord and brainstem, where the anterior horn cells and cells of the nuclei of the motor cranial nerves show a diminution of size and number. There are secondary degenerative changes in anterior roots and nerves and marked evidence of denervation atrophy in the voluntary muscle groups.

A number of clinical forms have been described, the chief distinctions being the age of onset and the rate of progression.

Progressive infantile spinal atrophy (Werdnig-Hoffman disease) is a uniformly fatal disease inherited as an autosomal recessive trait. The earliest signs can be noted at or shortly after birth, or the onset may be delayed until somewhat later in the first year. Progressive evidence of lower motor neuron weakness and atrophy appears in trunk, neck, pelvis, and shoulder girdles. The extremities are involved later, but the distal musculature of the hands and feet is frequently spared. Hypotonia and weakness progress to atrophy and paralysis. Areflexia is present. There is no evidence of sensory loss or cerebellar ataxia. Mentality is not disturbed. Facial musculature is often spared, but the tongue is frequently atrophic and demonstrates prominent fasciculations. Some cases present with the clinical picture of arthrogryposis multiplex. Death almost always occurs in about two years as a result of intercostal paralysis and intercurrent respiratory infection.

There is an intermediate form of infantile progressive spinal atrophy in which the disease process is manifest at birth but progresses much less rapidly, sometimes appearing to have become stationary. Death usually occurs in the middle of the second decade.

Wohlfart, Kugelberg, and Welander have described a more slowly progressive variant of Werdnig-Hoffmann's disease. Since it is slowly progressive and primarily involves the girdle musculature, the *Kugelberg-Welander syndrome* has been descriptively called heredofamilial juvenile muscular atrophy simulating muscular dystrophy. Although of recessive inheritance, this condition may occur sporadically or be found in a family where the more usually fatal type is present. The course is slower and relatively favorable. The patient, having acquired normal gait patterns, gradually develops weakness in the lower extremities with subsequent involvement of the upper extremities. Paresis is maximal in the girdle musculature, and the deep tendon reflexes are lost. Fasciculations are characteristically absent.

The "floppy infant" or "limp child" syndromes can result from nonprogressive brain lesions as well as involvement of peripheral nerve and muscle. These disorders must be distinguished from Werdnig-Hoffmann's disease, which superficially has a similar clinical picture of hypotonia. Atonic diplegia and Down's syndrome, examples of nonprogressive brain lesions, have hypotonia with preservation of deep tendon reflexes and significant intellectual impairment. Polyneuritis can be distinguished by the occasional demonstration of sensory impairment, elevated cerebrospinal fluid protein content, and a decreased nerve conduction velocity time. Congenital myopathies (benign congenital myopathy, central core disease, nemaline myopathy) are differentiated by preservation of reflexes and muscle biopsy. Myasthenia gravis often presents with hypotonia and weakness, bulbar signs, and extraocular muscle impairment. These physical findings lessen or disappear with intravenous edrophonium (Tensilon). The term "benign congenital hypotonia" has been applied to children with hypotonia in early infancy who subsequently show improvement and ultimately may have little or no motor weakness.

Oppenheim's disease or amyotonia congenita is no longer considered a clinical entity and probably encompassed many disorders with hypotonia.

Closely related to the spinal atrophies is *familial juvenile amyotrophic lateral sclerosis.* This is a rare disorder and usually occurs later in the juvenile period. It is more closely allied to adult amyotrophic lateral sclerosis and to the familial form of that disease. In contrast to Werdnig-Hoffmann's disease, the onset is later in life and tends to manifest itself earlier by weakness and atrophy of the small muscles of the hands and feet with later involvement of the proximal musculature. A further important clinical differentiation is the presence of overactive reflexes and persistently pathologic plantar responses. The pathology is a combined degeneration of both upper and lower motor neurons.

Progressive bulbar paralysis of childhood (*Fazio-Londes disease*) is a rare familial form of progressive atrophy in which the cranial nerve motor nuclei are prominently involved.

Cranial and Peripheral Nerve Degenerations

Leber's optic atrophy represents a heredodegenerative disorder involving for the most part a single cranial nerve. This sex-linked recessive disorder may occasionally be transmitted as an autosomal recessive or dominant trait. Symptoms may begin as early as 5 years of age. Puberty appears to be the usual time of onset of progressive loss of central vision which is characteristic of the disease. Early, the optic discs may be slightly edematous. Finally, temporal pallor is marked, due to the severe involvement of the papillomacular bundle. In some cases spasticity, mental retardation, ataxia, and seizures have been described. Total blindness occurs rarely. No treatment is available.

Peroneal muscular atrophy (neuromuscular atrophy, Charcot-Marie-Tooth disease) has a strong familial tendency. All modes of inheritance have been reported in addition to sporadic nonfamilial cases. Males are somewhat more affected than females. The onset is almost always in childhood, shortly after the sixth year. The age of onset and rate of progression have a strong tendency to be constant in a given family. The rate of progression is usually very slow, and orthopedic management of the bilateral footdrop is frequently of great value.

Degenerative pathologic changes are found in both peripheral nerves and spinal cord. Anterior horn cells, anterior roots, dorsal roots and ganglia, pyramidal tracts, the dorsal columns, and Clark's column are degenerated. The muscles show severe atrophy secondary to denervation.

The outstanding clinical feature of this syndrome is the symmetrically distributed atrophy of the feet and lower legs which results in the virtually pathognomonic "stork-leg" appearance. Bilateral footdrop results in the typical high-stepping gait and the characteristic slapping sound as the foot flops to the floor unhindered by dorsal flexion. Later the muscles of the hands and forearms may become atrophic. The thigh, upper arms, and proximal muscle groups are usually spared. Paresthesias, cramps, and pain are occasionally reported. Diminished touch, pain, and temperature sensation may be noted, particularly in the distribution of the peroneal nerve. Achilles tendon reflex is absent, but other reflexes are often spared.

Signs and symptoms more characteristic of either Friedreich's ataxia or the progressive spinal atrophies may be observed in some cases and serve to reemphasize the close interrelationship of the entire group of spinal cord degenerations. *A hypertrophic neuropathic form of Charcot-Marie-Tooth disease* with "stork-leg" and high-arched feet with hammer toe is inherited as an autosomal dominant.

A number of other forms of heredodegenerative peripheral neuropathies are more rarely encountered in children. The *hypertrophic interstitial neuritis of Dejerine-Sottas* is characterized by a grossly palpable enlargement of the peripheral nerves. The peripheral nerve involvement is asymmetric and affects several single peripheral nerves such as the median nerve, resulting in a carpal tunnel syndrome together with a peroneal palsy causing a drop foot. This combination of multiple single nerves has been called "mononeuritis multiplex." One form of hypertrophic interstitial neuritis manifests itself during the first year of life with profound interference with learning to walk. A familial form of recurrent brachial neuritis has been reported and is occasionally seen in children. Hereditary neuropathy with interstitial neuritis and nerve deafness (*Alport's syndrome*) is a rare condition first suspected bcause of deafness in childhood. Hereditary polyneuritis associated with retinitis pigmentosa and ataxia (*Refsum's syndrome*) and progressive hereditary sensory radicular neuropathy have also been reported in children.

Congenital indifference to pain may occur on a familial basis. All sensation is appreciated, but the patient is indifferent to pain. Severe and normally painful injuries are not painful to the child. Multiple fractures, neurotrophic joint changes, burns, and infections are common. Child rearing is hazardous and difficult.

Refsum's syndrome is an autosomal recessively inherited condition otherwise known as heredopathia atactica polyneuritiformis. A symmetric chronic polyneuritis and ataxia with other cerebellar signs are the principal neurologic findings. Retinitis pigmentosa is a common feature. Occasionally neurogenic hearing loss and anosmia are noted. Often electrocardiographic abnormalities are found. Epiphyseal dysplasia with pes cavus and shortening of the metacarpals and metatarsals may be seen. Ichthyosis of the skin is frequently present. Cerebrospinal fluid protein is increased without pleocytosis.

The onset is in childhood but may be delayed into the second or third decade. The course is essentially progressive with some tendency to relapses and remission. No therapy is available.

Pathologically an interstitial hypertrophic polyneuropathy is associated with posterior column degeneration and anterior horn cell degeneration. There is patchy demyelination of the brainstem and cell loss in the olivary, red, vestibular, cochlear, vagal, and dentate nuclei.

Biochemical studies by Klenk and by Kahlke have shown an accumulation of an unusual branched-chain fatty acid, 3,7,11,15,-tetramethyl hexadecanoic acid (phytanic acid), in the fatty acids of phospholipid and cholesterol ester fractions of plasma and in liver and kidney. The accumulation of phytanic acid is the result of faulty alpha oxidation of phytanic acid to alpha-hydroxyphytanic acid. Dietary restriction of phytanic acid precursors has therapeutic promise.

Hereditary sensory neuropathy associated with spinal cord disease has been described as having its onset in adolescence. These cases are distinguished from hereditary sensory radicular neuropathy by virtue of the presence of spinal cord pathology. Familial lumbosacral syringomyelia may also occur and must be distinguished from the purely neuropathic syndromes. In the Anrade form of primary amyloidosis the neuropathy may strongly suggest lumbar syringomyelia.

The Neurocutaneous Syndromes

Since skin and nervous system have a common embryologic origin from the ectodermal layer, it is not surprising that there is a large number of neurologic conditions associated with cutaneous manifestations. Again the familial and hereditary nature of these disorders argues for a genetic origin and a basic enzymatic or metabolic defect as the primary pathogenic feature, although biochemical data are lacking.

Tuberous sclerosis (adenoma sebaceum, epiloia, Bourneville-Pringle's disease) is inherited as a dominant autosomal trait, the expression of which is dependent upon the presence or absence of a modifying gene. This accounts for the marked variability of expression noted in clinical practice (Table 15 and Fig. 38A, B, C, D, E, and F).

The full syndrome is characterized by seizures, mental deficiency, and adenoma sebaceum with foci of intracranial calcification, particularly in the periventricular region, although they may be scattered throughout the hemispheres. The seizures are most often infantile spasms in the very young child and the grand mal type in the older child; any variant of convulsive disorder may be seen. In the full syndrome, mental deficiency is generally of a severe degree. However, cases of tuberous sclerosis with normal or near-normal intellectual capacity are seen. The characteristic skin lesions, fibroangiomatous nevi, have been mislabeled adenoma sebaceum. The sebaceous glands are only involved secondarily. Fibroangiomatous nevi may be present during the first year of life, but more commonly are not noted until about the age of 4 or 5. These lesions take the form of discrete pink or yellowish papules located principally on the face and in the so-called butterfly distribution on the bridge of the nose, the malar prominences, and along the nasal-labial folds. They may also occur on forehead, neck, and trunk. Individual lesions remain static, gradually growing redder and eventually becoming brownish. They do not itch nor do they suppurate; these features serve to distinguish them from acne vulgaris and seborrheic dermatitis. Other skin lesions consist of raised plaquelike flesh-colored lesions, which may be found anywhere on the body, and the "shagreen patches," which are slightly pigmented and raised and resemble coarse-grained leather. These are found principally on the trunk and lower extremities. Fibromas of the scalp are seen on occasion, as are areas of depigmentation. These latter may be one of the earliest ectodermal manifestations of tuberous sclerosis. If present, the subungual fibroma, a flesh-colored sessile growth emerging from the groove of the nailbed, is quite characteristic. Several types of retinal lesions may be observed. One is a small, flat, white or yellowish phakoma or spot on or close to the optic nerve head. These may be multiple. A second lesion seen in the fundus is a raised cluster of translucent white tissue. Systemic involvement may include multiple small fibroadenomas of the kidney, rhabdomyoma of the heart, and myomas of the uterus and vagina.

The brain contains many small firm sclerotic nodules (tubera) which are chiefly in the cortex but may be found in all parts of the central nervous system. They may project into the ventricle causing deformities which can be detected by pneumoencephalography (Fig. 38D). Hydrocephalus with increased intracranial pressure may develop as a result of one of these masses blocking the ventricular system. These nodules contain giant-sized haphazardly arranged cells, at times appearing to be astrocytic and at other times resembling ganglion cells. Adjacent to these collections of giant glial cells may be found degeneration of nerve cells and fibers and often cavity formation. Dense astrocytic gliosis is also seen.

The diagnosis can be established on the basis of the triad of seizures, mental deficiency, and adenoma sebaceum. In infancy, tuberous sclerosis should be suspected when infantile spasms coexist with depigmented skin lesions. In such children a careful evalu-

TABLE 15. *Tuberous Sclerosis—Clinical and Pathologic Manifestations*

Skin	Depigmented nevi Adenoma sebaceum Shagreen patch Lipoma Subungual fibroma
Brain	Convulsions Retardation Intracranial calcifications
Eye	Retinal phakoma
Bone	Skull: areas of sclerosis Phalanges: areas of rarefaction; thickening of the cortex
Heart	Rhabdomyoma
Lung	"Honeycomb"
Kidney	Polycystic or angiomyolipoma

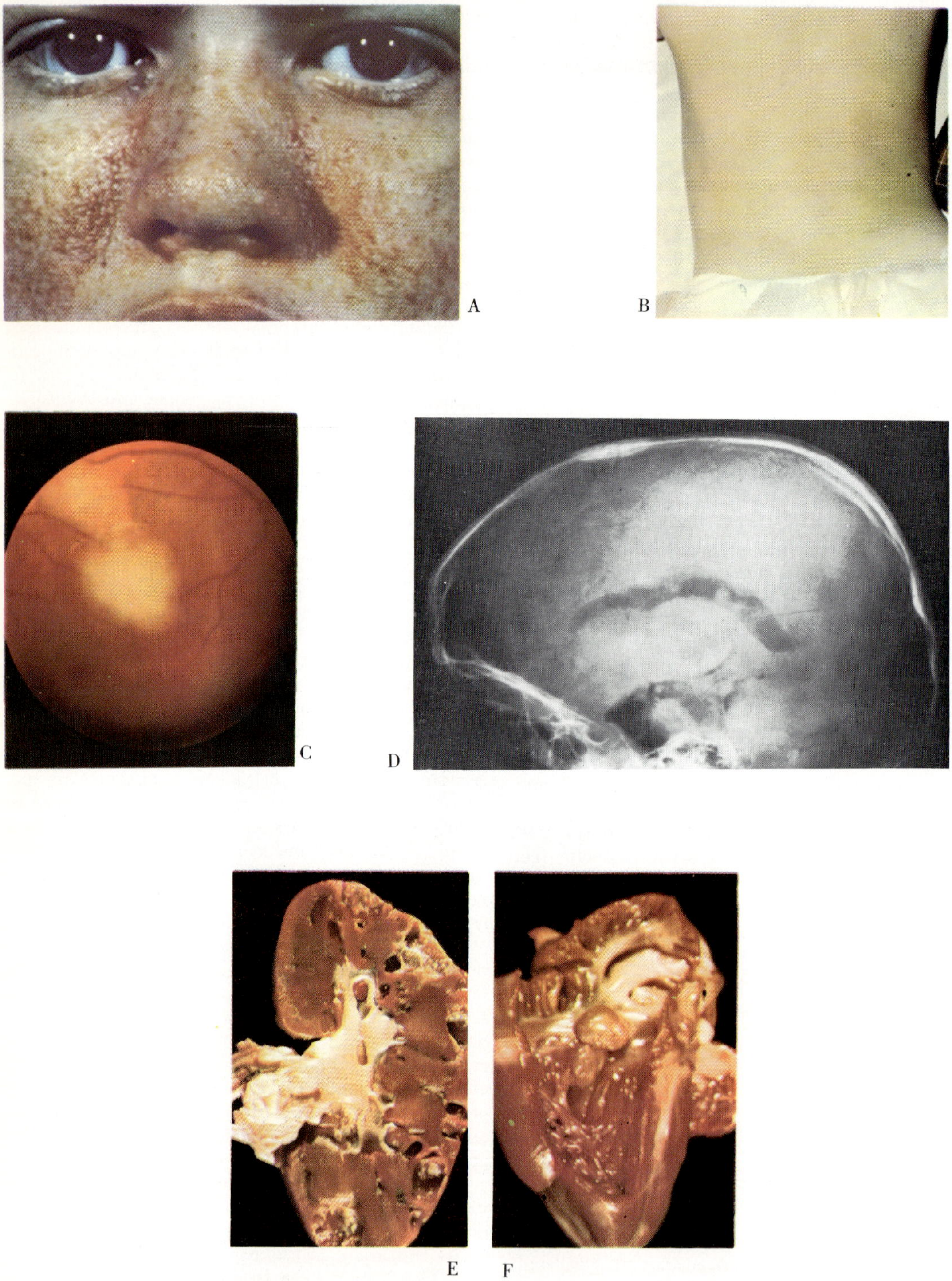

Fig. 38. Tuberous sclerosis. *A*. Adenoma sebaceum. *B*. Depigmented nevi. *C*. Retinal phakoma. *D*. Pneumonencephalogram demonstrating gliotic nodules projecting into ventricle ("candle dripping"). *E*. Polycystic kidney. *F*. Rhabdomyoma of heart.

TABLE 16. *Neurofibromatosis—Clinical and Pathologic Manifestations*

Soft Tissue	Café-au-lait nevus Fibroma molluscum	
Neurologic	Peripheral nerve	Neurofibroma Plexiform neuroma
	Nerve roots	Intradural neurofibroma
	Spinal cord	Syringomyelia Tumors—ependymoma
	Cranial nerves	Optic nerve glioma Acoustic neuroma
	Brain	Convulsions Mental deficiency Brain tumors
Bone	Scoliosis Congenital bowing and pseudarthrosis Posterosuperior orbital wall defects. Unilateral pulsating exophthalmos Disorders of bone growth Macrocephaly	
Congenital anomalies	Spina bifida Anomalies of vertebral segmentation Pes cavus Rib deformities	

ation of the family may reveal other cases of this disorder. X-rays of the skull often show intracranial calcifications. X-rays of the hands and feet may show small cystic lesions in the distal phalanges. Pneumoencephalography may outline the many glial nodules in the walls of the ventricles, giving what has been called "candle-guttering" with the effect of dripping wax.

Treatment is entirely symptomatic and is focused largely on the control of the convulsive disorder and management of the mentally defective child. Care should be taken in giving the prognosis in an infant or young child, since such great variation is seen in the neurologic as well as dermatologic aspects of this disorder.

Neurofibromatosis (von Recklinghausen's disease) is inherited as an autosomal dominant trait with marked variability of expression: while the characteristic pathology consists of neurofibromas of the peripheral, spinal, and cranial nerves, meningiomas and gliomas of the spinal cord and brain do occur. The condition includes the following manifestations (Table 16): multiple soft tumors beneath the skin (fibroma molluscum), multiple tumors situated along nerve trunks (neurofibromas), and pigmentation of the skin. Varying degrees of mental deficiency may occur. The peripheral neurofibromas are found along the course of nerve trunks, subcutaneous nerves, and cranial nerves. The auditory nerve is very frequently involved. The optic nerve is a frequent site of astrocytoma and less commonly meningioma. Within the spinal cord ependymomas, astrocytomas, and diffuse gliomas are seen. Pheochromocytomas are seen in the adult age group.

Clinically a common sequence is for excessive pigmentation to be noted during infancy; the characteristic superficial skin lesions make their appearance in childhood or puberty; individual lesions grow slowly, with puberty and pregnancy apparently exercising an accelerating effect. Siblings, parents, and other members of the family will often show the typical skin lesions. These cutaneous manifestations may take two forms, "café-au-lait" spots and pigmented nevi (Fig. 39). The pigmented nevi appear at an earlier age and are in no way different from the common moles, save in their number. The "café-au-lait" lesions are fewer in number and tend to be distributed along the paths of the cutaneous nerves. They are roughly oval in outline, with the long axis parallel to the nerve.

The tumors may be confined to the subcutaneous tissues or may be predominantly within the bony confines of the central nervous system. The most common histologic lesion is the benign neurilemmoma. Fibromas are also present, and sarcomatous degeneration may occur in the adult. When the tu-

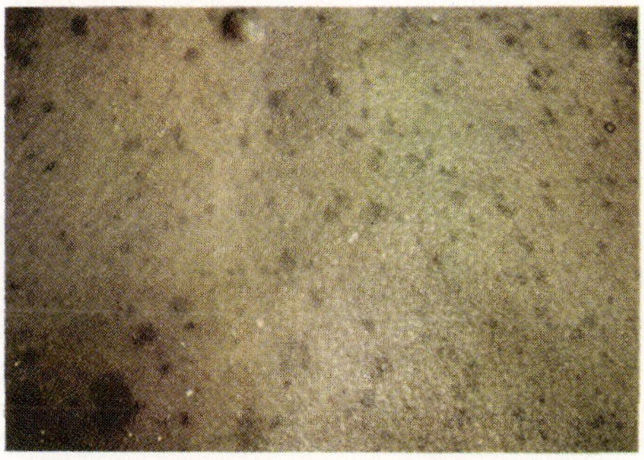

Fig. 39. Neurofibromatosis. Café-au-lait nevus.

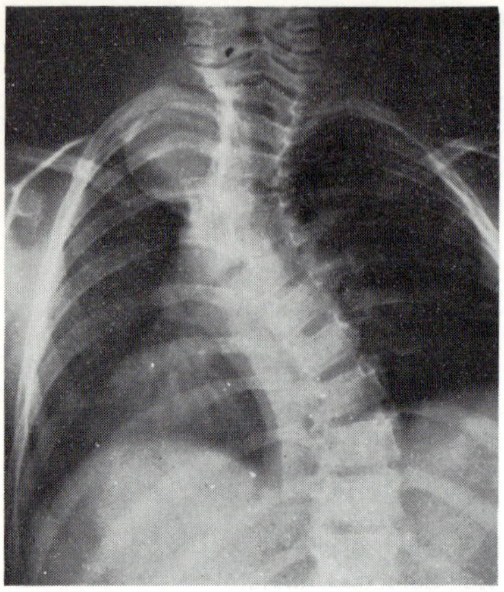

Fig. 40. Neurofibromatosis. Scoliosis and characteristic apical lesion.

TABLE 17. *Encephalotrigeminal Angiomatosis (Sturge-Weber-Dimitri Disease)—Clinical and Laboratory Manifestations*

Skin	Port-wine facial nevus usually in trigeminal nerve distribution
Neurologic	Convulsions Hemiparesis Hemianopia Mental retardation
Ocular	Glaucoma
Laboratory	Skull x-ray: "trolley track" calcifications EEG: focal abnormalities Carotid arteriogram: vascular anomalies or thromboses

mors occupy bone they produce localized areas of rarefaction, or they may give rise to thickening or excessive linear growth of the long bone. The pendulous masses of fibrous tissue and skin are more characteristic of the adult form of neurofibromatosis and are rarely seen in children.

Neurofibromatosis must be differentiated from tuberous sclerosis. In the former, the lesions tend to involve the peripheral outflow of the central nervous system, whereas in the tuberous sclerotic patient, the central lesions are the primary pathology. Mental deficiency is much more frequent with tuberous sclerosis than it is with neurofibromatosis. Epilepsy may occur in both, but it is a very common complication in tuberous sclerosis and is relatively rare in neurofibromatosis. As in tuberous sclerosis, a parent may have a relatively benign form of the disease, whereas the child can be very severely involved from the neurologic point of view.

A great variety of signs and symptoms may occur in neurofibromatosis, depending upon the location of the lesions. Optic nerve tumors within the orbit may lead to progressive exophthalmos with optic atrophy. Astrocytomas of the third ventricle and hypothalamus may be associated with neurofibromatosis and result in the symptom complex of diabetes insipidus, adiposity, genital maldevelopment, or precocious puberty. The lesions may present themselves as intramedullary tumors of the spinal cord. In some families, bilateral acoustic nerve tumors may be the prominent feature with few skin manifestations.

The diagnosis is often aided by x-ray studies which may reveal large "scalloped" neural foramina in the spine, scoliosis (Fig. 40), or enlarged optic foramina if optic nerve tumors are present. With auditory nerve tumors, an enlarged internal auditory canal may be apparent on roentgenologic study. The diagnosis is best made on the basis of the nature of the cutaneous manifestations and evidence of multiple peripheral nerve lesions.

Therapy is surgical removal of the offending neurofibromas, but it must be recalled that no definitive cure can be expected owing to the multiple nature of the lesions. Surgery should only be carried out when a particular lesion becomes a major symptomatic problem for the patient. Definitive treatment is not possible. A conservative therapeutic policy seems advisable.

Polyostotic fibrous dysplasia (Albright's syndrome) is important in the differential diagnosis of neurofibromatosis. In this condition large areas of tan or brown, irregularly outlined pigmentation appear on the skin and are associated with precocious puberty in the female.

Encephalotrigeminal angiomatosis (Sturge-Weber-Dimitri syndrome). This syndrome (Table 17) includes a port-wine vascular nevus often in the distribution of the first division of the trigeminal nerve (Fig. 41); convulsions, often focal and involving the contralateral side; contralateral hemipa-

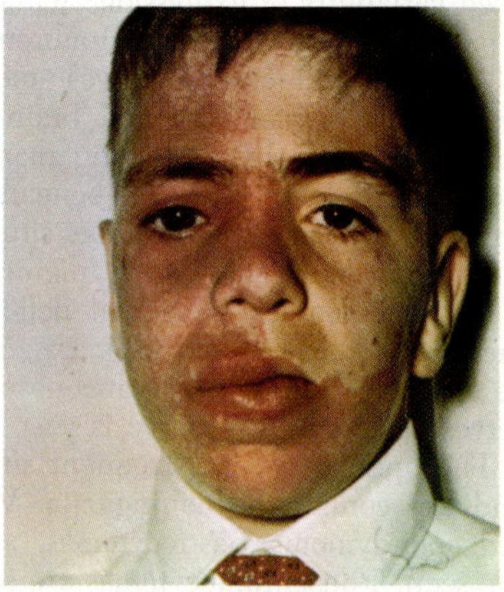

Fig. 41. Encephalotrigeminal angiomatosis. Characteristic port-wine facial nevus in distribution of trigeminal nerve. Note involvement of both sides of face.

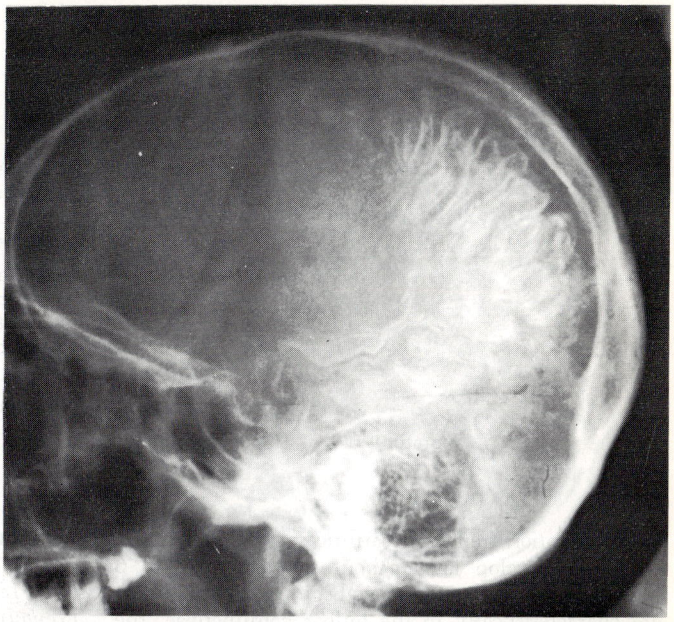

Fig. 42. Encephalotrigeminal angiomatosis. Skull x-ray showing characteristic intracranial calcification.

resis; and occasionally homonymous hemianopsia. Ipsilateral intracranial calcifications are found by x-ray. These calcifications are characteristically in paired lines, often called "trolley tracks" (Fig. 42). Additional symptomatology includes increased intraocular tension caused by angiomatous involvement of the uveal tract. This may give rise to enlargement of the involved globe. Approximately two-thirds of the children with this condition are mentally retarded, and somewhat more than 50 percent have convulsive disorders. A hemiparesis is less common.

There is great variability in the severity of the individual symptoms, and in some instances one or another may be missing entirely. Hemangiomas may be found in various parts of the body as well as on the face and rarely in the fundi.

The intracranial lesion is an angiomatous one which involves the meninges in the area supplied by the first division of the trigeminal nerve and sometimes also the superficial vessels occupying the sulci over the convexity, particularly in the occipital and parietal regions. This may cause atrophy of the underlying brain tissue, and the degenerative changes in cerebral tissue lying just below the gyral surface are frequently followed by the characteristic calcifications. The demonstration of intracranial calcifications limited to the convexity of the brain and showing the characteristic gyral pattern is almost pathognomonic. The diagnosis is usually made from the physical findings alone. Electroencephalography may show suppression of activity on the side which contains the nevus, and pneumoencephalography may reveal some cortical atrophy with dilation of the lateral ventricle on the involved side.

Therapy is entirely symptomatic, although early surgical intervention has been successful occasionally.

The differential diagnosis should include the Wyburn-Mason syndrome, in which telangiectasia or hypertrophic angiomas may appear on the face. However, in this condition there is the constant association of cirsoid angioma of the retina and mesencephalic aneurysmal angiomas. The syndrome of Van Bogaert-Divry is a combination of diffuse cortical meningeal angiomatosis in which dementia, severe convulsive disorder, pyramidal and extrapyramidal motor symptoms, and congenital poikiloderma with multiple telangiectasia are found.

Several other conditions must be mentioned in relation to the vascular malformations involving the central nervous system. *Von Hippel-Lindau's disease,* a disorder limited to adults, is characterized by hemangioblastomas of the cerebellum, liver, pancreas, and kidneys. Skin lesions are not seen in this condition, which is inherited as a dominant trait. *Neurocutaneous melanosis* consists of multiple pigmented nevi, often in the "bathing trunk" distribution (see Fig. 11), widely scattered over the surface of the skin. Intracranially, multiple pigmented and nonpigmented nevi are found in the meninges and in perivascular areas of brain and cerebellum. Multiple pia-arachnoid telangiectases are associated with the nevi. Progressive hydrocephalus is the clinical manifestation most often noted. *Disseminated hemangiomatosis* of the skin and multiple cerebral, pontine, and cerebellar hemangiomas have been reported to occur in familial distribution. Macrocephaly and pseudopapilledema may be associated with the multiple cutaneous strawberry hemangiomas.

Ataxia-telangiectasia (Louis-Bar) (Table 18) is a recessively inherited, progressive ataxia in which oculocutaneous telangiectasia is a diagnostic feature. Ataxia becomes evident when the child begins to

TABLE 18. *Ataxia-Telangiectasia—Clinical and Laboratory Manifestations*

Inheritance	Autosomal recessive
Clinical	Onset 1½-3 years—Neurologic Progressive cerebellar ataxia and/or choreoathetosis Speech—slow and dysarthric Parkinsonian facies
	At 4-6 years of age—Telangiectasis Bulbar conjunctiva Butterfly area of face Elbows and knees
	At any age—Infections Primary sinopulmonary
Laboratory	Hypogammaglobulinemia

walk; intention tremor, dysarthric speech, and choreoathetosis develop later. About the age of 4 to 6 years, the telangiectatic lesions begin to appear. These are characteristically in the bulbar conjunctivae, the "butterfly" area of the face, and the external ear (Fig. 43). Later, the antecubital and popliteal fossae and creases of the neck also show the telangiectatic lesions. Frequent upper respiratory infections are another characteristic of the disease. These are believed to be due to a decreased serum gamma-1A globulin. The course is slowly progressive, and most children are incapacitated by the time they reach adolescence. The oldest surviving patient was 25 years of age.

Pathologically there is a primary and diffuse cortical cerebellar degeneration. The Purkinje cells are chiefly affected. The white matter is essentially spared. There are some changes in dentate and olivary nuclei, but the rest of the central nervous system appears to be relatively spared. The thymus has been reported as abnormally small and tonsils and adenoids virtually absent. Several patients have died of lymphoreticular malignancies. Excessive amino-aciduria with large amounts of a peptide containing proline and hydroxyproline has been reported.

Hemangiectatic hypertrophy of a limb (Klippel-Trenaunay syndrome) may be associated with ichthyosis, mental deficiency, and a convulsive disorder. Differential diagnosis from other forms of neurocutaneous syndromes and in particular neurofibromatosis should be made.

A variety of other dermatologic conditions are associated with central nervous system malfunction. Spastic paraparesis in cases of juvenile acanthosis nigricans has been reported. Ichthyosis, mental deficiency, and epilepsy are described in combination as *Rud's syndrome*. In some cases retinal degeneration and genital hypoplasia are noted. The combination of spastic diplegia, mental deficiency, and congenital ichthyosis is reported as an autosomal recessive trait under the term *Sjögren-Larsson's syndrome*. *Anhidrotic* or *hypohidrotic* ectodermal dysplasias may be associated with mild to moderate mental retardation. Follicular keratosis has been reported in association with mental deficiency (*Darier's disease*).

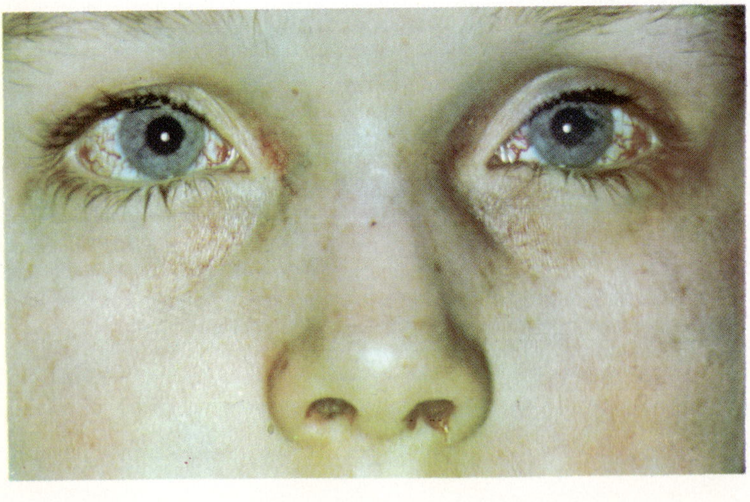

Fig. 43. Ataxia-telangiectasia. Typical bulbar conjunctival telangiectasia in 13-year-old boy. (Courtesy of Drs. E. Boder and R. P. Sedgwick.)

Incontinentia pigmenti (Bloch-Sulzberger's syndrome) has been reported as a familial disorder. Most cases are sporadic. There appears to be a definite prevalence in females. Typically during the neonatal period groups of vesicles occur in a linear distribution along the extremities. As these disappear, the linear verrucal skin lesions begin to show the characteristic gray-blue to brown pigmentation which is distributed in wavy lines, giving an appearance similar to the pattern of marble. In some cases the preliminary vesicular and verrucous lesions apparently do not occur. Alopecia and dental defects are also frequently seen. From a neurologic point of view, mental deficiency, spasticity, and hemiparesis occur. A convulsive disorder is frequent, and microcephaly is not uncommon. Pneumoencephalography usually shows ventricular dilation. In at least one case showing skin lesions almost exclusively confined to one side, the ipsilateral cerebral ventricle was more dilated than that on the side of the noninvolved skin. Congenital generalized melanoleucoderma (Naegeli's syndrome) may be confused with incontinenta pigmenti.

Linear nevus sebaceus is associated with a convulsive disorder and mental retardation. The skin lesion consists of very closely placed papules formed by thickening and hyperkeratosis of the epidermis with marked hyperplasia of the sebaceous glands. The lesion characteristically starts as an oval-shaped area in the center of the forehead extending as a fine line over the midline of the nose to the upper lip. Neurologic examination is normal, but the electroencephalogram shows focal discharges of high-voltage spikes in the parietal and occipital regions. Seizures and mental retardation are the prominent symptoms.

Ectodermal dysplasia (anhidrotic type) is a sex-linked recessive condition in which the brain damage, seizures, and mental retardation are probably due to repeated episodes of high temperatures. The features are aplasia of sweat, sebaceous, and mucous glands with hypotrichosis. Small, wide-spaced teeth with peg-shaped incisors are present.

The basal cell nevus syndrome, an autosomal dominant disorder, consists of brown, slightly raised, hard basal cell nevi appearing anywhere on the skin. These may appear in childhood and may later degenerate to basal cell carcinomas. Cysts of the jaw, hypertelorism, and lamellar calcification of the falx cerebri make up the complete syndrome. Mental deficiency, hydrocephalus, agenesis of the corpus callosum, and medulloblastomas have been reported with the disorder.

Supportive Therapy and Management of the Progressive Degenerative Diseases

Although no specific curative or definitive treatment can be offered in the diseases previously discussed, much can be accomplished by way of supportive therapy for both patient and family.

The problems of management can be divided into those pertaining to the patient and those which primarily concern the parents. Frank, sympathetic, and direct discussion with the parents should include a careful explanation of the definitive diagnosis, the course of the disease, the prognosis for life, and an offer of genetic counseling and supportive psychiatric assistance. Enlisting the aid of trained social workers and visiting nurses is often extremely helpful. In the less rapidly progressive disorders and where mental retardation, ataxia, spasticity, visual impairment, and seizures occur in a variety of combinations, the parents will need help in educational placement. School systems and teachers should be given adequate interpretations of the handicaps and instruction in their management.

The increasing incapacity of the child leads to serious problems in feeding, prevention of infection and decubiti, fluid and electrolyte balance, prevention of contractures, and bowel and bladder care. Gavage feedings almost always become necessary in the storage diseases and in the diffuse sclerosis. Too high a caloric intake is to be avoided in order to facilitate skin care and maintenance of good positioning. Passive exercise, footboards, and frequent scheduled turning are also indicated. Paralytic ileus is a common complication. Enemas and suppositories are often required. Urinary and fecal incontinence demand extra attention to skin care. In the terminal stages, machine aspiration will be needed. With careful instruction, most of these maintenance procedures can be carried out in a home environment and thus obviate the necessity for long and expensive hospitalization. In the terminal stages, hospitalization is essential.

In the spinocerebellar, spinal, and neuromuscular disorders where progression is slower, physical therapy, occupational therapy, and occasionally judicious orthopedic intervention may be helpful. However, parents, orthopedists, and patients should not be led to believe that such therapy is definitive and must come to understand the fundamentally progressive nature of the disorder.

Anticonvulsant therapy is often more difficult in the degenerative diseases than in other forms of symptomatic or idiopathic epilepsy, but the same basic principles apply as in all forms of seizure disorders. Myoclonic seizures are difficult to control, and exclusion of as many sensory stimuli as possible may be helpful, particularly in the "stimulus-sensitive" forms of myoclonus. Phenobarbital and Dilantin continue to be the most useful anticonvulsants. Paradione, Tridione, Zarontin, Valium, and occasionally the milder forms of tranquilizing drugs may be helpful in controlling the myoclonic activity.

In the phakomatous group of diseases a careful watch for the development of secondary glaucoma must be maintained. In many of the neurocutaneous syndromes the development of secondary malignancies and increased intracranial pressure should be a source of constant concern for the attending physician.

The treatment and management of the progressive degenerative diseases of the central nervous system represent a challenge for physicians as well as auxiliary personnel in nursing, physical therapy, occupational therapy, and psychologic and educational services. These patients and especially their parents present some of the most difficult physician-patient relationship problems to be faced in pediatric practice.

REFERENCES

Aita, J. A. Neurocutaneous Diseases. Springfield, Ill., Charles C Thomas, Publ., 1966.

Freeman, J. M., and McKhann, G. M. Degenerative diseases of the central nervous system. *In* Advances in Pediatrics. Chicago, Year Book Medical Publishers, 1969, Vol. 16.

Gellis, S. S., and Feingold, M. Atlas of Mental Retardation Syndromes. Washington, D.C., U.S. Govt. Printing Office, 1968.

Gibbs, C. J., Jr., and Gajdusek, D. C. Infection as the etiology of spongiform encephalopathy (Creutzfeldt-Jakob Disease). Science, 165:1023, 1969.

McKusick, V. A. Mendelian Inheritance in Man, 2nd ed. Baltimore, Johns Hopkins Press, 1968.

Stanbury, J. B., Wyngaarden, J. B., and Fredrickson, D. S., eds. The Metabolic Basis of Inherited Disease, 2nd ed. New York, McGraw-Hill Book Co., 1966.

CEREBROMACULAR DEGENERATION

Brady, R. O. Genetics and the sphingolipidoses. Med. Clin. N. Amer., 53:827, 1969.

Brown, N. J., Corner, D. B., and Dodgson, M. C. H. A sceond case in the same family of congenital familial cerebral lipoidosis resembling amaurotic family idiocy. Arch. Dis. Child., 29:48, 1954.

Derry, D. M., Fawcett, J. S., Anderman, F., and Wolfe, L. S. Late infantile systemic lipidosis. Neurology, 18: 340, 1968.

Donahue, S., Zeman, W., and Watanabe, I. Electron microscopic observations in Batten's disease. *In* Inborn Errors of Sphingolipid Metabolism. New York, Pergamon Press, Inc., 1966.

Hagberg, B., Hultquist, G., Ohman, R., and Svennerholm, L. Congenital amaurotic idiocy. Acta Paediat. (Uppsala), 54:116, 1965.

Harlem, O. K. Juvenile cerebroretinal degeneration (Spielmeyer-Vogt): Blood and EEG findings in a family of 10 members. Amer. J. Dis. Child., 100:918, 1960.

Jatzkewitz, H., and Sandhoff, K. On a biochemically special form of infantile amaurotic idiocy. Biochem. Biophys. Acta, 70:354, 1963.

Jervis, G. A. Juvenile amaurotic idiocy. Amer. J. Dis. Child., 97:663, 1959.

Kanof, A., Aronson, S. M., and Volk, B. W. Clinical progression of amaurotic family idiocy. Amer. J. Dis. Child., 97:656, 1959.

Kristensson, K., and Sourander, P. Occurrence of lipofuscin in inherited metabolic diseases affecting the nervous system. J. Neurol. Neurosurg. Psychiat., 29: 113, 1966.

Knudson, A. G., and Kaplan, W. D. Genetics of sphingolipidoses. *In* Aronson, S. M., and Volk, B. W., eds., The Sphingolipidoses. New York, Academic Press, Inc., 1962, pp. 395-411.

Korey, S. R., and Stein, A. Studies in Tay-Sachs disease. III. Biochemistry. B. Catabolism of gangliosides and related compounds. J. Neuropath. Exp. Neurol., 22: 67, 1963.

Landing, B. H., Silverman, F. N., Craig, J. M., Jacoby, M. E., Lahey, M. E., and Chadwick, D. L. Familial neurovisceral lipidosis. Amer. J. Dis. Child., 108:503, 1964.

Merritt, A. D., Smith, S. A., Strouth, J. C., and Zeman, W. Detection of heterozygotes in Batten's disease. Ann. N.Y. Acad. Sci., 155:860, 1968.

Norman, R. M., and Wood, N. Congenital form of amaurotic family idiocy. J. Neurol. Psychiat., 4:175, 1941.

Okada, S., and O'Brien, J. S. Generalized gangliosidosis: Beta-galactosidase deficiency. Science, 160:1002, 1968.

——— and O'Brien, J. S. Tay-Sachs disease: Generalized absence of a beta-D-N-hexosaminidase component. Science, 165:698, 1969.

Rayner, S. Juvenile Amaurotic Idiocy in Sweden. Uppsala Institute for Medical Genetics of the University of Sweden, 1962.

Suzuki, K. Cerebral GM_1-gangliosidosis: Chemical pathology of visceral organs. Science, 159:1471, 1968.

——— Suzuki, K., Rapin, I., Suzuki, Y., and Ishii, N. Juvenile GM_2-gangliosidosis. Neurology, 20:190, 1970.

——— Suzuki, K., and Kamoshita, S. Chemical pathology of GM_1-gangliosidosis (generalized gangliosidosis). J. Neuropath. Exp. Neurol., 28:25, 1969.

Svennerholm, L. Gangliosides. J. Lipid Res., 5:145, 1964.

——— The chemical structure of normal human brain and Tay-Sachs gangliosides. Biochem. Biophys. Res. Commun., 9:436, 1962.

Vogt, B. W., Aronson, S. M., and Saifer, A. Fructose-1-phosphate adolase deficiency in Tay-Sachs disease. Amer. J. Med., 36:481, 1964.

——— Schneck, L., Saifer, A., and Aronson, S. M. Tay-Sachs Disease. New York, Grune and Stratton, Inc., 1964.

——— et al. G_5 ganglioside variant of systemic late infantile lipidosis. Arch. Path., 87:393, 1969.

Wolfe, L. S., Callahan, J., Fawcett, M. S., Andermann, F., and Scriver, C. R. GM_1-gangliosidosis without chondrodystrophy or visceromegaly: Beta-galactosidase deficiency with gangliosidosis and the excessive excretion of a keratan sulfate. Neurology, 20:23, 1970.

Zeman, W., and Donahue, S. Fine structure of the lipid bodies in juvenile amaurotic idiocy. Acta Neuropath., 3:144, 1963.

NIEMANN-PICK DISEASE

Brady, R. O. The spingolipidoses. New Eng. J. Med., 275:312, 1966.

Crocker, A. C., and Farber, S. Niemann-Pick's disease: A review of 18 patients. Medicine, 37:1, 1958.

Forsythe, W. E., McKeown, E. F., and Neill, D. W. Three cases of Niemann-Pick's disease in children. Arch. Dis. Child., 34:406, 1959.

GAUCHER'S DISEASE

Banker, B. Q., Miller, J. Q., and Crocker, A. C. The cerebral pathology of infantile Gaucher's disease. *In* Aronson, S. M., and Volk, B. W., eds., Cerebral Sphingolipidoses. New York, Academic Press, Inc., 1962.

Kampine, J. P., Brady, R. O., Kanfer, J. N., Feld, M., and Shapiro, D. Diagnosis of Gaucher's disease and Niemann-Pick's disease with small samples of venous blood. Science, 155:86, 1967.

Maloney, A. F. J., and Cumings, J. N. A case of juvenile Gaucher's disease with intraneuronal lipid storage. J. Neurol. Neurosurg. Psychiat., 23:207, 1960.

Stein, M., and Gardner, L. I. Acute infantile Gaucher's disease. Pediatrics, 27:491, 1961.

PROGRESSIVE FAMILIAL MYOCLONIC EPILEPSY (UNVERRICHT'S DISEASE)

Aigner, B. R., and Mulder, D. W. Myoclonus. Arch. Neurol., 2:600, 1960.

Gilbert, G. J., McEntee, W. J., and Glaser, G. H. Familial myoclonus and ataxia; pathophysiologic implications. Neurology, 13:365, 1963.

Harriman, D. G. F., Millar, J. H. D., and Stevenson, A. C. Progressive familial myoclonic epilepsy in three families: its clinical features and pathological basis. Brain, 78:325, 1955.

Janeway, R., Ravens, J. R., Pearce, L. A., Odor, D. L., and Suzuki, K. Progressive myoclonus epilepsy with Lafora inclusion bodies: I. Clinical, genetic, histopathologic and biochemical aspects. Arch. Neurol., 16: 565, 1967.

Odor, D. L., Janeway, R., Pearce, L. A., and Ravens, J. R. Progressive myoclonus epilepsy: II. Studies of ultrastructure. Arch. Neurol., 16:583, 1967.

Van Heycop Ten Ham, M. W., and DeJager, H. Progressive myoclonus epilepsy with Lafora bodies, clinical-pathological features. Epilepsia, 4:95, 1963.

FARBER'S DISEASE

Abul-Haj, S. K., Martz, D. G., Douglas, W. F., and Geppert, L. J. Pathogenesis of Farber's disease. J. Pediat., 61:221, 1962.

Farber, S. A lipid metabolic disorder—disseminated "lipogranulomatosis." Amer. J. Dis. Child., 84:499, 1952.

Prensky, A. L. et al. Ceramide and ganglioside accumulation in Farber's lipogranulomatosis. Proc. Soc. Exp. Biol. Med., 126:725, 1967.

FABRY'S DISEASE

Brady, R. O. et al. Enzymatic defect in Fabry's disease; ceramidetrihexosidase deficiency. New Eng. J. Med., 276:1163, 1967.

Kocen, R. S., and Thomas, P. K. Peripheral nerve involvement in Fabry's disease. Arch. Neurol., 22:81, 1970.

Low, H. O. C., and Reske-Nielsen, E. The central nervous system in Fabry's disease. Arch. Neurol., 25:351, 1971.

Matalon, R., Dorfman, A., Dawson, G., and Sweeley, C. C. Glycolipid and mucopolysaccharide abnormality in fibroblasts of Fabry's disease. Science, 164:1522, 1969.

Rahman, A. N., and Lindenberg, G. The neuropathology of hereditary dystopic lipidosis. Arch. Neurol., 9:373, 1963.

Wise, D. et al. Angiokeratoma corporis diffusum: Clinical study of eight affected families. Quart. J. Med., 31:177, 1961.

CEREBRAL CHOLINESTEROSIS

Jervis, G. A. Degenerative encephalopathy of childhood (cortical degeneration, cerebellar atrophy, cholesterinosis of basal ganglia). J. Neuropath. Exp. Neurol., 16: 308, 1957.

Van Bogaert, L., Scherer, H. J., and Epstein, E. Une Forme Cerebrale de la Cholesterinose Generaliseé. Paris, Masson et Cie, 1937.

Wolman, M., Sterk, V. V., Gott, S., and Frenkel, M. Primary familial xanthomatosis with involvement and calcification of the adrenals. Pediatrics, 28:742, 1961.

HELLER'S DISEASE

Dietze, H. J. Dementia infantilis, Heller. Amer. J. Ment. Defic., 68:193, 1963.

Korey, S. R., and Winograd, H. Biochemical alterations in a case of Heller's disease. Amer. J. Dis. Child., 97: 668, 1959.

HURLER'S DISEASE (GARGOYLISM)

Berry, H. K., and Spinanger, J. Paper spot test useful in study of Hurler's syndrome. J. Lab. Clin. Med., 55: 136, 1960.

Foly, K. M., Danes, B. S., and Bearn, A. G. White blood cell cultures in genetic studies on the human mucopolysaccharidoses. Science, 164:424, 1969.

Fratantoni, J. C., Hall, C. W., and Neufeld, E. F. Hurler and Hunter syndromes: Mutual correction of the defect in cultural fibroblasts. Science, 162:570, 1968.

——— et al. Intrauterine diagnosis of Hurler and Hunter syndromes. New Eng. J. Med., 280:686, 1969.

Hambrick, G. W., Jr. Skin changes in Hurler's syndrome. Arch. Derm., 85:455, 1962.

Ho, M. W., and O'Brien, J. S. Hurler's syndrome: Deficiency of a specific beta-galactosidase isoenzyme. Science, 165:611, 1969.

Lindsay, S., Reilly, W. A., Gotham, T. J., and Skahen, R. Gargoylism, study of pathologic lesions and clinical review of twelve cases. Amer. J. Dis. Child., 76:239, 1948.

McKusick, V. A. et al. The genetic mucopolysaccharidoses. Medicine, 44:6, 445, 1965.

Muir, H., Miltwoch, U., and Bitter, T. Diagnostic value of isolated urinary mucopolysaccharides and lymphocytic inclusions in gargoylism. Arch. Dis. Child., 38: 358, 1963.

Renuart, A. W. Screening for inborn errors of metabolism associated with mental deficiency or neurologic disorders or both. New Eng. J. Med., 274:384, 1966.

Sanfilippo, S. J., Podosin, R., Langer, L., and Good, R. A. Mental retardation associated with acid mucopolysacchariduria (hepartin sulfate). J. Pediat., 63: 837, 1963.

GLYCOGEN STORAGE DISEASE

Hug, G., Garancis, J. C., Schubert, W. K., and Kaplan, S. Glycogen storage disease types II, III, VIII, IX. A biochemical and electron microscopic analysis. Amer. J. Dis. Child., 111:457, 1966.

Smith, H. L. et al. Type II glycogenosis. Amer. J. Dis. Child., 3:475-481, 1966.

PROGRESSIVE DEGENERATION OF CEREBRAL GRAY MATTER

Alpers, B. J. Progressive cerebral degeneration of infancy. J. Nerv. Ment. Dis., 130:442, 1960.

Blackwood, W., Buxton, P. H., Cumings, J. N., Robertson, D. J., and Tucker, S. M. Diffuse cerebral degeneration in infancy (Alper's disease). Arch. Dis. Child., 38:193, 1963.

Dreifuss, F. E., and Netsky, M. G. Progressive poliodystrophy. The degenerations of cerebral gray matter. Amer. J. Dis. Child., 107:649, 1964.

Dunn, H. G., and Dolman, C. L. Necrotizing encephalomyelopathy. Neurology, 19:536, 1969.

Greenhouse, A. H., and Neuberger, K. T. The syndrome of progressive cerebral poliodystrophy. Arch. Neurol., 10:47, 1964.

Kamoshila, S., Aguilar, M. J., and Landing, B. H. Infantile subacute necrotizing encephalomyelopathy. Amer. J. Dis. Child., 116:120, 1968.

Leigh, D. Subacute necrotizing encephalomyelopathy in an infant. J. Neurol. Neurosurg. Psychiat., 12:216, 1951.

Richter, R. B. Infantile subacute necrotizing encephalopathy with predilection for the brain stem. J. Neuropath. Exp. Neurol., 16:281, 1957.

Robinson, F., Solitare, G. B., Lamarche, J. B., and Levy, L. L. Necrotizing encephalomyelopathy of childhood. Neurology, 17:472, 1967.

Tom, M. I., and Rencastle, N. B. Infantile subacute necrotizing encephalopathy. Neurology, 12:624, 1962.

DEMYELINATING DISEASES

Adams, R. D., and Richardson, E. P. The demyelinating diseases of the human nervous system. *In* Folch-Pi, J., ed., Chemical Pathology of the Nervous System. New York, Pergamon Press, Inc., 1961, pp. 162-191.

Korey, S. R. Glia, lipogenesis and formation of myelin. Arch. Neurol., 2:140, 1960.

Poser, C. M. Leukodystrophy and the concept of dysmyelination. Arch. Neurol., 4:323, 1961.

PELIZAEUS-MERZBACHER DISEASE

Gerstl, B., Malamud, N., Hayman, R. B., and Bond, P. R. Morphological and neurochemical study of Pelizaeus-Merzbacher disease. J. Neurol. Neurosurg. Psychiat., 28:540, 1965.

Zeman, W., DeMyer, W., and Falls, H. F. Pelizaeus-Merzbacher disease. J. Neuropath. Exp. Neurol., 23: 334, 1964.

Zerbin-Rudin, E., and Peiffer, J. Eingenetischer Beitrag Zur Frage Der Spotform Der Pelizaeus-Merzbacherschen Krankheit. Humangenetik, 1:107, 1964.

METACHROMATIC LEUCODYSTROPHY

Abraham, K., and Lampert, R. Intraneuronal lipid deposits in metachromatic leukodystrophy. Neurology, 13:686, 1964.

Aurebeck, G., Osterberg, K., Blau, M., Chou, S., and Nelson, E. Electron microscope observations in metachromatic leukodystrophy. Arch. Neurol., 11:273, 1964.

Austin, J. H. et al. Metachromatic leukodystrophy. Arch. Neurol., 18:225, 1968.

——— et al. Metachromatic form of diffuse cerebral sclerosis. VI. A rapid test for the sulfatase A deficiency in metachromatic leukodystrophy (MLD) urine. Arch. Neurol., 14:259, 1966.

Bass, N. H., Witmer, E. J., and Dreifuss. F. E. A pedigree study of metachromatic leukodystrophy: Biochemical identification of the carrier state. Neurology, 20: 52, 1970.

Hagberg, B., and Svennerholm, L. Metachromatic leukodystrophy. A generalized lipidosis. Acta Pediat. Scand., 49:690, 1960.

Mehl, E., and Jatzkervitz, H. Cerebroside 3 sulfate as a physiological substrate of arylsulfatase A. Biochem. biophys. Acta, 151:619, 1968.

Ogawa, K. Late infantile metachromatic leukodystrophy. The nature of the chromotope. Arch. Neurol., 4:418, 1961.

Schutta, H. S., Pratt, R. T. C., Metz, H., Evans, K. A., and Carter, C. D. A family study of the late infantile and juvenile forms of metachromatic leucodystrophy. J. Med. Genet., 3:86, 1966.

GLOBOID-CELL LEUCODYSTROPHY (KRABBE'S DISEASE)

Austin, J. Studies in globoid (Krabbe's) leukodystrophy. Arch. Neurol., 9:207, 1963.

——— et al. Defective sulfatide synthesis in Krabbe's disease (globoid leukodystrophy). Trans. Amer. Neurol. Ass., 92:175, 1967.

D'Agostina, A. M., Sayre, G. P., and Hayes, A. B. Krabbe's disease. Arch. Neurol., 8:82, 1963.

Hagberg, B., Sourander, P., and Svennerholm, L. Diagnosis of Krabbe's disease. Arch. Neurol., 8:82, 1963.

Norman, R. M., Oppenheimer, D. R., and Tingey, A. H. Histological and chemical findings in Krabbe's leukodystrophy. J. Neurol. Neurosurg. Psychiat., 24:223, 1961.

SPONGY SCLEROSIS (CANAVAN'S DISEASE)

Buchanan, D. S., and Davis, R. L. Spongy degeneration of the nervous system. Neurology, 15:207, 1965.

Hogan, G. R., and Richardson, E. P., Jr. Spongy degeneration of the nervous system (Canavan's disease). Pediatrics, 35:284, 1965.

Van Bogaert, L., and Bertrand, I. Spongy Degeneration of the Brain in Infancy. Amsterdam, North-Holland Publishing Co., 1967.

ZuRhein, G. M., Eichman, P. L., and Puletti, F. Familial idiocy with spongy degeneration of the central nervous system of van Bogaert-Bertrand. Neurology, 10:998, 1960.

SUDANOPHILIC (NEUTRAL FAT, ORTHOCHROMIC) FAMILIAL LEUCODYSTROPHY

Gerstl, B., Rubenstein, L. J., Eng, L. F., and Tavaststjerna, M. Neurochemical study of a case of sudanophilic leucodystrophy. Arch. Neurol., 15:603, 1966.
Gordon, N., and Marsden, H. B. Diffuse cerebral sclerosis and adrenal atrophy. Develop. Med. Child Neurol., 8:719, 1966.
Van Bogaert, L., Edgar, G. W. F., and Karcher, D. Type orthochromotique (à substance soudanophile) diffus de la leucodystrophie familiale. Acta Neuropath. (Berlin), 1:289, 1961.

ALEXANDER'S DISEASE

Friede, R. L. Alexander's disease. Arch. Neurol., 11:414, 1964.

DEMYELINATING SCLEROSIS

Gall, J. C., Jr., Hayles, A. B., Siekert, R. G., and Keith, H. M. Multiple sclerosis in children. A clinical study of 40 cases with onset in childhood. Pediatrics, 21:703, 1958.
Greevic, N. Concentric lacunar leukoencephalopathy. Arch. Neurol., 2:266, 1960.
Kennedy, C., and Carter, S. Relation of optic neuritis to multiple sclerosis in childhood. Pediatrics, 28:377, 1961.
Low, N. L., and Carter, S. Multiple sclerosis in childhood. Pediatrics, 18:24, 1956.
McAlpine, D., Compston, N. D., and Lumsden, C. E. Multiple Sclerosis. Edinburgh, E. & S. Livingston, Ltd., 1955.
Multiple Sclerosis and the Demyelinating Diseases. Res. Publ. Ass. Res. Nerv. Ment. Dis., Baltimore, Williams and Wilkins Co., 1950, Vol. 28.
Stansbury, F. C. Neuromyelitis optica (Devic's disease); presentation of 5 cases with pathologic study, and review of the literature. Arch. Ophthal., 42:292, 1949.

SCHILDER'S DISEASE

Bowman, L. Diffuse Sclerosis (Encephalitis Periaxialis Diffusa). Baltimore, William Wood & Co. (a division of Williams and Wilkins Co.), 1934.
Poser, C. M., and Van Bogaert, L. Natural history and evolution of the concept of Schilder's diffuse sclerosis. Acta Psychiat. Scand., 31:285, 1956.
Zeman, W., and Whieldon, J. A. Clinical considerations in "Schilder's disease." Amer. J. Dis. Child., 104:635, 1962.

SUBACUTE SCLEROSING PANENCEPHALITIS (SSPE)

Chen, T. T. et al. Subacute sclerosing panencephalitis: Propagation of measles virus from brain biopsy in tissue culture. Science, 163:1193, 1969.
Gibbs, C. J., and Gajdusek, D. C. Infection as the etiology of spongiform encephalopathy (Creutzfeldt-Jakob disease). Science, 165:1023, 1969.
Jabbour, J. T. et al. Subacute sclerosing panencephalitis: a multidisciplinary study of eight cases. J.A.M.A., 207:2248, 1969.
Katz, M. et al. Transmission of an encephalitogenic agent from patients with SSPE to ferrets. Amer. Pediat. Soc. (Abstr.), May, 1968.
Lombroso, C. T. Remarks on the EEG and movement disorder in SSPE. Neurology, 18:69, 1968.
Metz, H., Gregorion, M., and Sandifer, P. Subacute sclerosing panencephalitis, a review of 17 cases with special reference to clinical diagnostic criteria. Arch. Dis. Child., 39:554, 1964.
Rustigan, R. Persistent infection of cells in culture by measles virus. J. Bact., 92:1792, 1966.

DEGENERATIONS OF THE BASAL GANGLIA

Bearn, A. G. Wilson's disease. *In* Wyngaarden, J. B., and Fredrickson, D. S., eds., The Metabolic Basis of Inherited Disease. New York, McGraw-Hill Book Co., 1966.
Byers, R. K., and Dodge, J. A. Huntington's chorea in children, report of four cases. Neurology, 17:587, 1967.
Cooper, I. S. Dystonia reversal by operation on basal ganglia. Arch. Neurol., 7:132, 1962.
DeMyer, W., Harter, D. H., and Zeman, W. Familial spasticity, hyperkinesia and dementia. Clinico-pathologic observations and comments on the nosology of Hallervorden-Spatz disease. Acta Neuropath. (Berlin), 4:28, 1964.
Denny-Brown, D. Diseases of the basal ganglia and subthalamic nuclei. *In* Christian, H. A., ed., Oxford Medicine. New York, Oxford Univ. Press, 1946.
——— Wilson's disease. New Eng. J. Med., 270:1149, 1964.
Goodman, R. M., Hall, C. L., Terango, L., Perrine, G. A., Jr., and Roberts, P. L. Huntington's chorea. Arch. Neurol., 15:345, 1966.
Hunt, J. R. Dyssynergia cerebellaris myoclonica, primary atrophy of the dentate system. Brain, 44:440, 1921.
Jervis, G. A. Huntington's chorea in childhood. Arch. Neurol., 9:50, 1963.
Johnson, W., Schwartz, G., and Barbeau, A. Studies on dystonia musculorum deformans. Arch. Neurol., 7:301, 1962.
Kerteaz, A. Paroxysmal kinesigenic choreoathetosis. Neurology, 17:680, 1967.
Mount, L. A., and Reback, S. Familial paroxysmal choreoathetosis. Arch. Neurol. Psychiat., 44:841, 1940.
Porter, H. Tissue copper proteins in Wilson's disease. Arch. Neurol., 11:341, 1964.
Pryles, C. V., Livingston, S., and Ford, F. R. Familial paroxysmal choreoathetosis of Mount and Reback. Pediatrics, 9:44, 1952.
Sternlieb, I., and Scheinberg, I. H. Diagnosis of Wilson's disease in asymptomatic patients. J.A.M.A., 183:747, 1963.
——— and Scheinberg, I. H. Penicillamine therapy for hepato-lenticular degeneration. J. A. M. A., 189:748, 1964.
Szanto, J., and Gallyas, F. A study of iron metabolism in neuropsychiatric patients (Hallervorden-Spatz disease). Arch. Neurol., 14:438, 1966.
Zeman, W., Koelbling, R., and Pasamanick, B. Idiopathic

dystonia musculorum deformans. II. The formes frustes. Neurology, 10:1068, 1960.

POLYMORPHOUS NEUROABIOTROPHIES

Dow, R. S., and Moruzzi, G. Physiology and Pathology of the Cerebellum. Minneapolis, Univ. Minnesota Press, 1958.
Greenfield, J. G. Spinocerebellar Degenerations. Springfield, Ill., Charles C Thomas, Publ., 1954.
Jervis, G. A. Early familial cerebellar degeneration. J. Nerv. Ment. Dis., 11:398, 1950.
Schut, J. W. The Hereditary Ataxias, Genetics and the Inheritance of Integrated Neurological and Psychiatric Patterns. Res. Publ. Ass. Res. Nerv. Ment. Dis., Vol. 33. Baltimore, Williams and Wilkins Co., 1954.

SPINOCEREBELLAR DEGENERATIONS

Alter, M., Talbert, O. R., and Croffead, G. Cerebellar ataxia, congenital cataracts, and retarded somatic and mental maturation. Report of cases of Marinesco-Sjögren syndrome. Neurology, 12:836, 1962.
Anderson, B. Marinesco-Sjögren syndrome. Develop. Med. Child. Neurol., 7:249, 1965.
Bergstedt, M., Johansson, S., and Miller, R. Hereditary spastic ataxia with central retinal degeneration and vestibular impairment. A clinical report on a family. Neurology, 12:124, 1962.
Mier, M., Schwartz, S. O., and Boshes, B. Acanthocytosis, pigmentary dysgenesis in three brothers. New Eng. J. Med., 271:593, 1964.
Thieffry, S., Arthuis, M., and Bargeton, E. Quarante cas de maladie de Werdnig-Hoffman avec onze examens anatomiques. Rev. Neurol., 93:621, 1955.
Walton, J. N. The "floppy" infant. Cereb. Palsy J., 2:10, 1960.
Wilson, S. A. K., and Bruce, A. N., eds., Neurology. Baltimore, Williams and Wilkins Co., 1955, Vol. 2, pp. 1126-1134, 1156-1167.

PERONEAL MUSCULAR ATROPHY

Austin, J. H. Observations on the syndrome of hypertrophic neuritis (the hypertrophic interstitial radiculoneuropathies). Medicine, 35:187, 1956.
Cammermeyer, J. Symposium on peripheral neuropathies. J. Neuropath. Exp. Neurol., 15:340, 1956.
Denny-Brown, D. Hereditary sensory radicular neuropathy. J. Neurol. Neurosurg. Psychiat., 14:237, 1951.
Dyck, P. J., Lambert, E. H., and Mulder, D. W. Charcot-Marie-Tooth disease: nerve conduction and clinical studies of a large kinship. Neurology, 13:1, 1963.
Gordon, N., and Hudson, R. E. Refsum's syndrome; heredopathia atactia polyneuritiformis; a report of three cases, including a study of the cardiac pathology. Brain, 82:41, 1959.
Jacob, J. C., Andermann, F., and Robb, J. P. Heredofamilial neuritis with brachial predilection. Neurology, 11:1025, 1961.
Khalifeh, R. R., and Zellweger, H. Hereditary sensory neuropathy with spinal cord disease. Neurology, 13: 405, 1963.
Schwartz, G. A., and Liu, C. N. Hereditary (familial) spastic paraplegia; further clinical and pathological observations. Arch. Neurol. Psychiat., 75:144, 1956.
Schwartz, J. F., Rowland, L. P., Eder, H., Marks, P. A., Osserman, E. F., Hirschberg, E., and Anderson, H. Bassen-Kornzweig syndrome: Deficiency of serum β-lipoprotein. Arch. Neurol., 8:438, 1963.
Thilenius, O. G., and Grossman, B. J. Friedreich's ataxia with heart disease in children. Pediatrics, 27:246, 1961.

BRAINSTEM AND SPINAL CORD DEGENERATIONS

Brandt, S. Werdnig-Hoffmann's Infantile Progressive Muscular Atrophy. Copenhagen, E. Munksgaard, 1950.
Dubowitz, V. The Floppy Infant. Clinics in Developmental Medicine No. 31. London, Spastics International Medical Publications, 1969.
Gomez, M. R., Clermont, V., and Bernstein, J. Progressive bulbar paralysis in childhood (Fazio-Londes' disease). Arch. Neurol., 6:317, 1962.
Fenechel, G. M. The Spinal Muscular Atrophies in Motor Neuron Diseases. Norris, F. H. J., and Kurland, Lt., eds. New York, Grune & Stratton, 1969.
Green, J. B. Familial amyotrophic lateral sclerosis occurring in four generations. Neurology, 10:960, 1960.
Merritt, H. H. Hereditary optic atrophy (Lebei's disease). Arch. Neurol. Psychiat., 24:775, 1930.
Plott, D. M. Congenital laryngeal abductor paralysis due to nucleus ambiguus degeneration of the retina and ataxia neuropathy: A genetically determined syndrome with associated metabolic disorder. Blood, 16:1586, 1960.
Klenk, E., and Kahlke, W. Uber das Vorkommen der 3, 7, 11, 15-Tetramethylhexadecansaure (Phytan saure) in den Cholesterinestern and anderen Lipoidfraktionen der Organe bei einem Krankheitsfall unbekannter Genese (Verdacht auf Heredopathia atactica polyneuritiformia). Z. Physiol. Chem., 333:133, 1963.
Kugelberg. E., and Welander, L. Heredo familial juvenile muscular atrophy simulating muscular dystrophy. Arch. Neurol., 75:500, 1956.
Magee, K. R. Congenital indifference to pain. Arch. Neurol., 9:635, 1963.
Ogden, T. E., Robert, F., and Carmichael, E. A. Some sensory syndromes in children: indifference to pain and sensory neuropathy. J. Neurol. Neurosurg. Psychiat., 22:267, 1959.
Refsum, S. Heredopathia atactica polyneuritiformis reconsideracion. World Neurol., 1:334, 1960.
——— Salmonsen, L., and Skatvedt, M. Heredopathia atactica polyneuritiformis in children. J. Pediat., 35: 335, 1949.
Richterich, R., van Mechelen, P., and Rossi, E. Refsum's disease (heredopathia atactica polyneuritiformis): An inborn error of lipid metabolism with storage of 3, 7, 11, 15-tetramethyl hexadecanoic acid. Amer. J. Med., 39:230, 1965.
Schwartz, A. R. Charcot-Marie-Tooth disease. Arch. Neurol., 9:623, 1963.
Steinberg, D., Mize, C., and Herndon, J. Phytanic acid in patients with Refsum's syndrome and response to dietary treatment. Arch. Intern. Med., 125:75, 1970.
Taylor, R. A. Heredofamilial mononeuritis multiplex with brachial predilection. Brain, 83:113, 1960.

NEUROCUTANEOUS SYNDROMES

Alexander, G. L., and Norman, R. M. The Sturge-Weber Syndrome. Bristol, John Wright & Sons, Ltd., 1960.

Blassingille, B., Sr. A rare form of ectodermal dysplasia. Mental retardation, congenital skin disorder and congenital spastic disorder. Neurology, 9:384, 1959.

Bowen, R. Hereditary ectodermal dysplasia of the anhidrotic type. Southern Med. J., 50:1018, 1957.

Burke, E. C., Winkelmann, R. K., and Strickland, M. K. Disseminated hemangiomatosis. Amer. J. Dis. Child., 108:418, 1964.

Chao, D. H. C. Congenital neurocutaneous syndromes in childhood. I. Neurofibromatosis. J. Pediat., 55:189, 1959.

——— Congenital neurocutaneous syndromes in childhood. II. Tuberous sclerosis. J. Pediat., 55:447, 1959.

——— Congenital neurocutaneous syndromes in childhood. III. Sturge-Weber disease. J. Pediat., 55:635, 1959.

Critchley, M., and Earl, C. J. C. Tuberous sclerosis and allied conditions. Brain, 55:311, 1932.

Crowe, F. W., Schull, W. J., and Neel, J. V. A Clinical, Pathological and Genetic Study of Multiple Neurofibromatosis. Springfield, Ill., Charles C Thomas, Publ., 1956.

Davidson. K. C. Cranial and intracranial lesions in neurofibromatosis. Amer. J. Roentgen., 98:550, 1966.

Feurstein, R. C., and Mims, L. C. Linear nevus sebaceus with convulsions and mental retardation. Amer. J. Dis. Child., 104:675, 1962.

Gold, A. P., and Freeman, J. M. Depigmented nevi: the earliest sign of tuberous sclerosis. Pediatrics, 35: 1003, 1965.

Gunther, M., and Penrose, L. S. Genetics of epiloia. J. Genet., 31:413, 1935.

Gutmann, L., and Lemli, L. Ataxia-telangiectasia associated with hypogammaglobulinemia. Arch. Neurol., 8:318, 1963.

Hartwell, S. W., Pickrell, K., and Quinn, G. Congenital anhidrotic ectodermal dysplasia. Clin. Pediat., 4:383, 1965.

Hilal, S. K., Solomon, G. E., Gold, A. P., and Carter, S. Primary cerebral arterial occlusive disease in children. Part II: Neurocutaneous syndromes. Radiology, 99:87, 1971.

Howell, J. B., Anderson, D. E., and McClendon, J. L. The basal cell nevus syndrome. J.A.M.A., 190:274, 1964.

Kofman, O., and Hyland, H. H. Tuberous sclerosis in adults with normal intelligence. Arch. Neurol. Psychiat., 81:43, 1959.

Kuster, F., and Olbing, H. Incontinentia pigmenti. Report on nine cases in one family and on one necropsy investigation. Ann. Paediat. (Basel), 202:92, 1964.

McPherson, A., and Auth, T. L. Bloch-Sulzberger syndrome (incontinentia pigmenti). Arch. Neurol., 8:332, 1963.

Meszaros, W. T., Guzzo, F., and Schorsch, H. Neurofibromatosis. Amer. J. Roentgen., 98:557, 1966.

Paine, R. S., and Efron, M. L. Atypical variants of the "ataxia telangiectasia" syndrome. Develop. Med. Child. Neurol., 5:14, 1963.

Paulson, G. W., and Lyle, C. B. Tuberous sclerosis. Develop. Med. Child. Neurol., 8:571, 1966.

Peterson, R. D. A., Kelley, W. D., and Good, R. A. Ataxia-telangiectasia, its association with a defective thymus, immunological deficiency disease and malignancy. Lancet, 1:1189, 1964.

Pollard, J. J., and New, P. F. J. Hereditary cutaneomandibular polyoncosis. A syndrome of myriad basal-cell nevi of the skin, mandibular cysts, and inconstant skeletal anomalies. Radiology, 82:840, 1964.

Riley, H. D., Jr., and Smith, W. R. Macrocephaly, pseudopapilledema and multiple hemangiomata: previously undescribed heredo-familial syndrome. Pediatrics, 26:293, 1960.

Rosenthal, I. R., Markowitz, A. S., and Medenis, R. Immunologic incompetence in ataxia-telangiectasia. Amer. J. Dis. Child., 110:69, 1965.

Sedgwick, R. P., and Boder, E. Progressive ataxia in children with particular reference to ataxia telangiectasia. Neurology, 10:705, 1960.

Solitare, G. B., and Lopez, V. F. Louis-Bar's syndrome (ataxia-telangiectasia). Neurology, 17:23, 1967.

Thibault, J. W., and Manuelidis, E. E. Tuberous sclerosis in a premature infant: Report of a case and review of the literature. Neurology, 20:139, 1970.

Van Bogaert, L. Pathologie des angiomatoses. Acta Neurol. Psychiat. Belg., 50:526, 1950.

Warin, R. P., and Walske, M. M. Juvenile acanthosis nigricans in twins with neurological changes including spastic paraparesis. Proc. Roy. Soc. Med., 56:303, 1963.

Weber, F. P. Hemangiectatic hypertrophy of limbs, congenital plebarteriectasis and so-called congenital varicose veins. Brit. J. Child. Dis., 25:13, 1918.

Wilcox, J. C. Melanomatosis of the skin and central nervous system in infants. A congenital neurocutaneous syndrome. Amer. J. Dis. Child., 57:391, 1939.

Chapter 5
TUMORS OF THE CENTRAL NERVOUS SYSTEM

ABE M. CHUTORIAN

Brain Tumors

Brain tumors are surpassed in incidence only by leukemia as a cause of neoplasia in children. Exceedingly rare in the first year of life, the frequency of their occurrence remains fairly constant during each succeeding year. Some series indicate a significantly higher occurrence rate of medulloblastomas and ependymomas in boys than in girls, but otherwise there are no striking differences in sex incidence.

Important differences exist between children and adults as regards both the type and location of the tumors. Gliomas account for 75 percent of intracranial neoplasms in children, compared with 45 percent in adults. In children, 50 to 60 percent of brain tumors are infratentorial (cerebellar, fourth ventricular, and brainstem), whereas in adults they are chiefly supratentorial. Finally, 75 percent or more of brain tumors in children occur in the midline (third and fourth ventricle, optic chiasm, and brainstem). Many of the differences are accounted for by the high incidence of astrocytomas and medulloblastomas in children. The former arise predominantly, and the latter almost exclusively, in the posterior fossa. These differences are further accentuated by the fact that craniopharyngiomas and optic gliomas mostly affect children, whereas meningiomas, pituitary adenomas, acoustic neurinomas, and metastatic tumors occur chiefly in adults.

Many intracranial neoplasms in children can only be treated palliatively. It is also frequently impossible to differentiate on clinical grounds, or even following contrast radiographic studies, between those which can and those which cannot be totally extirpated. Furthermore, many relatively slowly growing neoplasms which cannot be totally removed may be associated with prolonged survival in the absence of severe neurologic deficit. For these reasons, specific diagnosis and appropriate treatment are eminently worthwhile.

CLINICAL MANIFESTATIONS. When a child presents with manifestations of increased intracranial pressure plus focal neurologic deficit, the possibility of brain tumor should be given serious consideration. In the following discussion of symptoms and signs an attempt is made to emphasize early factors that should alert the physician to suspect a cerebral neoplasm. Early diagnosis can often lead to effective therapy and a good prognosis.

Increased Intracranial Pressure. The classical symptoms and signs of increased intracranial pressure are headache, vomiting, diplopia, papilledema, enlarged cranium, and, late in the course, lethargy and somnolence.

Headache. Headache in children is rarely of localizing value, and furthermore there is frequently nothing to distinguish the character of the headache associated with brain tumor from that encountered in other illnesses. Perhaps the most important clinical feature is that the headache associated with tumor tends to remit and exacerbate. Presumably the remissions are associated with transient accommodation of increased intracranial pressure by ventricular dilation or spread of cranial sutures, with or without increased girth of the cranial vault. Thus at one or more points in the course of the illness, headache will be absent for variable and often considerable periods of time.

An intermittent headache, which recurs with increasing frequency and severity, which occurs after a prolonged period of recumbency, at night or on arising in the morning, and which is exacerbated by coughing or straining at stool, should arouse suspicion of increased intracranial pressure. Manifestations of these phenomena in younger or relatively inarticulate children may simply be marked irritability or even constipation due to reluctance to strain at stool.

With rare exceptions, headache tends to occur frontally or occipitally but is not of localizing value; it is seen with equal frequency in supratentorial and infratentorial tumors.

Cranial enlargement. When neoplasms arising in midline structures begin their growth early in life, obstructive hydrocephalus will occur; it cannot be readily differentiated from hydrocephalus due to other causes, such as aqueductal stenosis. Such midline tumors are usually in the posterior fossa.

Vomiting. Vomiting due to increased intracranial pressure is variable and intermittent in character and tends to occur on arising; it may or may not be associated with a headache. It may be an irritative phenomenon in the absence of increased intracranial pressure early in the course of posterior fossa neoplasms. In such instances it may be difficult to delineate the cause of the vomiting, but its recurrent nature should suggest an intracranial cause.

Diplopia and strabismus. Double vision is the result of a sixth nerve palsy. This is a nonspecific finding of increased intracranial pressure and does not have localizing value. Diplopia may not be apparent despite the presence of paralytic strabismus, the chief reason being the rapidity with which suppression of binocular vision occurs by central or peripheral mechanisms in children. Hence, it is more common for a parent to report a tendency on the part of the child to tilt the head to one side or to turn the head laterally to view objects near the central field of vision in compensation for some degree of abducens paresis and associated internal strabismus. Another mechanism of suppression of binocular vision involves partial closure of one eye, which may be interpretated as involuntary ptosis until each eye is examined separately while the other is covered.

Papilledema. Although choking of the discs may or may not be present with increased intracranial pressure, it may be the only sign that intracranial pressure is elevated. It is, therefore, especially important to obtain adequate visualization of the fundi in the presence of unexplained vomiting and headache. This examination is often difficult in uncooperative younger children, in whom sedation and dilation of the pupils will often be necessary.

It is unusual in children for optic atrophy to occur as a result of increased intracranial pressure early in the course of neoplasms arising distant from the optic chiasm. Optic atrophy may be the result of direct chiasmatic compression or infiltration (e.g., craniopharyngioma, chiasmal glioma) or the result of chronic increased intracranial pressure, where gliosis of the optic nerve prevents the development of edema.

The differentiation of papilledema from pseudopapilledema and papillitis (optic neuritis) is of diagnostic importance. In pseudopapilledema the blind spot may be normal in size, and it is usually possible to detect frank or buried drusen at some point along the disc margin. In papillitis, there is acute loss of vision and pain on ocular movement with central or paracentral scotomas on visual field plots.

Focal Neurologic Signs. Brain tumors may produce focal neurologic signs of localizing significance with or without manifestations of increased intracranial pressure.

Nystagmus. Nystagmus on fixation of gaze within the range of binocular vision is of particular importance in connection with intracranial neoplasms. However, its localizing value is limited, for either irritative or destructive lesions involving cerebellovestibular pathways in the same location may produce nystagmus whose quick and slow components are in the opposite direction. Furthermore, unilateral cerebellar hemisphere lesions may produce bilateral manifestations by virtue of compression across the midline, while lesions located entirely within the brainstem may produce nystagmus which is indistinguishable from that due to cerebellar lesions. If there are coarse movements on deviation of the eyes in one direction and fine rapid nystagmus, or none, on gaze in the opposite direction, the lesion is very apt to be on the side to which coarse nystagmus occurs.

Nystagmus may occur simply on the basis of increased intracranial pressure; it is also produced by many drugs, including phenobarbital and Dilantin. The presence of true vertigo in association with nystagmus indicates peripheral labyrinthine disturbance; in children it is rarely associated with neoplasia.

Pendular nystagmus on forward gaze with marked visual deficit occurs, as a rule, in the first two years of life and may be associated with peripheral or cortical blindness, congenital optic atrophy, or tumors in the chiasmatic region. It is also seen as a congenital phenomenon, in which case it may be unilateral or bilateral, without defective vision.

Vertical nystagmus implies intrinsic brainstem disease but may be produced by lesions causing brainstem compression. It may also occur as a drug-induced phenomenon.

A paretic ocular muscle may undergo nystagmoid movements when moving the globe in the direction of its major action.

Opticokinetic nystagmus is a normal phenomenon encountered in following a moving object such as a rotating drum. Diminution or absence of this phenomenon in one direction implies a lesion of the contralateral parietal lobe and hence is frequently, but not always, associated with hemianopia.

Impaired vision. The visual fields and acuity of young children are notoriously difficult to measure accurately. It is, therefore, mandatory for the physician to pursue vigorously the diagnostic evaluation of visual deficit in a child. Unless there is clearly full refractive correction of defective vision —and this is rarely documented in younger children —the possibility of a lesion within or in the neighborhood of the optic nerves, chiasm, tracts, or radiations must be kept in mind. For reasons that are not entirely clear, fully one-third of children with optic gliomas, and not infrequently children with craniopharyngiomas, have their visual deficit at least partially corrected with lenses for a variable period prior to diagnosis.

Visual field defects, generally bitemporal hemianopia, may be seen in optic atrophy without neoplasia but more often are a reflection of chiasmal compression by craniopharyngioma, chiasmal glioma, teratoma, or other tumors of the chiasmal area. Homonymous defects in the visual field may be seen with any lesion involving the optic pathways behind the chiasm.

Cranial neuropathy. Cranial nerve involvement occurs as one of the first symptoms in 20 to 25 percent of children with brain tumor. Abducens paresis may be expected if intracranial pressure is increased; it is of no localizing value.

Supranuclear palsies are manifested chiefly by involvement of facial musculature, the tongue, or as pseudobulbar palsies. In a supranuclear facial paresis, the muscles of the forehead are spared, and orbicularis oculi muscles are *relatively* intact. Supranuclear lesions involving pathways to the hypoglossal nuclei result in weakness of the tongue with deviation to the contralateral side, but the atrophy and fasciculations characteristic of a nuclear lesion are absent. In pseudobulbar palsy, although swallowing and handling of secretions may be significantly impaired, the gag reflex and movements of the uvula are fully intact, differentiating this from bulbar palsy, where the reflex arc is impaired.

Nuclear palsies (e.g., bulbar palsy) occur as a result of brainstem tumors, in which case multiple cranial nerves are usually involved. Differentiation from intrinsic cranial neuropathies encountered in poliomyelitis, polyneuritis, meningitis, and other conditions such as myasthenia gravis and Möbius' syndrome does not, as a rule, present any difficulty. In brainstem gliomas, the pyramidal tracts and cerebellar outflow pathways are almost invariably involved, giving rise to a characteristic complex of symptoms and signs which will be discussed more fully in a later section (p. 96).

The cranial nerves may be involved in infranuclear palsy anywhere along their course within the brainstem or along the base of the brain to their respective destinations. Nasopharyngeal carcinomas, chondrosarcomas, rhabdomyosarcoma, lymphosarcomas, and chordomas are the neoplasms which characteristically involve multiple cranial nerves successively in their extramedullary course. They do not commonly have sufficient bulk early in their course to produce other signs and symptoms by compression of the base of the brain or brainstem.

Head tilt (Fig. 44). Abnormal posturing of the head is seen in association with extraocular muscle paresis, particularly of the superior oblique muscle, in which case it serves as a compensatory mechanism for the production of optimal binocular vision.

Lesions of the pathway from the flocculonodular lobe of the cerebellum to the vestibular nuclei are apt to produce head tilt, with the occiput tilted toward the side of the lesion. However, nuchal rigidity with some degree of head tilt occurs in association with posterior fossa neoplasms as a result of either traction upon the dura and lower cranial nerves or displacement of the cerebellar tonsils. In the latter instance, the head tilt is not of localizing value. It is well to remember that posterior fossa tumors abutting on the ventricular or subarachnoid spaces may produce cerebrospinal fluid pleocytosis and an elevated

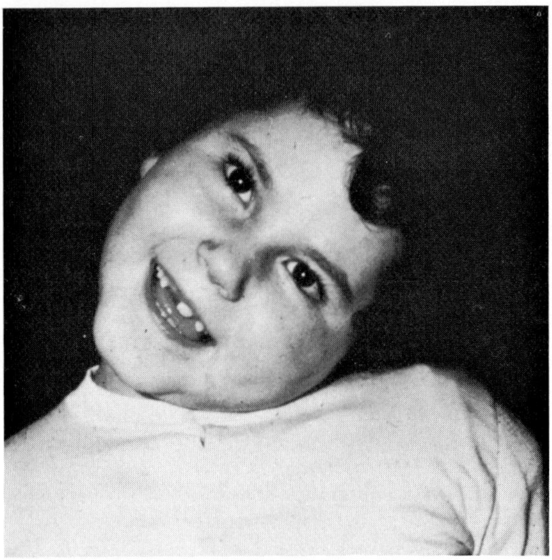

Fig. 44. Extreme head tilt in a girl with a posterior fossa tumor.

protein content, which in association with nuchal rigidity may lead to a diagnosis of meningitis. The normal sugar and bacteriologic studies will militate against this diagnosis, but on occasion the difficulty of diagnosis is compounded by the presence of low-grade fever and, in the case of extensive subarachnoid seeding of a tumor, such as medulloblastoma, by a fall in the cerebrospinal fluid sugar.

Personality change. Personality change is hardly to be considered specific to intracranial neoplasia. However, nonspecific changes such as irritability, apathy, emotional lability, pallor, and fatigue may be early symptoms of brain tumor in children. Their presence should alert the physician to the possibility of such a lesion.

Ataxia. Incoordination of the axial musculature is frequently referred to as titubation. Ataxia caused by cerebellar neoplasm involves the axial musculature when the tumor is vermian or midline. Cerebellar hemisphere tumors produce ataxia in the ipsilateral extremities. False localization is not uncommon because of contrecoup effects or simultaneous involvement of the midline and hemispheral structures.

Ataxia is a common manifestation of brainstem gliomas due to involvement of the cerebellar pathways. The unsteadiness in such instances may be axial and/or of the extremities.

Ataxia by itself is not a valuable localizing sign. It may be seen in aqueductal insufficiency, presumably as a result of transmission of increased intracranial pressure to cerebellar pathways anywhere from the frontal lobes to the brainstem. Unilateral incoordination may result from a frontal lobe, thalamic, or cerebellar hemisphere neoplasm, and it may not be possible on clinical grounds to ascertain the source.

Ataxia may also be caused by proprioceptive defects produced by peripheral nerve, root, or posterior column lesions. In this instance, the ataxia is aggravated by eye closure.

Other causes of ataxia include degenerative, metabolic, and infectious or parainfectious central nervous system disorders. The latter include "acute cerebellar ataxia," characterized by its relatively acute onset, course, and absence of increased intracranial pressure (see p. 8).

Focal pyramidal deficit. Upper motor neuron lesions of a slowly progressive type are usually first manifested in children by subtle changes of handedness, posture, and dexterity which are not a source of distress and therefore are often overlooked until the appearance of frank paralysis or marked spasticity. Examination usually reveals a combination of increased deep tendon reflexes, altered superficial reflexes, and Babinski or other pathologic reflexes, and some degree of spasticity. Frank weakness may or may not be manifest, but a tendency to disuse or abnormal postures of the suspected extremity often occur.

The chronicity of a lesion or its acute onset will help differentiate "congenital," vascular, traumatic, and toxic lesions from neoplastic causes. Since pyramidal deficit implies a cerebral, brainstem, or spinal cord lesion, the presence of parietal lobe phenomena is helpful in ascertaining the site of the lesion. If the child is old enough to cooperate, testing for corticosensory discriminations, visual field defects (hemianopia), and opticokinetic nystagmus may be helpful.

Although pyramidal tract deficit is rare in association with cerebellar tumors or neoplasms in the chiasmatic area, it is encountered occasionally when there is brainstem compression and/or infiltration.

Seizures. Generalized, psychomotor, and focal motor or sensory seizures may be the initial symptom of cerebral hemisphere neoplasms in children. In some instances, the seizures persist for years before the diagnosis becomes evident. Seizures in the pediatric age group are more likely the result of static lesions or metabolic factors. For this reason selective criteria must be adopted to rule out or establish the presence of a cerebral neoplasm in an individual case.

Seizures are considered an unusual manifestation of posterior fossa tumors. Ictus infratentorialis refers to the intermittent decerebrate posture observed in some children with posterior fossa neoplasms or other lesions. It is perhaps not a true convulsive phenomenon, though its exact nature is not fully established. The best evidence currently is that such episodes are due to interruption of vermian or anterior lobe cerebellar stimuli to reticular nuclei. When the episodes are accompanied by cyanosis, respiratory irregularity, and alteration of consciousness, impending cerebellar herniation through the foramen magnum may be suspected. The occurrence of convulsions in children with medulloblastoma is most readily explained by the presence of cerebral hemisphere tumor implants.

At times the only explanation available is that cortical irritability is increased by the presence of increased intracranial pressure or cerebral edema.

Hypothalamic and Endocrine Dysfunction. Tumors giving rise to disturbances of hypothalamic and endocrine function include craniopharyngiomas, optic and other gliomas, anterior third ventricular dermoids, teratomas, and ectopic or "metastatic" pinealomas. Peculiarly, the manifestations differ very significantly among the different tumor types, despite the large bulk and apparently similar compressive effects of the different lesions. Thus, the occurrence of sexual and somatic infantilism is the rule in craniopharyngioma, whereas in chiasmal glioma, sexual change is uncommon. Any sexual abnormality in chiasmal glioma is apt to involve sexual precocity, the same being true also of pineal tumors and teratomas.

The diencephalic syndrome of infancy is characterized by emaciation and recurrent vomiting in a euphoric, alert baby. The lesion is usually an astrocytoma arising in the anterior third ventricle. The syndrome characteristically occurs before the tumor has produced macrocephaly or other manifestations of raised intracranial pressure.

All tumors occurring in the hypothalamic region share the propensity to produce early and progressive optic atrophy due to involvement of the optic chiasm.

DIAGNOSTIC PROCEDURES. Ancillary procedures of value in the diagnosis of brain tumors include:

1. Skull radiography
2. Electroencephalography
3. Echoencephalography
4. Radioisotopic brain scanning
5. Cerebrospinal fluid analysis
    a. Pressure, cells, protein, sugar
    b. Enzymes
    c. Millipore filtration for identification of tumor cells
6. Intracranial contrast radiography
    a. Pneumoencephalography
    b. Ventriculography
    c. Cerebral angiography

The various procedures will be discussed with specific reference to the diagnosis of different tumors.

TREATMENT. Specific therapy includes surgery, roentgen therapy, chemotherapy, and drugs employed to reduce increased intracranial pressure. Surgical and roentgen therapy are discussed separately for individual tumors.

Chemotherapy remains a palliative procedure of limited value in the treatment of intracranial tumors in children. Current experimentation with the use of intracarotid or intrathecal chemotherapy is not of sufficiently established value to be routinely recommended. However, various investigators have reported chemotherapeutic remissions of variable duration with the use of sequential intravenous vincristine therapy or intrathecal methotrexate. The chief indication for such treatment at the present time is clinical relapse following maximum permissible surgery and radiotherapy for glioblastoma, ependymoma, and medulloblastoma. The *prophylactic* potential of chemotherapy has not been reliably explored.

The use of adrenocortical steroids for the relief of increased intracranial pressure in children with brain tumor is recommended in selected cases. Dramatic results are sometimes obtained, and symptoms of increased intracranial pressure associated with cerebral edema are improved in the majority of patients. Variable but significant improvement of focal neurologic deficit has also been observed. The most frequent indication for the use of adrenocortical steroids is the occurrence of signs and symptoms of increased intracranial pressure during a course of roentgen therapy, when decompressive surgery either has already been performed or, for various reasons, is being avoided.

In older children, dexamethasone, 4 to 8 mg intravenously, may be given, followed with 2 mg intramuscularly four times daily for several days. Under ordinary circumstances, attempts to taper and discontinue the drug over a period of one to two weeks should be made. Corticosteroid therapy is of value postsurgically as well as preoperatively in selected cases. Patients who develop a *sterile* meningitis, often accompanied by a significant febrile reaction, following either posterior fossa surgery or the communication of a cystic lesion with the ventricular or subarachnoid space, may show striking remission of cerebrospinal fluid pleocytosis, hypoglycorrhea, fever, and meningeal signs after corticosteroid administration. Needless to say, bacterial infection should be ruled out prior to such therapy.

The value of steroid therapy in patients with neoplasms of the posterior fossa must be weighed against the increased risk of intestinal ulceration in these children.

In more acute situations demanding urgent treatment of increased intracranial pressure, parenteral urea or mannitol should be used and may be lifesaving. The combined use of dexamethasone and mannitol tends to prevent "rebound" of pressure which is characteristic following urea, and to a lesser extent mannitol.

Tumors of the Cerebellum

Astrocytoma

INCIDENCE. Approximately 25 percent of all brain tumors in children are cerebellar astrocytomas. The peak age incidence is 5 to 8 years, but no age group is excepted.

CLINICAL MANIFESTATIONS. Symptoms and signs in this group are not distinctive enough to differentiate them accurately from other posterior fossa neoplasms. They include:

1. Signs and symptoms of increased intracranial pressure, including headache, vomiting, abducens paresis, and papilledema
2. Ataxia, predominating in or confined to one side in the case of a cerebellar hemisphere astrocytoma
3. Nystagmus, sometimes of localizing value
4. Head tilt

Within this symptom complex there is considerable variation. Thus in some, a cystic astrocytoma confined to one hemisphere may produce ipsilateral intention tremor and ataxia before any other phenomena become evident, while in others it may result in signs of impending herniation of the cerebellar tonsils, with pyramidal deficit added as a result of brainstem compression, and possible impairment of vision due to chronic papilledema.

The course of cerebellar astrocytoma in children is insidious in onset, slow in progression, and relatively benign in outlook. The variation in duration of symptoms is, however, great enough to make this picture an unreliable criterion of the diagnosis. The majority have symptoms for two to seven months prior to diagnosis, some for as long as several years, contrasting sharply with medulloblastoma, where the majority are symptomatic less than two months prior to diagnosis.

DIAGNOSIS. Papilledema and spread of the cranial sutures on radiograms of the skull are common findings. Tumor calcification is rare. Occasionally local occipital rarefaction of bone or enlargement of the opening which admits the occipital emissary vein will suggest the presence of a slowly growing cerebellar astrocytoma.

Ventriculography will establish more precisely the location of the tumor but not the precise tumor type, which is established at the time of suboccipital craniotomy.

Brachial and vertebral angiography, which provide information concerning the posterior fossa circulation, have assumed a limited, but growing, value in the diagnosis of posterior fossa mass lesions. These studies are most helpful in patients whose cerebellar deficit is so minimal that doubt exists in relation to the location of the neoplasm. The advantage provided by such study is the absence of disturbance of cerebrospinal fluid dynamics while diagnostic information is obtained. These studies are not routinely required.

Radioisotope brain scanning generally tends to be unreliable for the localization of posterior fossa tumors because of the high uptake of isotope by the occipitocervical musculature and the lateral sinuses.

THERAPY AND PROGNOSIS. In approximately one-third of the cases, the tumor is located entirely within one cerebellar hemisphere. These tumors are apt to be cystic, the cysts being quite large in relation to the solid portion of the tumor, which may consist of a small mural nodule in the wall of the cyst. In other cases, solid tumor tissue surrounds a cyst. Surgical extirpation of these tumors is eminently successful, and many patients have been cured by total surgical removal of the tumor. In some instances in which the solid portion of the tumor predominates, "gross total" removal may be accomplished, but the fate of the patient may not be determined for many years because of the slowly growing character of these neoplasms.

The solid, midline astrocytomas tend to extend deeply toward cerebellar peduncles, aqueduct of Sylvius, and brainstem. The surgical results are, therefore, far less satisfactory than with the cystic tumors, but years of freedom from symptoms may follow decompression and partial extirpation of these more solid midline tumors. Partly because of their inherently slow growth and protracted course there is no proof that the growth of these tumors is altered by radiotherapy, which is therefore frequently withheld, especially following removal of a cystic cerebellar hemisphere astrocytoma. However, there is definite evidence that radiotherapy does affect astrocytomas of the brainstem and of the optic nerve and chiasm, which are similar histologically to many cerebellar astrocytomas. Furthermore, of 150 patients with cerebellar astrocytoma treated at Columbia-Presbyterian Medical Center, 93 had subtotal tumor excision and irradiation, with an average interval of seven years to the time of tumor recurrence. This compares favorably with other series, in which subtotal removal has not been followed by radiotherapy and the average interval to tumor recurrence is cited as three years. We therefore recommend radiotherapy for patients in whom it is believed tumor tissue has been left behind following surgery.

Postoperatively intravenous fluids are rarely required after 24 to 48 hours, but during this period it is best to use physiologic solutions to provide the usual maintenance requirements of water and electrolytes. Reduction of water and electrolytes postoperatively, as frequently advocated, is not believed necessary; in fact, it may prolong the postoperative recovery period.

Following removal of a cerebellar astrocytoma, the cerebellar deficit is characteristically aggravated, and ataxia and tremor are more pronounced. There is progressive improvement in these symptoms over weeks to months following surgery, and persistent symptoms are rarely disabling. The degree of residual deficit is variable; often it cannot be discerned without careful neurologic examination. Postoperative hydrocephalus secondary to aseptic inflammatory changes in the meninges is not infrequently encountered.

Medulloblastoma

INCIDENCE. Of the posterior fossa tumors in children, medulloblastoma is the most frequent, comprising approximately 40 percent. There is a tendency for males to outnumber females in the ratio of about 3 to 2. The peak age incidence is approximately 3 to 5 years.

CLINICAL MANIFESTATIONS. The symptoms and signs of medulloblastoma are similar to those described for cerebellar astrocytoma. However, the onset is typically more acute, and despite the short history the complete picture of an advanced posterior fossa neoplasm is more apt to be encountered. The signs will be more characteristic of a midline cerebellar neoplasm (i.e., early obstructive hydrocephalus and prominent ataxia of axial musculature). Seizures are not common in medulloblastomas, their occurrence reflecting cerebral implantation of tumor. Similarly, in advanced cases with extensive seeding of a tumor along the subarachnoid space, the picture of a polyneuropathy may supervene, with loss of tendon reflexes, root pain, paresthesias, and cranial nerve involvement. The course is rapid and the outlook for long-term survival generally poor.

DIAGNOSIS. As in cerebellar astrocytoma, the majority of plain radiograms of the skull will show cranial suture spread or other x-ray evidence of increased intracranial pressure. Ventriculograms rarely admit air into the fourth ventricle because of frequent obstruction of the rostral end of this cavity, with the production of symmetrically dilated lateral and third ventricles. At times, air will enter a massively dilated fourth ventricle which is largely occupied by tumor.

The indications for angiography and the limitations of brain scanning are as described for the diagnosis of astrocytomas.

Medulloblastomas tend to shed their actively growing cells and seed them from their site of origin in the roof of the fourth ventricle throughout the subarachnoid space. Tumor implants become a source of further seeding. It is thus possible to make a diagnosis of recurrence or seeding of medulloblastoma in some cases by detecting tumor cells in millipore filtrates of cerebrospinal or ventricular fluid.

THERAPY AND PROGNOSIS. Since medulloblastoma cannot be differentiated with certainty from other cerebellar neoplasms without a tissue diagnosis, all of these patients should have a craniotomy. The tumor is characteristically bulky, and considerable portions must be removed in order to reestablish free flow of cerebrospinal fluid through the fourth ventricle. It is never possible to extirpate the tumor completely by surgical means.

The tumor is highly radiosensitive. Because of the strong proclivity of the neoplasm to seed tumor cells through the neuraxis, radiotherapy is initially routinely directed to the entire neuraxis. In general the outlook for long-term survival is poor. Seventy percent do not live more than three years. Newer techniques in radiation therapy are resulting in longer survivals.

Comments on chemotherapy have been made in the introductory section on treatment (p. 93).

Tumors of the Fourth Ventricle

Ependymoma

INCIDENCE. The third most frequent infratentorial neoplasm in children is the ependymoma. The tumor comprises approximately 10 percent of all posterior fossa tumors in children. Although the size of individual series of patients with ependymomas is not large, there does seem to be a tendency to male preponderance (2:1) and relatively early age of onset. Clinically these tumors resemble the picture of medulloblastoma more than that of astrocytoma. Choroid plexus papillomas and other lateral ventricle ependymomas are far less frequent.

The duration of symptoms is intermediate between that of medulloblastoma and astrocytoma, as is the ultimate outlook for survival. The average duration of symptoms prior to diagnosis is two to three months.

The point of attachment of the tumor is almost always the floor of the fourth ventricle, which is frequently filled with tumor, and early signs and symptoms of obstructive hydrocephalus are to be expected. However, the ependymoma is apt, more than other posterior fossa tumors, to be associated with repeated vomiting as the earliest manifestation, due to direct stimulation of emetic centers underlying the site of origin of the tumor. Apart from this tendency, the tumor on rare occasions arises in one of the lateral recesses of the fourth ventricle and grows out into cerebellopontine angle, producing combined ipsilateral selective cranial nerve involvement and cerebellar signs which in the adult would be more likely to signify the presence of an acoustic neurinoma or cerebellopontine angle meningioma.

The tumor otherwise produces the symptoms and signs described for the other posterior fossa neoplasms, including those associated with increased intracranial pressure, ataxia, nystagmus, and head tilt. On occasion, ependymomas extend intraspinally from the posterior fossa and may even seed to more distant sites in the subarachnoid space, but this tendency is far less marked than in medulloblastoma. Consequently, radiotherapy is not routinely directed to the entire neuraxis.

DIAGNOSIS. As is the case with medulloblastoma and astrocytoma, the majority of children with ependymomas show cranial suture separation and/or other signs of increased intracranial pressure.

Microscopically ependymomas show extensively distributed flecks of calcium, but this is only occasionally of sufficient extent to be of diagnostic help on plain radiograms of the skull.

The diagnosis is more apt to be confused with subacute meningitis than in the case of the other posterior fossa tumors, with the exception of the rare reticulum cell sarcoma, leptomeningeal carcinomatosis, and other similar neoplasms.

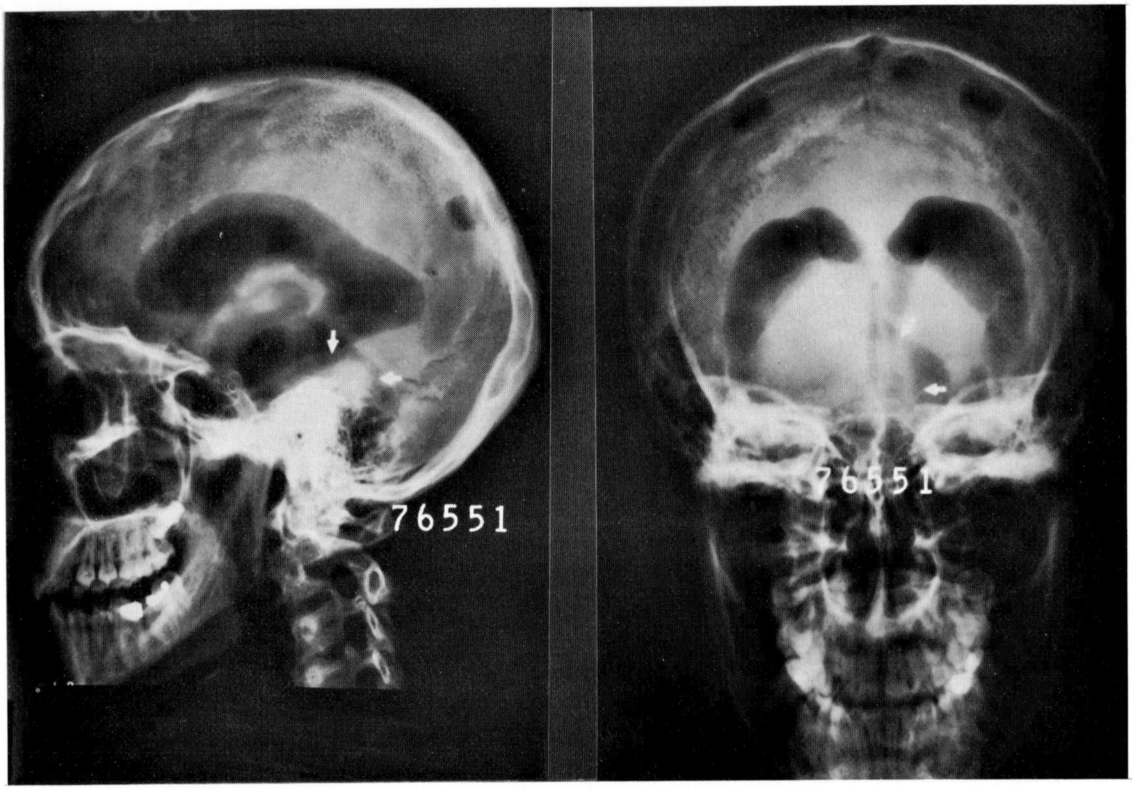

Fig. 45. Ventriculogram of a child outlining the ventricular system and demonstrating a large defect in the fourth ventricle (arrows). The defect and the displacement shown are due to the presence of an ependymoma.

The diagnosis ultimately depends upon the findings at craniotomy following ventriculography (Fig. 45). The indications for angiography and the limitations of brain scanning are as described for the diagnosis of astrocytomas.

THERAPY. Ependymomas are inseparable from vital structures in the floor of the fourth ventricle. Surgery is, therefore, limited to the bulk of the tumor beyond the floor of the ventricle and is aimed chiefly at reestablishing free circulation of the cerebrospinal fluid.

X-ray therapy is directed to the posterior fossa after surgery. Comments on chemotherapy have been made in the introductory section under treatment (p. 93).

PROGNOSIS. The immediate postoperative mortality is not high if the surgeon recognizes the inadvisability of excessive manipulation or extensive dissection because of the attachment of the tumor. In the rare cerebellopontine angle tumor, total excision is theoretically possible but even then is not ordinarily achieved.

Survival beyond the postoperative period is variable and is generally intermediate in duration between the rapidly advancing medulloblastoma and very slowly growing astrocytoma. Survival thus varies from several months to 10 years or longer, usually lasting several years.

Tumors of the Brainstem

Brainstem Gliomas

INCIDENCE. Brainstem gliomas occur almost exclusively in children, though no age group is exempted; they constitute approximately 10 percent of all intracranial tumors in children. The average age of onset is approximately 6½ years. The duration of symptoms is typically 3 to 5 months but may be considerably longer or shorter.

CLINICAL MANIFESTATIONS. This tumor, which presents with one of the most characteristic clinical pictures, is at the same time unfortunately one of the least amenable to effective therapy, except of a transient and palliative nature.

The onset of neurologic symptoms and signs is usually insidious, and increased intracranial pressure is infrequent, except as a late manifestation.

Because of their location, these tumors are apt to interfere early in the course of their growth with the function of cranial nerve nuclei, pyramidal tracts, and cerebellar pathways, giving rise to a characteristic triad of symptoms and signs.

1. Cranial Nerve Nuclei. Early in the clinical course there may be an isolated cranial nerve deficit; later multiple involvement is the rule. Although any cranial nerve nucleus may be affected, the most common are: VII, 90 percent; IX and X, 80 percent; V (sensory), 60 percent; and VI, 55 percent.

Since the tumor (astrocytoma or less often glioblastoma) is infiltrative in nature, "skip lesions" are common, and bilateral involvement of different cranial nerves is the rule.

Paresis of conjugate gaze, the most important sign localizing the lesion within the brainstem, occurs in more than half of the patients.

2. Pyramidal Tracts. Signs of pyramidal tract involvement occur in 80 to 90 percent of the children. Symptomatically, these may be masked by the more prominent ataxic manifestations or may present chiefly as subtle changes in gait, handedness, or posture of an extremity.

Hemiparesis is associated with reflex preponderance, and an extensor plantar response is the usual picture; frequently, however, bilateral reflex changes and rarely weakness of all extremities are seen.

3. Cerebellar Pathways. Both truncal and extremity ataxia are found in the majority of children, indicating involvement chiefly of corticopontocerebellar fibers coursing through the brainstem. Horizontal nystagmus is present in over half of the patients and vertical nystagmus in almost a third.

Other Signs. Occasionally nuchal rigidity and urinary retention occur and confuse the picture. Papilledema occurs at some time during the course in approximately a third of the patients. Sensory deficits occur uncommonly, and basal ganglia manifestations, such as tremor and choreoathetosis, are rare.

DIAGNOSIS. In keeping with the typical absence of symptoms and signs of increased intracranial pressure, the cerebrospinal fluid pressure is normal. Similarly, the cerebrospinal fluid cell count, protein, and sugar are normal. Rarely, growth of the tumor impinging on the leptomeninges will produce a low-grade pleocytosis and elevated cerebrospinal fluid protein.

Plain radiographs of the skull are usually unrewarding. In those instances, therefore, in which intracranial pressure is believed to be normal (the majority), pneumoencephalography is performed. The typical findings in brainstem tumor include posterior and upward displacement of the aqueduct of Sylvius and the fourth ventricle, best seen in the lateral view (Fig. 46). The pontine cistern is, characteristically, narrowed by the increased bulk of the tumor-bearing pons. Ventricular dilation of mild degree is often present but is rarely of striking proportion.

THERAPY. Craniotomy is seldom, if ever, indicated in patients with brainstem gliomas. The typical pneumoencephalographic findings, together with the clinical picture, are sufficiently diagnostic as a rule to justify radiotherapy. In our experience, one or more courses of radiotherapy are associated with an average survival time of 12 months. Almost all the patients manifest significant improvement between 3 and 6 weeks after the onset of therapy, which currently consists of 4,000 r delivered as a single tumor dose over 28 days. Typically, there is incomplete clearing of cranial nerve palsies, pyramidal signs, and ataxic phenomena. In some instances, improvement is quite dramatic, in others only slight. Relapse may be expected in the majority within 6 months. In a very few instances, survival with useful function extends to several years or longer.

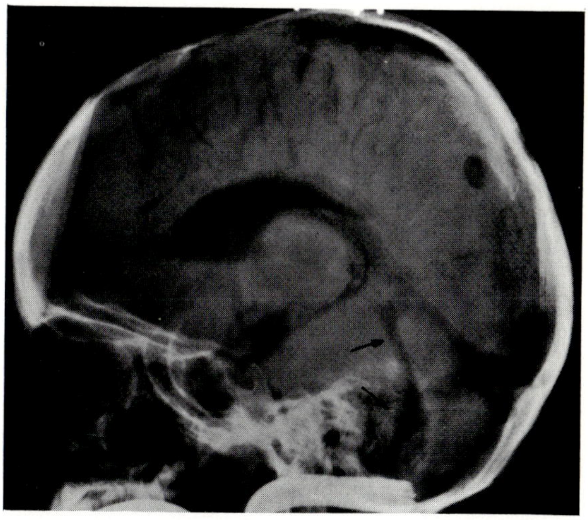

Fig. 46. Pneumoencephalogram of a child with a large tumor of the pons. Posterior displacement and bowing of the aqueduct and fourth ventricle is shown. The distance from the posterior portion of the pituitary fossa to the floor of the fourth ventricle is nearly twice the normal measurement.

Tumors of the Third Ventricle

For the purpose of classification, tumors grouped in this area include pinealomas, colloid cysts, and hypothalamic gliomas. The latter produce the "diencephalic syndrome" of infancy. Suprasellar and chiasmatic tumors, which by virtue of their origin in the region of the anterior portion of the third ventricle may closely mimic signs and symptoms produced by tumors arising within the third ventricle, are discussed separately (p. 102).

Pinealomas

INCIDENCE. These rare tumors, which comprise less than 2 percent of all gliomas, occur chiefly (80 percent) in males; approximately one-third are in children under the age of 15 years. In this group, the average age of onset is 10 to 11 years.

CLINICAL MANIFESTATIONS. The most classical localizing sign of a pinealoma is paralysis of upward gaze (Parinaud syndrome), the first manifestation of which may be bilateral ptosis. This finding is indicative of pressure on the superior colliculi, above which the pineal gland protrudes. The inferior colliculi may also be involved, with the production of bilateral hearing loss. However, these signs have been produced by increased intracranial pressure in the absence of a tumor in the pineal area.

A further distinctive syndrome, produced uncommonly by pineal tumors, is that of macrogenitosomia praecox.

The other neurologic manifestations of pineal tumors are nonspecific. Increased intracranial pressure is produced by early obstruction of the aqueduct of Sylvius, which lies close beneath the colliculi. Ataxia, nystagmus, and nuchal rigidity occur in many of the patients, and pyramidal deficit results from pressure on the long tracts in the brainstem.

DIAGNOSIS. Calcification of the pineal gland, particularly if unusual in character or extensive, is sufficiently uncommon in children to suggest the diagnosis in the presence of the typical clinical picture.

Ventriculography is necessary to demonstrate the extent of the lesion and its effects. It may not be possible by this means to distinguish a pinealoma from tumors of the anterior lobe of the cerebellum or from the unusual vein of Galen malformations which occur in this area. The latter are associated with high-output cardiac failure in infancy, convulsions and psychomotor retardation in childhood, and hydrocephalus in the presence of an intracranial bruit. The diagnosis is established by arteriography.

TREATMENT. The infiltrative nature of pineal tumors precludes surgical removal. Shunting of cerebrospinal fluid, if possible by the Torkildsen procedure, is usually indicated, followed by deep roentgen therapy.

PROGNOSIS. Symptoms may be expected to abate following therapy, with freedom from recurrence averaging two to five years, after which time a second course of radiotherapy may be considered. Occasional patients enjoy many years of freedom from recurrence.

Colloid Cyst

These rare cysts arise, possibly from remnants of the paraphysis, in the anterior part of the third ventricle and produce symptoms by occluding the foramina of Monro. Although most of the patients have been diagnosed in adult life, approximately 50 percent have intermittent symptoms for as long as 10 years or more and have clearly had the onset of symptoms in childhood.

Since occlusion may be constant or intermittent, the symptoms may remit and exacerbate and at times are induced by flexion of the head and neck. Some patients present with unlocalized symptoms and signs of increased intracranial pressure, others have paroxysmal symptoms severe enough to lead to stupor or loss of consciousness, and a few undergo progressive dementia as a result of slowly progressive hydrocephalus.

The characteristic syndrome involves sudden severe headache, vomiting, and stupor, especially in association with changes in position which cause the tumor to occlude completely the foramina of Monro (head and neck flexion).

Endocrine symptoms have not been prominent. Several patients have shown transient glycosuria, especially during acute attacks. Scattered instances of obesity, weight loss, polyuria, polyphagia, and acromegaly have occurred.

Of 11 patients with colloid cysts surgically removed in the series of Cairns and Mosberg, 9 survivors were followed up to 15½ years; all were relieved of their preoperative headache and visual symptoms, with the exception of one with irreversible optic atrophy. Sudden death has occurred in about 20 percent of the patients. Occasionally an asymptomatic colloid cyst of the third ventricle is discovered at autopsy following death from unrelated cause.

Diencephalic Syndrome

The "diencephalic syndrome" is a rare symptoms complex described in young infants usually beginning at 2 to 5 months of age and associated with a glioma of the hypothalamus. The most striking features of the syndrome are the preservation of alertness and the presence of euphoria in the face of marked emaciation.

Emaciation is universal. Unusual alertness, wiry vigor, and hyperkinesias are common but are not necessarily striking in degree. Vomiting is usually present but is frequently of mild degree and does not as a rule account for the virtually total absence of subcutaneous fat. Optic atrophy and associated nystagmus, usually of the combined searching and oscillatory type, are common, as might be expected from the proximity of the tumor to the optic chiasm; these findings may, however, be absent despite advanced symptoms and signs.

Excessive diaphoresis, polyuria, and tremor are variable symptoms. Enlargement of the cranium has occurred but is not the rule. More often the head appears enlarged because of the wasted trunk and extremities. Acute peptic ulceration and gastric hemorrhage have occurred.

The occurrence of emaciation and excessive alertness in infants with hypothalamic tumor, rather than growth retardation, obesity, and other features more commonly associated with neoplasms of this region in older children, is unexplained. Marked emaciation does occur occasionally in older children with hypothalamic tumors and is not necessarily restricted to gliomas.

The diagnosis is confirmed by pneumoencephalography, which, because of the open fontanel, can be safely performed even in the presence of optic atrophy and the unusual instance of suspected hydrocephalus. Plain radiograms of the skull are not apt to be helpful, and the cerebrospinal fluid protein content is usually normal.

Because of the location of the neoplasm, surgical excision is impossible, and only roentgen therapy can be offered. The prognosis for long-term survival is poor, death usually occurring between 10 months and 2 years of age. Exceptional cases show a more striking response to radiotherapy and do well for many years.

Thalamic Tumors

Cerebral tumor is generally not considered in the differential diagnosis of extrapyramidal signs and symptoms in children. However, the existing literature has occasional reference to children with basal ganglia tumors and suggests that a Parkinsonlike syndrome may be produced by tumors involving one or both thalami. The actual frequency of tumors in this location in childhood is greater than the number of reported cases would suggest.

A rhythmic alternating tremor of one extremity is the common finding. Other manifestations include athetosis, torsion spasm, posturing, rigidity, and bradykinesia. More often, however, a thalamic tumor in a child is liable to masquerade as a tumor of either a cerebellar or cerebral hemisphere. Thus, a tremor indistinguishable from that produced by a cerebellar neoplasm or hemiparesis of varying degree may be the earliest or sole manifestation of a thalamic tumor in children. It is peculiar that despite the most profound hemiplegia associated with thalamic tumors in children, sensation may be completely intact even in older children, in whom it may be reliably tested. Signs and symptoms of increased intracranial pressure are frequently present, since the thalami form the major portion of the walls of the third ventricle.

These tumors are mainly astrocytomas and glioblastomas, and because of their inaccessible location the outlook is poor. In occasional instances, a cystic astrocytoma may be treated by partial excision and aspiration of the cyst, followed by radiotherapy, with a surprising number of years of remission.

Tumors of the Cerebral Hemispheres

INCIDENCE. It is generally stated that infratentorial tumors tend to predominate in children. However, experience in some large medical centers, including our own, indicates an approximately equal incidence of supratentorial and infratentorial neoplasms.

In general, approximately one-third of supratentorial tumors in children are gliomas of the cerebral hemispheres. There is no striking difference in the age or sex incidence. Half of the patients fall into the age group between 7 and 11 years.

CLINICAL MANIFESTATIONS. Personality change, a symptom difficult to document statistically with reliability, is probably the most common early manifestation of a cerebral hemisphere tumor in a child. In retrospect, intermittent irritability and/or listlessness virtually always antedate the more specific symptoms and signs which precipitate neurodiagnostic study.

Headache, vomiting, or both occur as early manifestations in 80 or 90 percent of the patients. However, headache without vomiting is much more common than in posterior fossa or midline supratentorial tumors (distal to midline channels of cerebrospinal fluid communication and to medullary vomiting centers). The diagnostic value of this symptom is, of course, related to the child's age and ability to verbalize.

Motor weakness occurs in over one-third of the patients. Focal pyramidal deficit is often demonstrated in the form of spasticity, hyperreflexia, and extensor plantar response in the absence of demonstrable weakness. Motor weakness may reveal itself in subtle fashion by change of handedness, reluctance to use an extremity, or unilateral abnormal posturing of the extremities on walking or performing other routine activities of daily living.

Convulsions are not present in the majority of patients with cerebral hemisphere tumors. Of 112 children with cerebral hemisphere tumors studied at the Columbia-Presbyterian Medical Center, 38 percent had seizures. Half of these children suffered from generalized convulsions. However, the seizures were frequently of mixed types with 80 percent having either focal or psychomotor attacks. Of considerable additional interest is the fact that one-third of this group of children with seizures and cerebral hemisphere tumors had convulsions for 3 to 10 years prior to diagnosis.

Papilledema of florid degree is not usually encountered but is present to some extent in the majority of patients at the time of diagnosis.

Aside from focal pyramidal deficit, other focal signs such as sensory deficit, visual field defects, and aphasic phenomena are rarely encountered, probably because of the large proportion of patients too young to cooperate reliably. The use of devices such as striped cloth or striped rotating drum to detect defects in opticokinetic nystagmus in children with parietal lobe tumors would increase the prevalence of this finding.

False localizing signs, particularly those ascribed to defects in cerebellar pathway function, have been discussed earlier. The findings on neurologic examination in children with cerebral hemisphere tumors are at times so sparse that a midline neoplasm or pseudotumor cerebri is suspected.

DIAGNOSIS. Ancillary studies are especially important for diagnosis in this group of patients because it is usually possible to localize the tumor precisely without resorting to ventriculography. The differential diagnosis includes space-occupying lesions of the hemisphere, such as subdural hematoma or hygroma, brain abscess, and, far less commonly

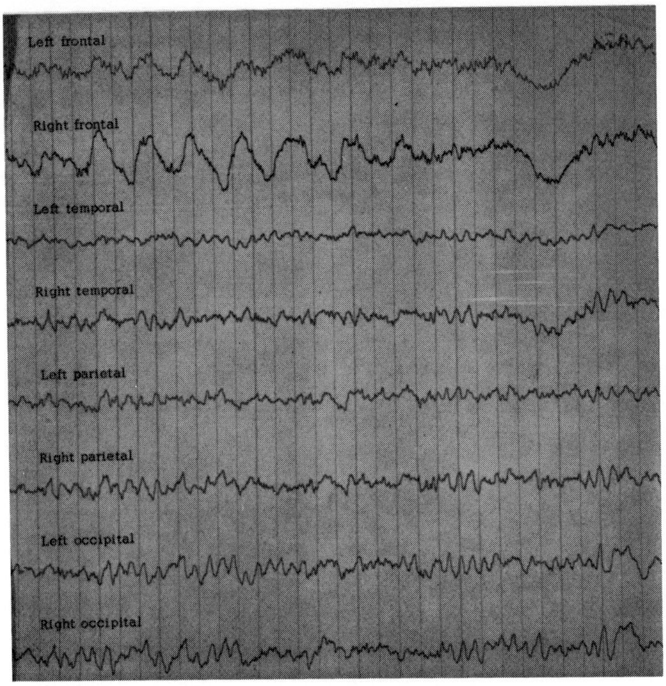

Fig. 47. Electroencephalogram showing a right frontal slow wave focus associated with an underlying astrocytoma.

in this country, parasitic or granulomatous lesions, such as hydatid cyst or tuberculoma. On occasion, an acute or subacute encephalitis, particularly herpes simplex encephalitis, will preferentially involve the temporal lobe to the extent of producing signs and symptoms of an expanding lesion within this structure. On rare occasions, a porencephalic cyst communicates with the subarachnoid space in ball-valve fashion so that a subarachnoid collection of fluid accumulates progressively and acts as a mass lesion.

In contradistinction to midline or posterior fossa neoplasms where the findings are nonspecific, consisting usually of generalized dysrhythmia which is maximal in the occipital regions, electroencephalography may be of definite localizing value in cerebral hemisphere tumors. The most consistent EEG abnormality is focal high amplitude slowing, though this is by no means diagnostic of a cerebral neoplasm (Fig. 47). The EEG is abnormal in over 90 percent of supratentorial tumors in children and is of localizing value in 75 percent. When the cerebral cortex is involved, localizing value approaches 90 percent.

Brain scanning for focal collection of radioisotope is of greatest value in the localization of cerebral hemisphere neoplasms. The diagnostic incidence approaches 90 percent in some large series as compared to approximately 60 percent for posterior fossa neoplasms. Evidence is accumulating to the effect that sequential scanning provides valuable information concerning tumor recurrence or extension following subtotal excision and/or radiotherapy. The use of technetium is currently favored for sequential scanning because of lower radiation exposure.

Plain radiograms of the skull are helpful in localizing cerebral hemisphere neoplasms when tumor calcification occurs (approximately 10 percent), or when local bony erosion is evident. The majority of patients show suture spread or other evidence of increased intracranial pressure, but somewhat less frequently and to a lesser extent than with posterior fossa neoplasms. Between one-fourth and one-third of plain radiograms of the skull are normal in children with cerebral hemisphere gliomas.

Echoencephalography (Fig. 48A and B) has been developed into a very useful tool for the detection of significant shifts of the midline cerebral structures created by any space-occupying lesion situated on one side of the midline. This diagnostic procedure is of particular value in children, since the pineal gland is rarely calcified in this age group. Ultrasound is deflected from normal midline structures in a characteristic manner, giving a prominent oscilloscopic deflection which can be photographed and measured in terms of distance from the right or left side of the cranial vault, after input of ultrasound from the appropriate side. Since structures in the vicinity of the third ventricle give rise to this deflection, lesions placed far anteriorly or posteriorly are less apt to give significant shifts, but the method has proved to be extremely useful as an initial screening procedure, entirely free of contraindications or complications. More than three-fourths of cerebral

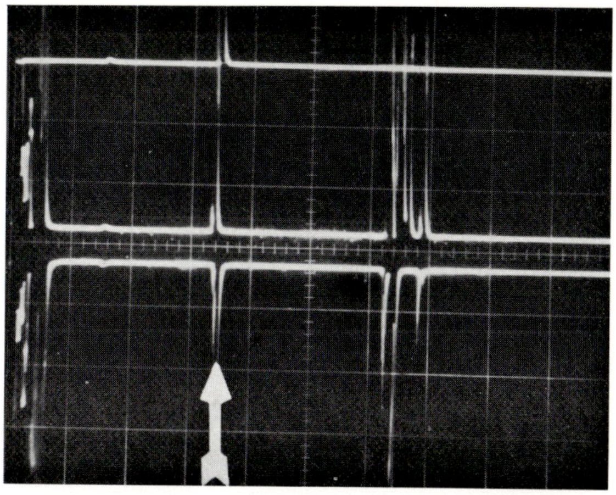

Fig. 48*A*. Normal echoencephalogram. Arrow indicates midline structures are in a normal position.

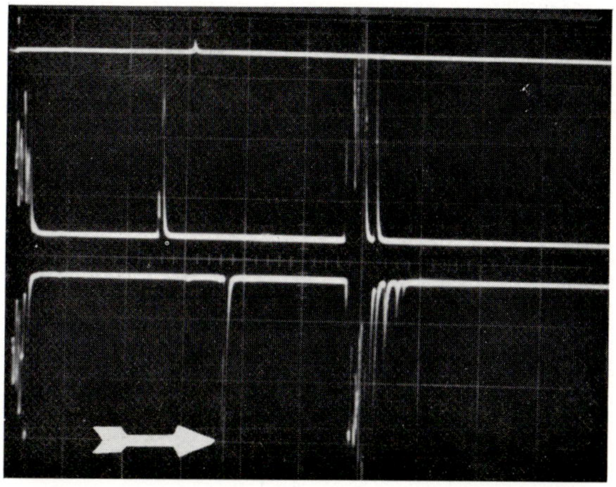

Fig. 48*B*. Abnormal echoencephalogram. Arrow indicates 10-mm shift of midline echoes from left to right. In this case due to a large left parietal lobe glioma in a 6-year-old boy.

hemisphere tumors are associated with a shift of the midline in excess of 2 mm, which is considered the upper limit of normal.

When signs of increased intracranial pressure are absent, lumbar puncture may be done and may reveal a moderate increase in cerebrospinal fluid pressure or in the protein content of the fluid. Cerebrospinal fluid enzymes may be elevated (e.g., transaminase, lactic dehydrogenase, phosphohexose isomerase). These findings are not specific and occur in other active lesions of the central nervous system.

Cerebral angiography is the contrast study of choice when focal findings or prior ancillary studies indicate the side of the lesion or when there is increased intracranial pressure without localizing signs. In experienced hands, percutaneous carotid angiography may be done under narcosis (combined secobarbital, meperidine, and chlorpromazine), obviating the need for and the risks of anesthesia. The advantages of angiography include demonstration of the vascular supply and the extent of vascularity of a given neoplasm, information of considerable importance to the neurosurgeon in planning the surgical approach.

Air contrast studies may be indicated as a supplement to angiography in order to amplify equivocal findings or to provide critical information not obtained by angiography.

TABLE 19. *Pathology of 104 Verified Cerebral Hemisphere Tumors*

Type of Tumor		Number
Astrocytoma (pure and mixed)		46
Solid	30	
Cystic	16	
Glioblastoma		13
Ependymoma		8
Meningioma		6
Sarcoma		5
Oligodendroglioma		4
Ganglioglioma		4
Malignant teratoma		2
Metastatic neuroblastoma		2
Choroid plexus papilloma		2
Miscellaneous		12
	Total	104

TREATMENT AND PROGNOSIS. Treatment and its outcome are in great part dependent on the histology of the tumor, though in general the results are disappointing. The histologic types encountered in 104 verified cerebral hemisphere tumors at the Columbia-Presbyterian Medical Center are outlined in Table 19. The different types will not be discussed separately.

Astrocytoma is the leading cerebral hemisphere tumor. It is far less commonly cystic than the cerebellar astrocytoma and only occasionally presents as a mural nodule in a large cyst. The tumor is so infiltrative in character that complete surgical excision is rarely, if ever, achieved, but many years of remission of symptoms can be achieved in a significant number of children. Obviously, the precise location of the tumor will dictate the extent of surgical excision possible. A tumor located within the motor and speech areas of the dominant cerebral hemisphere lends itself rather poorly to surgical intervention, whereas a tumor anteriorly placed in one frontal lobe can be attacked more radically.

Anticonvulsant medication is routinely recommended postoperatively for children with cerebral hemisphere neoplasms and is continued indefinitely when recurrence is expected, as it is in the majority. Otherwise, the indications for continuing anticonvulsant medication are the same as those employed in convulsions due to other causes.

TABLE 20. *Symptoms and Signs in 56 Patients with Optic Nerve Glioma*

	Initial	Presenting	Subsequent
Diminished visual acuity	28	39	53
Exophthalmos	25	27	29
Nystagmus	8	8	14
Strabismus	6	11	17
Field cut	1	1	12
Disk change			
Pallor			36
Pallor and blurring			11
Blurring			8
Increased intracranial pressure	3	13	15
Enlarged head	1	1	4
Multiple café-au-lait spots		2	12
Paresis		3	4

Tumors of the Optic Nerve and Chiasm

INCIDENCE. Tumors of the optic nerve and chiasm consist almost entirely of gliomas (astrocytomas), of which over 95 percent occur in children. Meningiomas of the dural sheath of the optic nerve are exceedingly rare in children, occurring approximately 20 times less frequently than optic nerve gliomas. At the Columbia-Presbyterian Medical Center between the years 1940 and 1964, 5 percent of 1,124 intracranial tumors in children under 16 years were optic nerve gliomas. Surprisingly, almost one-third of the patients have their earliest symptom under the age of 2 years, and as many as 10 percent in the first 6 months of life. The diagnosis, however, is characteristically delayed for one to several years after onset.

CLINICAL MANIFESTATIONS. Table 20 indicates the various symptoms and signs at the time of onset and of diagnosis.

The difference between the number of children or parents complaining of diminished visual acuity and those showing visual defects on examination reflects the tendency for children to tolerate occult visual deficit. Exophthalmos is a particularly early and frequent (96 percent) sign when the tumor is confined to one optic nerve, though 20 percent of patients with chiasmal gliomas also have some degree of proptosis. Nystagmus is related chiefly to the presence of severe visual deficit prior to the age of 4 years, more particularly prior to 2 years of age. Increased intracranial pressure is present only when the chiasm is involved and a large tumor has occluded the foramina of Monro. Multiple café-au-lait spots, the most common manifestation of neurofibromatosis, are present in approximately 25 percent of the children. Strabismus, when encountered, is not paretic in type but relates to defective fixation of a poorly seeing eye. Optic atrophy is an invariable finding. It may be confined to one optic nerve, despite early involvement of the chiasm.

DIAGNOSIS. The differential diagnosis in cases of optic nerve tumor includes other tumors of the orbit, particularly neurofibroma, and less frequently meningioma and retinoblastoma. The clinical and roentgenographic criteria outlined here make it clear that separation of these entities is possible in virtually every instance without resort to a tissue diagnosis. The most important differential point in regard to proptosis is that in optic glioma it is of mild degree, occurs in a straightforward axis with little lateral or vertical displacement of the globe, and is associated with a significant degree of optic atrophy and visual defect; other orbital tumors producing proptosis lead to more marked and bizarrely positioned protrusion of the globe, in the presence of remarkable preservation of vision, and usually absence of optic atrophy.

Chiasmal gliomas may be confused with other tumors arising in this area—craniopharyngioma, teratomas, dermoids, ectopic pinealomas, colloid cysts of the third ventricle, and hypothalamic gliomas. The characteristic features on plain radiograms of the skull are the most important means of differentiating chiasmal gliomas from other tumors in this region. They are indicated in Figures 49 and 50 and consist of enlarged optic foramina and typical deformity of the anterior clinoids. Helpful clinical features include multiple café-au-lait spots and the characteristic, though not invariable, absence of diabetes insipidus and growth retardation in children with chiasmal gliomas. Approximately 5 percent of children with chiasmal gliomas show endocrine changes which, if present, usually include precocious puberty.

Over 25 percent of children with optic gliomas are followed for one to three years after the onset of visual defects, strabismus, or nystagmus before the diagnosis is established. The optic disc pallor encountered is often ascribed to congenital optic atrophy. For unexplained reasons, the children may show some correction of visual acuity with appropriate refraction. Their age makes it impossible, in most instances, for

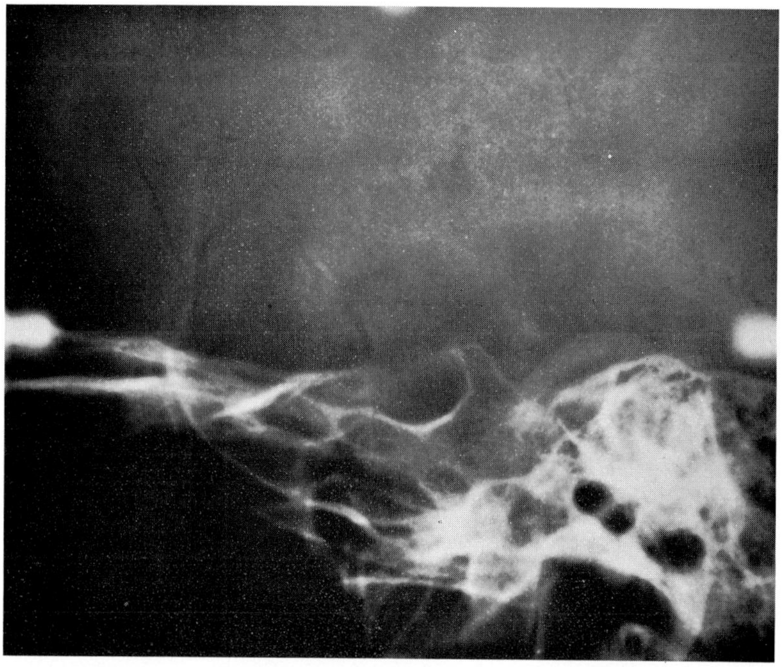

Fig. 49. J-shaped deformity of the sella in a 4-year-old boy with right optic nerve and chiasm glioma. A depression of the right lateral aspect of the chiasmatic sulcus with intact cortical margins is shown. The anterior clinoid process is thinned by the optic nerve tumor at the cranial porus of the right optic canal.

the ophthalmologist to be certain that full correction is achieved. It is, therefore, urged that when disc pallor of any degree is present, or visual defect is not fully corrected by refraction, the simple expedient of obtaining skull x-rays with adequate views of the optic foramina and sella turcica be considered.

The tools employed in the diagnosis or exclusion of optic nerve gliomas include, whenever possible, measurement of visual fields and acuity, careful examination of the fundi, x-rays of the skull, orbits, and optic foramina, and, in addition, intracranial pneumography. In the presence of a chiasmal glioma, pneumoencephalography reveals a filling defect in the anterior portion of the third ventricle, which is invaginated by the optic chiasm. Intracranial involvement of a single optic nerve may also be detected by intracranial pneumography but may be missed by this study if the chiasm is not involved.

TREATMENT. If it is suspected that an optic nerve glioma is confined to a single optic nerve, a combined transcranial operation with unroofing of the orbit, preferably performed by a neurosurgeon and ophthal-

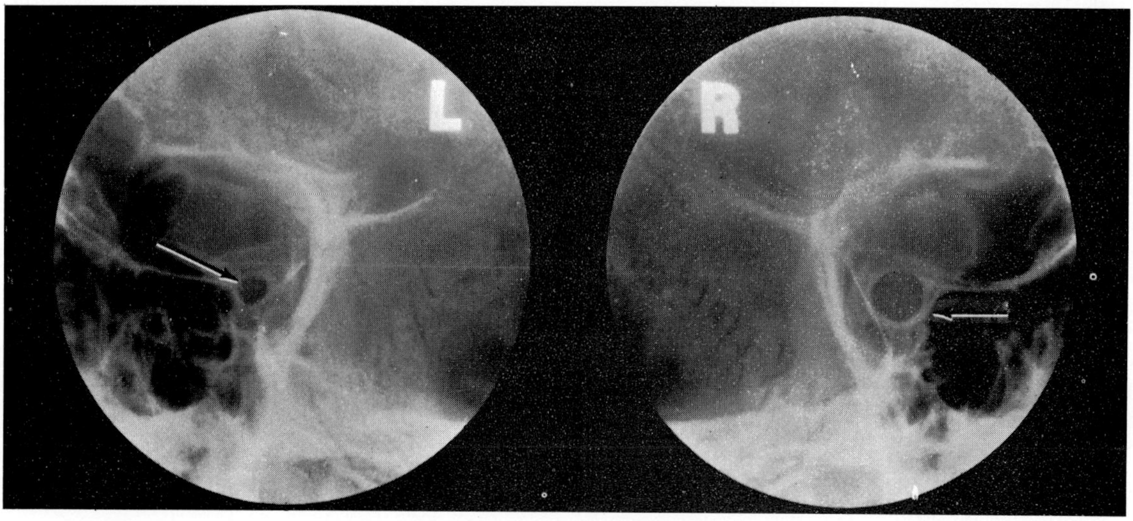

Fig. 50. Orbital and intracranial right optic nerve glioma in a 14-year-old boy. The normal left optic canal is oval and 5 mm in diameter. The right optic canal is enlarged to a circular lumen of 11 mm diameter with intact cortical margin.

mologist, is still indicated even if pneumography fails to reveal intracranial extension. In this manner, the tumor can be completely resected. It is almost always possible to preserve the globe, which subsequently serves as an excellent "natural prosthesis" and moves reflexly in conjugate fashion, directed by the eye with useful vision.

Chiasmal gliomas cannot be totally resected and are best treated by radiotherapy. It may be possible partially to resect a chiasmal glioma in order to reestablish cerebrospinal fluid communication when the foramina of Monro are obstructed, but more commonly ventricular shunting is indicated as an adjunct to radiotherapy. Transient diabetes insipidus may occur after surgery in this region and requires careful replacement therapy.

PROGNOSIS. Patients with proptosis seem to do well, regardless of whether the chiasm is involved. Undoubtedly this is because proptosis reflects origin of a very slowly growing tumor in the optic nerve. Those with gliomas confined to the optic nerve can be offered a complete cure in virtually every instance.

For unexplained reasons, in some patients with chiasmal gliomas, whose tumors are identical histologically with those proved by biopsy in patients who do well, the course is rapid and they succumb to their disease within a year of diagnosis. More than 80 percent of these patients who do poorly have had increased intracranial pressure at the time of diagnosis. However, as many as one-third of patients with chiasmal gliomas who have shown long-term survival with useful vision also had increased intracranial pressure when diagnosed.

The majority with chiasmal gliomas treated with radiotherapy may be expected to survive with little or no neurologic deficit and with useful vision for many years. The longest follow-up of a patient known to us with a chiasmal glioma, following biopsy of the lesion and radiotherapy, without evidence of clinical relapse, is 30 years.

Craniopharyngioma

INCIDENCE. The incidence of craniopharyngiomas is only slightly higher than that of all optic nerve gliomas but is severalfold that of chiasmal gliomas, with which they may occasionally, in atypical cases, be confused. Between 5 and 10 percent of all intracranial tumors in children are craniopharyngiomas. The majority of the children seen for the first time are between 7 and 12 years of age.

CLINICAL MANIFESTATIONS. The cardinal signs and symptoms of craniopharyngioma are: (1) increased intracranial pressure; (2) visual defects; (3) endocrine dysfunction; and (4) hypothalamic dysfunction.

Increased Intracranial Pressure. Increased intracranial pressure is due to upward extension of the tumor and obstruction of one or both foramina of Monro. The signs and symptoms of increased intracranial pressure are not distinctive, but it must be remembered that occasionally optic atrophy prevents the occurrence of papilledema. Almost always, however, papilledema and disc pallor are both present at the time of initial diagnosis.

Visual Defects. Visual acuity is usually diminished to a significant degree owing to chiasmatic compression and optic atrophy. Visual field defects are common and variable in type, though the typical finding, because of the midline position of the tumor, is bitemporal hemianopia. In very young, dull, or inarticulate children, it may be impossible to document the type or extent of visual deficit.

Endocrine Dysfunction. The observed deficits in endocrine function are due to diminished pituitary activity; the principal manifestations are growth retardation and sexual infantilism. Preoperatively, clinical manifestations of hypothyroidism are not to be expected.

While these children tend to tire easily and may be hypotensive, obesity of the "female" type is more common than cachexia, and florid panhypopituitarism is distinctly rare.

Hypothalamic Dysfunction. Diabetes insipidus is uncommon before surgical extirpation, but is encountered preoperatively in some patients.

Other signs and symptoms of hypothalamic involvement include growth retardation, somnolence, obesity, hypothermia or hyperthermia, hypertension or hypotension, inappropriate secretion of antidiuretic hormone, and alarming changes in vital signs. However, with the exception of somatic and sexual infantilism, these phenomena occur more often as postoperative complications than as part of the preoperative clinical picture.

DIAGNOSIS. Approximately three-fourths of children with craniopharyngiomas show diffuse flecks of calcification in the sella or suprasellar region in plain radiograms of the skull (Fig. 51). Enlargement of the sella is present in half of the cases, and more than half show nonspecific signs of increased intracranial pressure, such as suture spread or demineralization of the vault or clinoid processes. When calcification is absent, it is wise to obtain films of the optic foramina and to study the anterior clinoids for evidence of a chiasmal glioma. Other tumors occurring less commonly in this region include teratomas, dermoids, colloid cysts, and hypothalamic gliomas. Calcification may occur in dermoid tumors and teratomas but is rare in the other tumors.

It is essential to document the extent of endocrine disturbance. The urine osmolality, serum electrolytes, and preoperative blood pressure require special attention so that optimal correction may be made preoperatively. Bone age is determined by radiograms of the hemiskeleton or of the hand and wrist. Other endocrine functions may be estimated by the various tests of anterior and posterior pituitary, thyroid, and adrenal function; and postoperative comparison can be made when the condition stabilizes so that optimal replacement endocrine therapy can be offered.

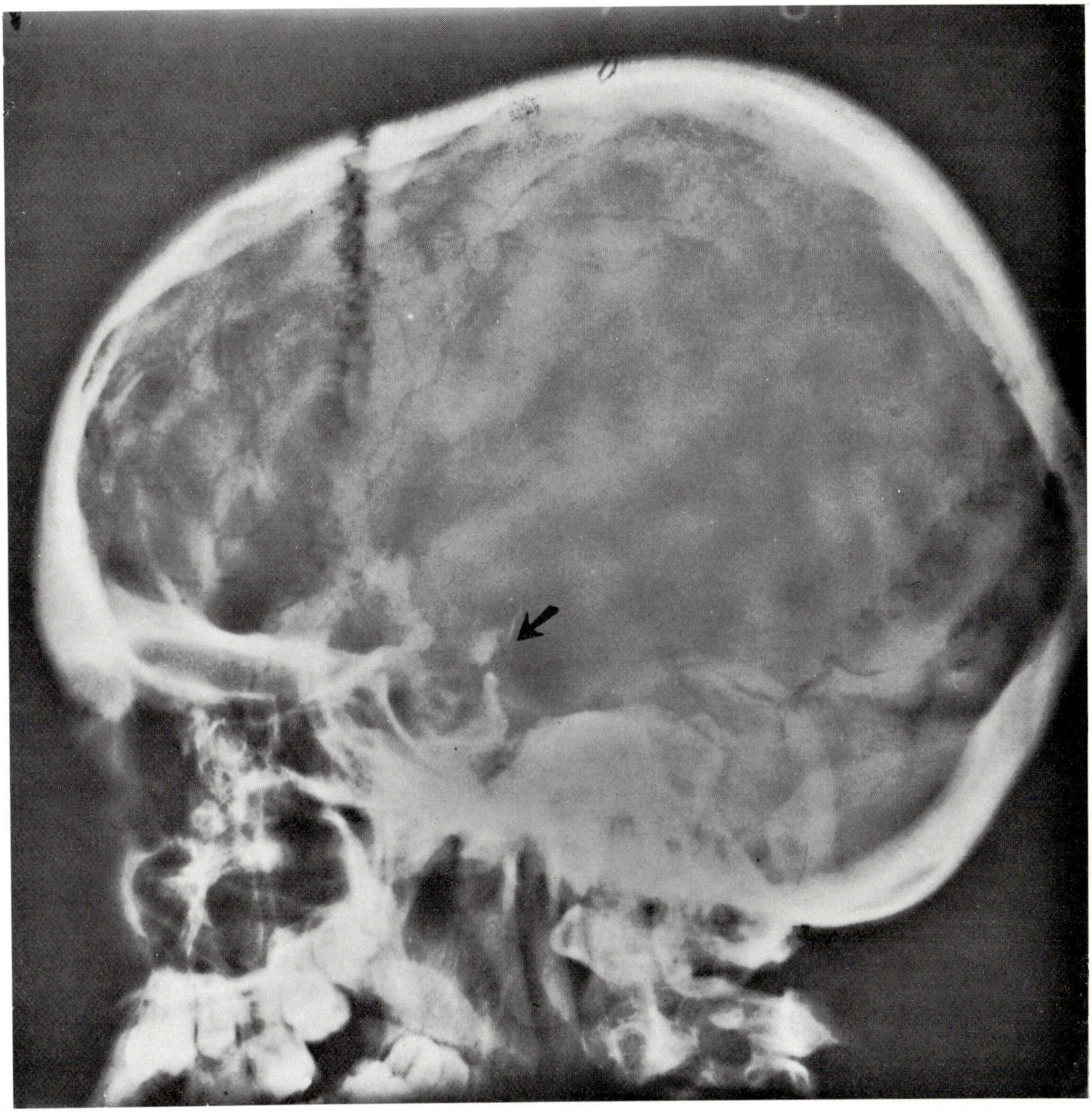

Fig. 51. Skull film of a child with craniopharyngioma showing sellar and suprasella calcifications (arrow), enlargement of the pituitary fossa, and separation of sutures.

The visual fields and acuity are carefully plotted, preoperatively and after stabilization, postoperatively, to permit comparison on subsequent examination for detection of recurrence.

The surgeon may or may not elect to perform ventriculography prior to surgical attack on the neoplasm. When the diagnosis seems secure, intracranial pneumography may be forgone. At times, cerebral angiography is performed so that optimal handling of stretched and distorted internal carotid and anterior cerebral vessels can be planned.

TREATMENT. Regardless of the results of endocrine study, cortisone should be given preoperatively and during surgery; its use has become the single largest factor in the marked increase in immediate postoperative survival and in the increase in the number of patients capable of having radical tumor removal. An average dose of cortisone is 50 mg on the evening prior to surgery and 50 mg on the morning of surgery. Approximately 100 mg of cortisone is given intravenously during surgery. On the first postoperative day, 100 mg of cortisone is administered, thereafter tapering the dose by 25 mg daily to a maintenance level of approximately 15 mg daily.

It is now believed possible for the experienced neurosurgeon to perform a gross total excision of the tumor in more than half of the patients. These tumors are encapsulated and almost always cystic to some extent. They may be located within the sella or entirely beyond the diaphragm of the sella in the pituitary stalk. The tumor capsule may adhere inseparably to the anterior cerebral or internal carotid vessels, the optic chiasm, or the hypothalamus. In such cases, only partial excision is possible and recurrence is invariable. However, dramatic remission of symptoms and restoration of vision may be achieved simply by aspiration of the "machinery-oil-like" fluid from a moderately sized or large cyst which has compressed surrounding structures.

The tumors, being squamous epitheliomas, are relatively radioresistant, but it is believed that radiotherapy may retard at least the rate of reaccumulation of cyst fluid.

In the immediate postoperative period, symptoms of diabetes insipidus may be severe, and careful attention to water and electrolyte balance is essential. For the first few days, replacement of water and electrolytes is generally advisable, without the use of vasopressin, because the immediate effects of surgery wane and diabetes insipidus is invariably lessened.

When the vasopressin is introduced, the aqueous parenteral preparation may be used, every 6 hours, if necessary.

Cortisone and thyroid replacement are often necessary, particularly when a radical tumor excision has been performed.

Accurate human growth hormone assays are now available, and human growth hormone can be secured in a limited amount. With this compound many children with previous growth retardation are showing reestablishment of normal growth curves. Normal pubescence may also be achieved by appropriate hormonal therapy, and even reproduction may be secured with the use of human chorionic gonadotropin.

The patient who has had excision of a craniopharyngioma must be followed with particular attention to visual fields and acuity and periodic skull x-rays for the detection of recurrence by extension of calcification or shift in the position clips placed at the time of surgery.

PROGNOSIS. Children treated prior to 1950 almost uniformly failed to survive. The long-term results of children treated more recently are being awaited but already are considerably more promising.

Even when total tumor excision is not possible, the interval from operation to recurrence may be many years, though occasionally it is less than a year. Repeated partial excision of solid tumor and capsule and cyst aspiration may keep such patients alive and functioning well for many years. Unfortunately, visual deficit often mounts with each insult, and the risk of postoperative morbidity and mortality is compounded.

Tumors of the Spinal Cord

Intraspinal tumors in infants and children are far less common than intracranial tumors, the ratio being approximately 1 to 5. Meningiomas and neurofibromas, relatively common in adults, are rarely encountered in children. Intraspinal lipomas, dermoid, and teratoid tumors, neuroblastomas, and intramedullary gliomas are the common intraspinal neoplasms in children. Approximately 20 percent of the tumors are of the dermoid and lipoma group, which are benign tumors of congenital origin. Gliomas and sarcomas each have a similar incidence, and together with the congenital group account for 60 percent of the total. Less common is the neuroblastoma which comprises 5 to 10 percent of intraspinal tumors in children.

Early diagnosis of intraspinal tumors in children is essential because of three considerations:

1. Irreversible neurologic deficit may occur when diagnosis is delayed, despite the otherwise favorable character of the neoplasm from the therapeutic point of view.
2. Intramedullary gliomas, contrary to popular belief, may at times either lend themselves to total surgical excision or respond dramatically to radiation therapy.
3. The lipoma, dermoid, and teratoid group of tumors, benign varieties of extramedullary tumors, may be associated, even after only partial excision, with prolonged relief of signs and symptoms.

CLINICAL MANIFESTATIONS. ***Disturbance of Gait and Posture.*** Disturbances of gait and posture are the most frequent symptoms of intraspinal tumors; in their presence an intraspinal neoplasm should always be considered. These changes may be due to weakness, spasticity, or compensatory posture to avoid pain. The most frequent disturbance of posture is a reluctance to flex the trunk; it may be present before frank neurologic deficit is detectable. There may be prominent paraspinal muscle spasm, a particularly important sign in the nonverbal or inarticulate child. The characteristic posture and gait of the child with a cervical intramedullary glioma are the flaillike drooping of the shoulders and reduced swing of the upper extremities due to segmental anterior horn cell involvement. Other abnormalities of gait depend upon the extremity involved and the degree to which changes of tone and power are pressed.

Pain. Pain is a common, but by no means universal, symptom of intraspinal tumor; it occurs as an initial complaint in approximately 50 percent of children. In the young child pain may be manifested by irritability and postural guarding. Older children frequently describe the pain as being accentuated by coughing, sneezing, or straining, as well as by flexion of the neck, trunk, or extension of the lower extremities.

Weakness. Approximately two-thirds of children with intraspinal tumors have some degree of weakness on initial evaluation. Functionally this may be evident only as a limp, easy fatigability, or reduced activity on one or more extremities. There is a flaccid paresis at the level of the lesion, below which the extremities are spastic. The weakness may be of the flaccid type below the level of the lesion when "spinal shock" occurs, as in rapidly evolving cord compression from neuroblastoma or other metastatic lesions.

Reflex Changes. Diminished deep tendon reflexes may be encountered within the limited segments occupied by tumor, due to encroachment on anterior horn cells, while hyperactive reflexes and extensor plantar responses are expected below the level of the lesion due to impairment of descending tracts. In "spinal shock," deep tendon reflexes are absent. Thus in intramedullary neoplasms of the cervical cord, diminished reflexes and loss of tone in the upper extremities are commonly associated with spasticity, hyperreflexia, and extensor plantar responses in the lower extremities. Absence or diminution of reflexes in the lower extremities is suggestive of a lesion of the cauda equina. An absent anal reflex is additional evidence of sacral cord or root involvement.

Impaired Bladder or Bowel Function. Bowel and bladder function may be impaired by involvement of descending tracts or by segmental loss of innervation in lumbosacral lesions. The result may be either a spastic, low-capacity bladder with frequency of urination, or a distended, atonic bladder with dribbling of urine. Laxity of the rectal sphincter and a diminished anal reflex with regressive bowel or bladder function are valuable objective signs in a child in whom the more subjective aspects of evaluation, such as sensory examination of the saddle area, are less reliable.

Sensory Impairment. In children the sensory examination is the most difficult and least reliable part of the neurologic examination. However, a careful examination may be rewarding even in an infant. Changes in facial expression or direction of attention may be helpful in fixing the level of a spinal cord lesion. Sensory deficits are ascertainable in one-third of children with intraspinal tumors, despite the fact that sensory complaints are rarely offered. There is often an absence or diminution of sweating below the level of the lesion, a valuable sign in this limited sensory examination in young children. The oft-cited tendency of intramedullary tumors to "spare" sacral sensation is particularly misleading in children.

Cutaneous and Skeletal Changes. Cutaneous or subcutaneous lesions may indicate an underlying neoplasm. Multiple café-au-lait spots in a child with spinal cord symptoms suggest the diagnosis of neurofibroma. In rare instances a single café-au-lait spot may mark the site of the tumor. A subcutaneous lipoma, nevus flammeus, dimple, sinus, or tuft of hair in the dorsal or lumbosacral region may be an innocent dermal anomaly; however, the presence of such a lesion in association with symptoms or signs of neurologic significance suggests the possibility of an underlying neoplasm of the lipomatous, dermoid, or teratoid type, with or without myelodysplasia and other anomalies.

Scoliosis may be a local manifestation of an intraspinal tumor or may be associated with neurofibromatosis even in the absence of any intraspinal tumor. However, an intraspinal tumor should be excluded in all patients with neurofibromatosis and scoliosis.

Miscellaneous Signs. Occasionally opsoclonus, with "polymyoclonia" or cerebellar ataxia, may be the only signs suggesting the possibility of an occult intraspinal ganglioneuroma or neuroblastoma.

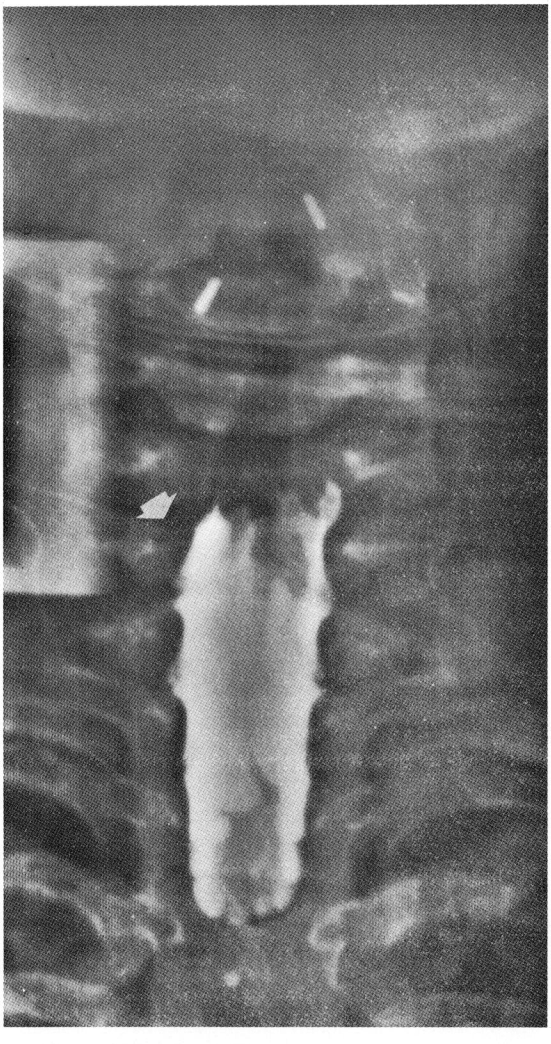

Fig. 52. Myelogram in a 4-year-old with complete spinal block due to an extradural compression. Neuroblastoma metastases to the cervical spine were demonstrated both radiographically and at surgery. The column of contrast material is seen to be displaced to the left (arrow) away from the pedicle of C-6. The cord is also seen to be displaced in the same direction. (Courtesy of Dr. Sadek Hilal.)

LABORATORY STUDIES. ***Cerebrospinal Fluid.*** Lumbar puncture is of considerable value in the diagnosis of spinal cord neoplasia. Radiographs of vertebral spines should always precede lumbar puncture. With suspected spinal cord lesions, careful manometric measurements should always be performed. The fluid may be slightly discolored or frankly xanthochromic. The cell count and sugar content are usually normal. In the presence of metastatic seeding (leptomeningeal sarcomatosis or carcinomatosis), there may be an increase in cells and a marked reduction in the sugar content. These findings, particularly when associated with nuchal rigidity, give rise to a picture that may be easily confused with bacterial meningitis. Cerebrospinal fluid protein is usually increased when a spinal cord tumor is present. In the presence of a complete subarachnoid block, the protein content is markedly elevated with an associated deep yellow discoloration (Froin syndrome).

Radiographic Studies. About two-thirds of children with intraspinal tumors have associated bony changes in the spine detectable on plain x-ray examination. Two significant findings suggesting an intraspinal tumor are widening of the interpedicular space and erosion of the pedicles. Myelography is the definitive diagnostic precedure and establishes the level of the lesion and its intramedullary or extramedullary location (Fig. 52).

DIFFERENTIAL DIAGNOSIS. The differential diagnosis of intraspinal tumors includes congenital defects (e.g., diastematomyelia), vascular malformations, tumors of the bony spine, and degenerative diseases. Diagnosis is often possible with a detailed history, careful neurologic examination, and the appropriate use of ancillary laboratory procedures.

TREATMENT. Therapy is largely dependent upon location of the tumor. Surgical extirpation is feasible for some extramedullary lesions; occasionally, partial removal and rarely total removal of an intramedullary tumor is possible. Decompressive laminectomy may give symptomatic relief.

Radiation therapy is utilized for inoperable tumors and as a supplement for radiosensitive mass lesions subtotally removed. Corticosteroid therapy may be of vital benefit in reducing cord edema associated with radiation therapy, or prior to surgical decompression.

REFERENCES

BRAIN TUMORS

Aron, B. S. Twenty years' experience with radiation therapy medulloblastoma. Amer. J. Roentgen, 105:37, 1969.

Bain, H. W., Darte, J. M. M., Keith, W. S., and Kruyff, E. The diencephalic syndrome of early infancy due to silent brain tumor: with special reference to treatment. Pediatrics, 38:473, 1966.

Bailey, P., Buchanan, D. N., and Bucy, P. C. Intracranial Tumors of Infancy and Childhood. Chicago, University of Chicago Press, 1939.

Bergstrand, C. G., Bergstedt, J., and Herrlin, M. M. Paediatric aspects of brain tumors in infancy and childhood. Acta Paediat. Scand., 47:688, 1958.

Bloom, H. J. G., Wallace, M. B., and Henk, J. M. The treatment and prognosis of medulloblastoma in children. Amer. J. Roetgen., 105:43, 1969.

Bouchard, J. J. Radiation Therapy of Tumors and Diseases of the Nervous System. Philadelphia, Lea and Febiger, 1966.

Bray, P. F., Carter, S., and Taveras, J. M. Brainstem tumors in children. Neurology, 8:1, 1958.

Cairns, H., and Mosberg, W. H., Jr. Colloid cyst of the third ventricle. Surg. Gynec. Obstet., 92:545, 1951.

Chang, C. H., Housepian, E. M., and Herbert, C., Jr. An operative staging system and a megavoltage radiotherapeutic technic for cerebellar medulloblastomas. Radiology, 93:1351, No. 6, 1969.

Cheek, W. R., and Taveras, J. M. Thalamic tumors. J. Neurosurg., 24:505, 1966.

Chutorian, A. M., Schwartz, J. F., Evans, R. A., and Carter, S. Optic gliomas in children. Neurology, 14: 83, 1964.

Cuneo, H. M., and Rand, C. W. Brain Tumors of Childhood. Springfield, Ill., Charles C Thomas, Publ., 1952.

Davidoff, L. M. Some considerations in the therapy of pineal tumors. Bull. N.Y. Acad. Med., 43:537, 1967.

Dods, L. A diencephalic syndrome of early infancy. Med. J. Aust., 1:222, 1967.

Fokes, E. C., and Earle, K. M. Ependymomas: clinical and pathological aspects. J. Neurosurg., 30:585, 1969.

French, L. A. The use of steroids in the treatment of cerebral edema. Bull. N.Y. Acad. Med., 42:30, 1966.

——— and Galicich, J. H. The use of steroids for control of cerebral edema. Clin. Neurosurg., 10:212, 1964.

Gold, L. H. A., and Loken, M. K. Retrospective evaluation of isotope images of the brain in 852 patients. Radiology, 92:1473, 1969.

Hammill, J. F., and Carter, S. Brain Tumors in Childhood, Practice of Pediatrics. Hagerstown, Md., W. F. Prior Co., Inc., 1966.

Jackson, I. J., and Thompson, R. K. Pediatric Neurosurgery. Springfield, Ill., Charles C Thomas, Publ., 1959.

Lampkin, B. C., Mauer, A. M., and McBride, B. H. Response of medulloblastoma to vincristine sulfate: a case report. Pediatrics, 39:761, 1967.

Lassman, L. P., Pearce, G. W., and Gang, J. Effect of vincristine sulfate on the intracranial gliomata of childhood. Brit. J. Surg., 53:9, 1966.

Low, N. L., Correll, J. W., and Hammill, J. F. Tumors of the cerebral hemispheres in children. Arch. Neurol., 13:547, 1965.

Matson, D. D. Craniopharyngioma. Clin. Neurosurg., 10:116, 1964.

——— Neurosurgery of Infancy and Childhood, 2nd ed. Springfield, Ill., Charles C Thomas, Publ., 1969.

McFarland, D., Horwitz, H., and Saenger, E., Medulloblastoma—a review of prognosis and survival. Brit. J. Radiol., 42:198, 1969.

Mealey, J., Jr., and Mishkin, F. S. Brain Tumor Scanning in Children. *In* Bakay, L., and Klein, D. M., eds., Brain Tumor Scanning with Radioisotopes. Springfield, Ill., Charles C Thomas, Publ., 1969.

Millichap, J. G., Bickford, R. G., Miller, R. H., and Backus, R. E. The EEG in children with intracranial tumors and seizures. Neurology, 12:329, 1962.
Newton, W. A., Jr., Sayers, M. P., and Samuels, L. D. Intrathecal methotrexate therapy for brain tumors in children. Cancer Chemother. Rep., 52:257, 1968.
Odom, G. L., Davis, C. H., and Woodhall, B. Brain tumors in children: clinical analysis of 164 cases. Pediatrics, 18:856, 1956.
Panitch, H. S., and Berg, B. O. Brain stem tumors of childhood and adolescence. Amer. J. Dis. Child., 119: 465, 1970.
Peirce, C. B. The efficacy of radiation therapy in the tretament of tumors of the brain and brain stem. Clin. Neurosurg., 10:195, 1964.
Planiol, T. Gamma-encephalography after ten years of utilization in neurosurgery. Progr. Neurol. Surg., 1:93, 1966.
Sassin, J. F., and Chutorian, A. M. Intracranial chordoma in children. Arch. Neurol., 17:89, 1967.
Tamaka, K., Ito, K., and Wagai, I. The localization of brain tumors by ultrasonic techniques (a clinical review of 111 cases). J. Neurosurg., 23:135, 1965.
White, P. T., and Ross, A. T. Inanition syndrome in infants with anterior hypothalamic neoplasms. Neurology, 13:974, 1963.
Zulch, K. J. Brain Tumors, Their Biology and Pathology. New York, Springer Publishing Co., Inc., 1957.

SPINAL CORD TUMORS

Coxe, W. S. Tumors of the spinal canal in children. Amer. Surg., 27:62, 1961.
Greenwood, J., Jr. Intramedullary tumors of the spinal cord; follow-up study after total surgical removal. J. Neurosurg., 20:665, 1963.
Haft, H., Ransohoff, J., and Carter, S. Spinal cord tumors in children. Pediatrics, 23:1152, 1959.
Hamby, W. B. Tumors in the spinal cord in childhood. J. Neuropath. Exp. Neurol., 3:397, 1944.
Matson, D. D., and Tachdjian, M. O. Intraspinal tumors in infants and children. Review of 115 cases. Postgrad. Med., 279, 1963.
Rand, R. W., and Rand, C. W. Intraspinal Tumors of Childhood. Springfield, Ill., Charles C Thomas, Publ., 1960.
Slooff, J. L., Kernahan, J. W., and MacCarty, C. S. Primary Intramedullary Tumors of the Spinal Cord and Filum Terminale. Philadelphia, W. B. Saunders Co., 1964.
Solomon, G. E., and Chutorian, A. M. Opsoclonus and occult neuroblastoma. New Eng. J. Med., 279:475, 1968.
Wood, E. H., Berne, A. S., and Taveras, J. M. The value of radiation therapy in the management of intrinsic tumors of the spinal cord. Radiology, 63:11, 1954.
Wyburn-Mason, R. The Vascular Abnormalities and Tumors of the Spinal Cord and Its Membranes. London, Henry Kimpton, 1944.

Chapter 6
PSEUDOTUMOR CEREBRI

MELVIN GREER

Pseudotumor cerebri refers to the neurologic syndrome characterized by increased intracranial pressure unassociated with focal signs of neural impairment, convulsions, alteration in mentation, or cerebrospinal fluid (CSF) changes. The signs and symptoms may otherwise be identical with those of any intracranial mass or hydrocephalus. The course is benign and the prognosis is usually good. Impairment of visual acuity as a consequence of persistent intracranial hypertension is the major problem.

ETIOLOGY. Pseudotumor cerebri is a syndrome of multiple causes in which the pathogenesis of the intracranial hypertension is often not apparent. Brain edema cannot be proved as the causative mechanism, and the absence of convulsions in addition to the presence of a normal mental state argue against this impression. Radioactive iodinated serum albumin studies after intrathecal injections suggest that a defect in CSF absorption is the underlying factor. In any single patient, it is essential to consider first the common causes of increased pressure: neoplasm, infection, congenital malformation, hematoma, and degenerative and toxic states. On the other hand, the history may suggest the presence of a benign cause.

A common cause of pseudotumor cerebri in children is obstruction of the intracranial venous drainage, secondary often to chronic mastoiditis and occlusion of the major draining lateral sinus (otitic hydrocephalus). Less common causes of intracranial hypertension secondary to blockage of venous drainage include obstruction of the sagittal sinus following traumatic skull fracture, sinus invasion by metastatic neuroblastoma, and vena cava obstruction secondary to surgery or to an intrathoracic mass. Under these conditions CSF absorption is impaired, the intracranial venous system is dilated, and increased pressure is the result.

Hormonal aberrations have been implicated in children with pseudotumor cerebri following corticosteroid therapy, in girls entering menarche, and in obese adolescent females. Hypoparathyroidism and hypophosphatasia also have been considered hormonal causes of the syndrome; however, adequate documentation of intracranial hypertension in the latter disorder is unavailable.

Pseudotumor cerebri also has been recognized in the adolescent female during severe iron-deficiency anemia of menstruation and following chronic vitamin A intoxication. In infancy, the syndrome has been described following the acute ingestion of massive quantities of vitamin A as well as after pro-

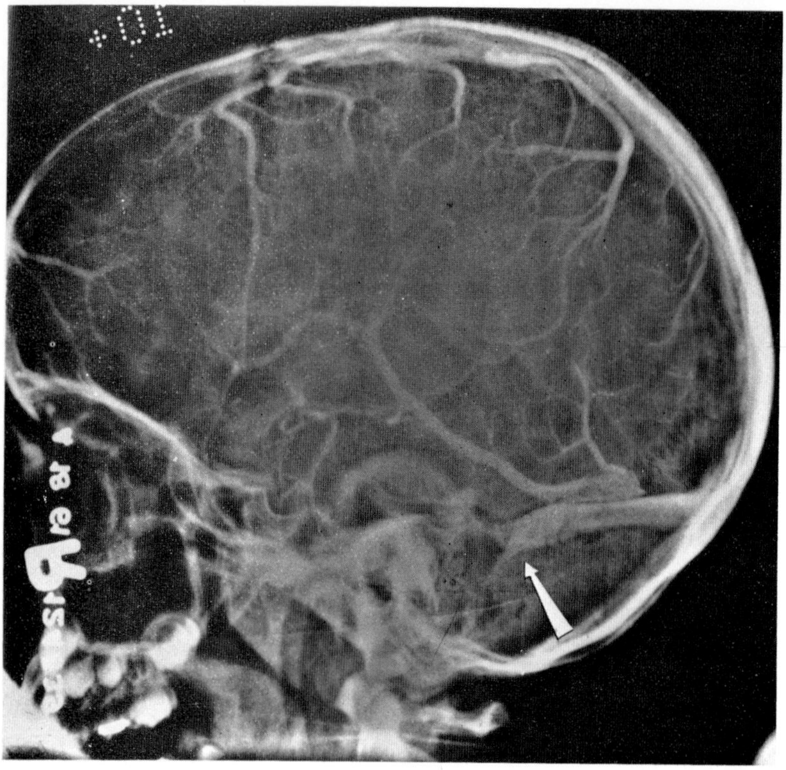

Fig. 53. Lateral sinus obstruction defined by venous phase of carotid arteriography in child with mastoiditis and pseudotumor cerebri. Arrow points to area of obstruction. (From Greer. *Neurology*, 12:472, 1962.)

longed vitamin A deficiency. However, signs such as fever, dehydration, diarrhea, irritability, and lethargy would indicate a toxic encephalopathy rather than a benign state as a result of deficiency or excess of vitamin A in infancy.

Nevertheless, it must be conceded that in some patients with intracranial hypertension, disturbance of mentation or seizures represent one end of the encephalopathy spectrum caused by an infectious, toxic, or metabolic process and, at the other end of the spectrum, the same underlying cause may be manifested by fewer overt signs of neural dysfunction and be considered a benign process.

A bulging fontanel accompanying fever in infancy has been termed meningism and is not unusual. Presumably it is related to an osmotic gradient between serum and CSF during fever which causes increased CSF volume. This may explain the intracranial hypertension described in roseola infantum. Afebrile infants who develop a bulging fontanel after being on tetracycline therapy for a few days and patients exhibiting intracranial hypertension after nalidixic acid therapy are two examples of iatrogenic causes of pseudotumor cerebri.

Other unexplained causes of pseudotumor cerebri in children include Sydenham's chorea, Aldrich's syndrome, and closed head trauma. Finally, there remain children with intracranial hypertension in whom no "etiology" can be found. This accounts for about one-third of all adequately studied children with pseudotumor cerebri.

CLINICAL MANIFESTATIONS. The presenting complaints include headache, nausea, vomiting, dizziness, blurred vision, and diplopia. The symptoms are intermittent and commonly exist for weeks. The examiner is struck by the child's well-being upon admission despite the florid papilledema and abducens nerve paresis which reflect the generalized increased pressure. There are no consistent signs of neurologic dysfunction, although mild unsteadiness of gait has often been described.

LABORATORY FINDINGS. Suture diastasis or erosion of the dorsum sella on skull roentgenography confirms the presence of intracranial hypertension. The electroencephalogram, echoencephalogram, and brain scan are normal, opposing the diagnosis of an encephalopathy or lateralized mass. Historical evidence suggesting mastoiditis or other extracranial diseases known to be related to intracranial hypertension calls for specific laboratory investigations such as mastoid x-rays, serum calcium, phosphorus, alkaline phosphatase, and vitamin A levels.

DIAGNOSIS. Carotid angiography (venous phase) may demonstrate intracranial venous sinus obstruction and, at the same time, exclude ventricular dilation (Fig. 53). If arteriography does not define sinus obstruction, a mass lesion, or ventricular dilation, pneumoencephalography may be performed. The air-filled

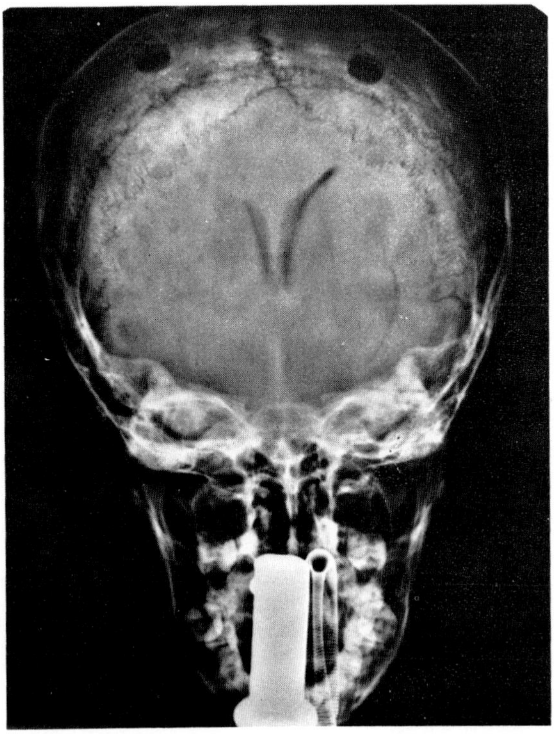

Fig. 54. Narrow lateral ventricles seen on ventriculogram (note burr holes) in child with pseudotumor cerebri in association with cessation of corticosteroid therapy for nephrosis.

ventricles commonly appear narrow (Fig. 54), and the CSF protein, sugar, and cell count are normal. Ventriculography has been commonly employed by the neurosurgeon as a diagnostic study of choice. In the presence of a mass lesion, of course, there exists a risk of cerebellar herniation and brainstem compression following pneumoencephalography; however, the more benign vascular study followed by air encephalography via the lumbar route lessens the trauma and risk attending ventricular puncture under general anesthesia in the child.

TREATMENT. Therapy is specific in the child whose intracranial hypertension is caused by lateral sinus obstruction (mastoidectomy, antibiotics), hypoparathyroidism (calcium, vitamin D), anemia of menstruation (iron, transfusion), drug intoxication (drug withdrawal), or possible adrenocortical insufficiency following cessation of corticosteroid therapy (reinstitution of corticosteroids).

In those children in whom no specific therapy for the increased pressure is available, the treatment is supportive. It is assumed that the illness in these instances is self-limiting. Indeed, in about one-half of the children in this group, the intracranial hypertension subsides spontaneously after air encephalography. The risk, however, of blindness because of persistent intracranial hypertension necessitates some treatment to reduce the pressure in those patients in whom spontaneous recovery is not immediate. This can be accomplished by serial lumbar punctures. Corticosteroids and carbonic anhydrase inhibitors have also been employed to lower the increased intracranial pressure; however, the response to these drugs has been neither reliable nor proved.

In a small percentage of children, neither repeated spinal taps nor corticosteroids are effective in maintaining a normal intracranial pressure. It is always advisable to repeat neuroradiologic studies if the symptoms and signs persist for more than three months. If intracranial pressure is still elevated, surgical treatment may be warranted. Ventricular or spinal shunting is much preferred to the crude subtemporal decompression procedure, since the latter entails a postoperative risk of temporal lobe trauma and seizures.

References

Bass, M. H. The relation of vitamin A intake to CSF pressure. Hospital, 24:713, 1957.

Beller, A. J. Benign post-traumatic intracranial hypertension. J. Neurol. Neurosurg. Psychiat., 27:149, 1964.

Chun, R. W. M., Smith, J., and Forster, F. M. Papilledema in Sydenham's chorea. Amer. J. Dis. Child., 101:641, 1961.

Collins-Williams, C. Idiopathic hypoparathyroidism with papilledema in a boy six years of age. Pediatrics, 5: 998, 1950.

Feldman, M. H., and Schlezinger, N. S. Benign intracranial hypertension associated with hypervitaminosis A. Arch. Neurol., 22:1, 1970.

Fields, J. P. Bulging fontanel: a complication of tetracycline therapy in infants. J. Pediat., 58:74, 1961.

Fraser, D., Yendt, E. R., and Christie, F. H. E. Metabolic abnormalities in hypophosphatasia. Lancet, 1: 286, 1955.

Greer, M. Benign intracranial hypertension. I. Mastoiditis and lateral sinus obstruction. Neurology, 12:472, 1962.

——— Benign intracranial hypertension. II. Following corticosteroid therapy. Neurology, 13:439, 1963.

——— Benign intracranial hypertension. IV. Menarche. Neurology, 14:569, 1964.

——— Benign intracranial hypertension. VI. Obesity. Neurology, 15:382, 1965.

——— Benign intracranial hypertension (pseudotumor cerebri). Pediat. Clin. N. Amer., 14:819, 1967.

——— Management of benign intracranial hypertension (pseudotumor cerebri). Clin. Neurosurg., 15:161, 1968.

——— Berk, M. S., and Williams, C. M. Dural metastasis, the cause of increased intracranial pressure in neuroblastoma. Amer. Pediat. Soc., 52, 1963 (Abstr.).

Hooper, R. Hydrocephalus and obstruction of the superior vena cava in infancy. Pediatrics, 28:792, 1961.

Marie, J., and See, G. Acute hypervitaminosis A of the infant. Amer. J. Dis. Child., 87:731, 1954.

Merritt, H. H., and Fremont-Smith, F. The Cerebrospinal Fluid. Philadelphia, W. B. Saunders Co., 1937.

Oliver, T. K., Jr. Chronic vitamin A intoxication: report of a case in an older child and review of the literature. Amer. J. Dis. Child., 95:57, 1958.

Oski, F. A. Roseola infantum. Amer. J. Dis. Child., 101:376, 1961.
Martin, J. P. Signs of obstruction of the superior longitudinal sinus following closed head injuries (traumatic hydrocephalus). Brit. Med. J., 2:467, 1955.
Rose, A., and Matson, D. D. Benign intracranial hypertension in children. Pediatrics, 39:227, 1967.
Schwaber, J. R., and Blumbert, A. G. Papilledema associated with blood loss anemia. Ann. Intern. Med., 55:1004, 1961.

Chapter 7
CEREBROVASCULAR DISEASES

ARNOLD P. GOLD, JAMES F. HAMMILL, and SIDNEY CARTER

Cerebrovascular diseases include all morbid processes, primary or secondary, in which the blood vessels of the brain are involved. Although no available classification of the various conditions is fully satisfactory, Table 21 has been found clinically useful.

Cerebrovascular accidents are most frequent in the elderly. Although they are generally considered a clinical rarity in childhood, they are actually not infrequent. Cerebrovascular diseases account for about 5 percent of admissions to a pediatric neurology service and 10 percent of pediatric pathology material. Children with congenital heart disease not uncommonly have cerebrovascular complications. Ten percent of patients with tetralogy of Fallot have cerebrovascular accidents, and 25 percent of all autopsied cardiac cases have evidence of cerebrovascular occlusion. These figures of incidence would be more impressive if they included children with blood dyscrasias. Spontaneous cerebral hemorrhage secondary to a hematologic disorder is not uncommon and is found in 50 percent of leukemic patients at necropsy. In the pediatric age group, arteriovenous malformations are 10 times as common as intracranial aneurysms and are the most common cause of primary subarachnoid hemorrhage.

Occlusive Vascular Disease

Arterial or venous occlusion deprives the brain of oxygen with resultant necrosis (encephalomalacia) of the surrounding tissue. If death does not result from this lesion, a process of repair occurs over the subsequent months with the formation of an astrocytic or fibroblastic scar. The ischemic area, or infarct, is the nonspecific end result of any type of occlusion; however, the changes in the blood vessels or surrounding brain may be highly specific. Arteriosclerosis in progeria, vascular changes in granulomatous arteritis (Takayasu's disease), and the lesions produced by blood dyscrasias, all have characteristic anatomic changes.

Dural Sinus and Cerebral Venous Thrombosis

Obstruction of venous drainage may lead to cerebral edema and hemorrhagic infarction of the brain. In some cases, thrombosis of venous sinuses may occur without causing any gross cerebral lesion because anastomoses of the cerebral venous system are often effective in bypassing the obstruction, and the integrity of the venous circulation is maintained.

Venous occlusion occurs most commonly following pyogenic infections of the face, mouth, mastoids, or leptomeninges. Cerebral venous thromboses may also develop in association with dehydration, debilitating and cachectic states, traumas, sickle-cell disease, or polycythemia. Less frequently venous occlusion is observed in Sturge-Weber-Dimitri syndrome, lead encephalopathy, metastatic neoplasia, or thrombotic thrombocytopenia.

CLINICAL MANIFESTATIONS. The clinical picture of venous thromboses is related to extent of involvement, rapidity of occlusion, and the nature of the primary disease.

Common manifestations include increased intracranial pressure, focal motor deficits, seizures, altered states of consciousness, and signs of circulatory stasis. Occlusion of a major lateral sinus may result in signs and symptoms of increased intracranial pressure without focal neurologic deficit. Those who develop focal signs may slowly recover or be left with a residual hemiparesis, seizures, or mental retardation. Superior sagittal sinus thrombosis is suggested by alternating hemiplegias and multifocal seizures. Signs of circulatory stasis may be pathognomonic for involvement of a specific vessel. Cavernous sinus thrombosis is characterized by exophthalmos of the homolateral eye, palpebral and conjunctival edema, and involvement of the third, fourth, fifth (first two branches), and sixth cranial nerves. Lateral sinus thrombosis may be accompanied by painful swelling in the mastoid region. Occlusion of the superior sagittal sinus results in venous distension over the scalp and eyelids.

LABORATORY FINDINGS. There is often a moderate polymorphonuclear leucocytosis and an elevated erythrocyte sedimentation rate. Changes in the cerebrospinal fluid vary according to the pathologic process. Unless there is an associated infection, the fluid, which may be under increased pressure, is usually clear and colorless with little or no pleocytosis. The Tobey-Ayer test, while not always reliable, may be of some value in the diagnosis of lateral sinus thrombosis. With this test, compression of the jugular vein on the affected side produces no rise in cerebrospinal fluid pressure, while compression of the normal side produces a prompt rise in pressure. The electroencephalogram may be normal, diffusely slow in the presence of increased intracranial pressure, or show marked abnormalities of a focal nature. Skull x-rays

TABLE 21. *Classification of Cerebrovascular Disease*

- Occlusive Vascular Disease
  - Dural sinus and cerebral venous thrombosis, associated with:
    - Meningitis
    - Infections of face, ears, or paranasal sinuses
    - Dehydration
    - Debilitating states (marantic)
    - Metastatic neoplasms, e.g., neuroblastoma
    - Congenital heart disease
    - Lead encephalopathy
    - Sturge-Weber-Dimitri syndrome (trigeminal encephaloangiomatosis)
  - Arterial thrombosis
    - Idiopathic or spontaneous, associated with:
      - Dissecting cerebral aneurysm
      - Arteriosclerosis (progeria)
      - Cyanotic congenital heart disease
      - Cerebral arteritis
        - Acute infectious diseases
        - Granulomatous (Takayasu's disease)
        - Syphilis
      - Collagen diseases
        - Polyarteritis nodosa
        - Lupus erythematosus
      - Blood dyscrasias: sickle-cell disease, polycythemia, thrombotic thrombocytopenia
      - Trauma to the carotid or cerebral arteries
      - Complications of arteriography
      - Extraarterial diseases
        - Retropharyngeal abscess
        - Mucomycosis
        - Tumors of the base of the skull
        - Craniometaphyseal dysplasia
  - Cerebral embolism, associated with:
    - Atrial fibrillation or other arrhythmias
      - Rheumatic heart disease
      - Congenital heart disease, right-to-left shunt
      - Coronary thrombosis
    - Acute or subacute bacterial endocarditis
    - Infarcted necrotic placental tissue
    - Air: complications of cardiac, neck, or thoracic surgery
    - Septic: pneumonia or lung abscess
    - Fat: complications of fractures of long bones
    - Tumor
- Intracranial Hemorrhage (includes intracerebral and subarachnoid)
  - Arteriovenus malformation or angioma
  - Intracranial aneurysm
  - Trauma
    - Cavernous sinus fistula
    - Subdural hemorrhage
    - Epidural hemorrhage
  - Blood dyscrasias
    - Leukemia
    - Thrombocytopenic purpura
    - Aplastic anemia
    - Hemophilia
    - Anaphylactoid purpura
  - Hypertension
  - Liver disease
  - Complications of anticoagulant therapy
  - Intracranial neoplasms
  - Deficiency syndromes
    - Vitamin B_1 deficiency (Wemicke encephalopathy)
    - Vitamin C deficiency (scurvy)
    - Vitamin K deficiency (hemorrhagic disease of the newborn)
  - Toxic or infectious encephalopathy

may be normal or show signs of increased intracranial pressure and mastoid disease. The site and extent of the thrombosis can often be confirmed by evaluating the venous phase of a carotid arteriogram.

Arterial Thrombosis

Cerebral arterial thromboses produce a variable clinical picture depending upon the rapidity of occlusion, the collateral circulation, and the maintenance of systemic blood pressure. The arterial occlusion usually occurs in a previously healthy child, although in some instances it is a complication of certain systemic diseases (Table 21).

CLINICAL MANIFESTATIONS. Depending upon the cause, the child demonstrates clinical phenomena of the underlying disorder as well as the neurologic changes secondary to the vessel involved.

Acute infantile hemiplegia characteristically appears in the first year or two of life. Unexplained or idiopathic hemiplegia is uncommon after the preschool period. The previously well youngster may suddenly develop fever, have a series of convulsions, and be left with a hemiplegia which may partially clear. In addition to the hemiplegia, there may be a cortical hemisensory loss, hemianopia, and aphasia. Recurrent focal motor seizures, often resistant to anticonvulsants, may complicate the subsequent course.

If the child is seen years after the onset, the involved extremities may be short, atrophic, and spastic. Arterial thrombosis may result in either cerebral hemiatrophy with a small head circumference or cerebral porencephaly with resultant macrocephaly. Seizures at the onset of the hemiparesis are more common in children under the age of 2 years and herald a poor prognosis for future seizures, hemiplegia, intellect, and behavior.

LABORATORY FINDINGS. Cerebrospinal fluid analysis during the acute episode is usually normal, but a slight leucocytic pleocytosis may be found a few weeks later. Electroencephalograms, occasionally normal, are characterized by a slow wave focus over the involved area. Radiologic studies are frequently of diagnostic importance. Early plain skull x-rays are normal. After a period of time, the x-rays may show the effect of cerebral hemiatrophy or porencephaly. The characteristic features of atrophy include thickening of the cranial vault, overdevelopment of the frontal and ethmoid sinuses, and elevation of the petrous pyramid of the temporal bone on the involved side. Porencephaly is suggested by the bulging and thinning of the cranial vault on the affected side and cephalofacial disproportion. Arteriography may demonstrate the arterial occlusion, and air contrast studies may show cerebral atrophy or a porencephalic cavity or fistula.

Cerebral Embolism

In embolism, a cerebral artery is occluded by a fragment of an organized thrombus, by bacteria, air, fat, or tumor. The middle cerebral artery or one of its branches is the vessel most frequently occluded. Cerebral embolic phenomena in childhood are usually of cardiac origin. Cyanotic congenital heart and rheumatic valvar disease may be responsible for this complication. Atrial fibrillation and other arrhythmias favor the formation of mural thrombi, fragments of which may then become detached. Emboli may result from the vegetations of bacterial endocarditis or from neck and thoracic surgery. In the newborn period, cerebral emboli may originate from liberated infarcted placental tissue. Arterial air embolism has been encountered with greater frequency since the advent of newer techniques in thoracic surgery. Fat embolism is usually associated with fractures of long bones.

CLINICAL MANIFESTATIONS. Cerebral embolism is characterized by acute onset without significant prodromata. Occasionally, premonitory symptoms of headache, vomiting, and lassitude occur. The clinical picture may be complete within seconds to minutes and may appear at any time of the day, unrelated to physical activity. Convulsions, transient loss of consciousness, and headache may be initially observed. Focal neurologic findings depend upon the cerebral artery occluded. Transient blindness is the most characteristic manifestation of air embolism.

Fat embolism has a characteristic clinical picture. Twelve to 48 hours after a long bone fracture, fever and pulmonary signs and symptoms appear with respiratory distress and blood-tinged sputum. This is then followed in a few hours by neurologic manifestations, petechial hemorrhages in the skin, fat in the retinal vessels, and free fat droplets in the urine.

LABORATORY FINDINGS. A moderate polymorphonuclear leucocytosis is frequently observed. Cerebrospinal fluid analysis and skull x-rays are usually normal. Electroencephalograms most commonly show a slow wave focus over the involved areas which tends to be persistent.

Intracranial Hemorrhage

Intracranial hemorrhage is the result of a defect in the integrity of cerebral blood vessels with extravasation of blood into one or more of the following: brain, ventricles, and subarachnoid, epidural, and subdural spaces. Trauma is the most frequent cause of hemorrhage, but not infrequently it may result from rupture of a vascular malformation or aneurysm or may be associated with infectious, toxic, metabolic, or neoplastic conditions (Table 21).

Despite the varied causes, clinical manifestations of hemorrhage are similar, and etiologic delineation is further complicated by the nonspecific finding of blood in the cerebrospinal fluid. Proper management is largely dependent upon delineation of the specific cause, which is possible only with a complete clinical history and adequate laboratory facilities.

Subarachnoid hemorrhage is characterized by signs and symptoms of increased intracranial pressure and meningeal irritation. The onset is usually dramatic with severe headache, vomiting, loss of consciousness, and convulsions. Fever, often a misleading feature, may be prominent, and systemic hypertension is not uncommon. Evidence of meningeal irritation is an early clinical manifestation with nuchal rigidity and Brudzinski and Kernig signs. The child with intracerebral bleeding may have evidence of blood in the subarachnoid space, in which case there may be the symptoms and signs previously mentioned as well as focal neurologic deficit. Secondary hydrocephalus may be a complication in those children who survive subarachnoid bleeding due to partial obliteration of the subarachnoid space.

The neonate with intracranial bleeding shows a more nonspecific picture with apathy or restlessness, cyanosis or pallor, bulging of the fontanels, respiratory distress, convulsions, a high-pitched cry, vomiting, poor suck, and an exaggerated or absent Moro reflex.

Children with intracranial hemorrhage may show a polymorphonuclear leucocytosis greater than 20,000 per mm^3, a normal or moderately elevated erythrocyte sedimentation rate, and a transient hyperglycemia, albuminuria, and glycosuria. The electroencephalographic changes with subarachnoid hemorrhage are similar to those seen in closed head injury; the tracing is diffusely abnormal with generalized slow activity which disappears as the clinical state of the child improves. Blood in the cerebrospinal fluid is the most conclusive evidence of intracranial bleeding. This must be clearly differentiated from the hemorrhage due to a traumatic lumbar puncture. Failure of the fluid to clear in successive test tubes or a xanthochromic supernatant in a hemorrhage older than two hours is diagnostic of bleeding antedating the lumbar puncture. The fluid is usually under increased pressure, the protein content is elevated, and white cells are in proportion to red cells.

Vascular Malformations

Vascular anomalies are the most common cause of *primary* subarachnoid hemorrhage in children and are at least 10 times as common as intracranial aneurysms.

The vascular malformations are usually classified as traumatic, infectious, or congenital. Traumatic or infectious causes are rarely seen because anatomically the cerebral vessels are unique and the principal cerebral arteries and veins are not in juxtaposition. The sole exception is the internal carotid artery in the cavernous sinus.

Arteriovenous malformations occur most frequently in two areas: deep midline (the area drained by the great vein of Galen) and hemispheric (the area supplied by major branches of the internal carotid artery).

DEEP MIDLINE ARTERIOVENOUS MALFORMATION. The malformation involving the Galenic system is a direct anastomosis between major cerebral arteries, most commonly the posterior cerebral or the superior cerebellar artery and the great vein. There is marked enlargement of the vein, forming a midline aneurysm which not infrequently compresses and displaces the aqueduct, the third ventricle, and the quadrigeminal plate.

The clinical manifestations can be divided into three groups depending upon the size of the shunt and the corresponding age at which symptoms first appear.

1. The symptomatic newborn infant has a shunt of arterial blood into the venous circulation of such magnitude that it results in peripheral congestion and congestive heart failure.

2. In infancy there is less blood shunted, with a paucity of clinical cardiac manifestations; however, cardiomegaly may be present. In this group, hydrocephalus is the most prominent clinical feature as the markedly distended vein of Galen displaces and compresses the aqueduct of Sylvius. An important sign in this age group is an intracranial bruit.

3. The older child has a still smaller shunt, and dilation of the vein of Galen is only moderate. There is neither cardiovascular dysfunction nor hydrocephalus, but headaches and episodes of subarachnoid hemorrhage are common. Because of the small size of the shunt, an intracranial bruit is rarely present in this age group.

Laboratory findings are variable and depend upon the magnitude of the arteriovenous shunt. The electrocardiogram, especially in the younger child, may show an intermediate axis or left axis deviation, and in this age group cardiomegaly may be present on chest x-ray. The cerebrospinal fluid is usually under increased pressure and not infrequently shows evidence of recent or old hemorrhage. Increased oxygen tension in jugular venous blood is an important simple diagnostic test.

Radiographic findings are frequently of diagnostic importance. Plain skull films in the younger child may show evidence of increased intracranial pressure. Air contrast studies suggest a vein of Galen malformation by demonstrating a posterior midline mass displacing the aqueduct downward. Cerebral angiography is the definitive diagnostic tool and demonstrates a midline collection of contrast material outlining the vein of Galen (Fig. 55).

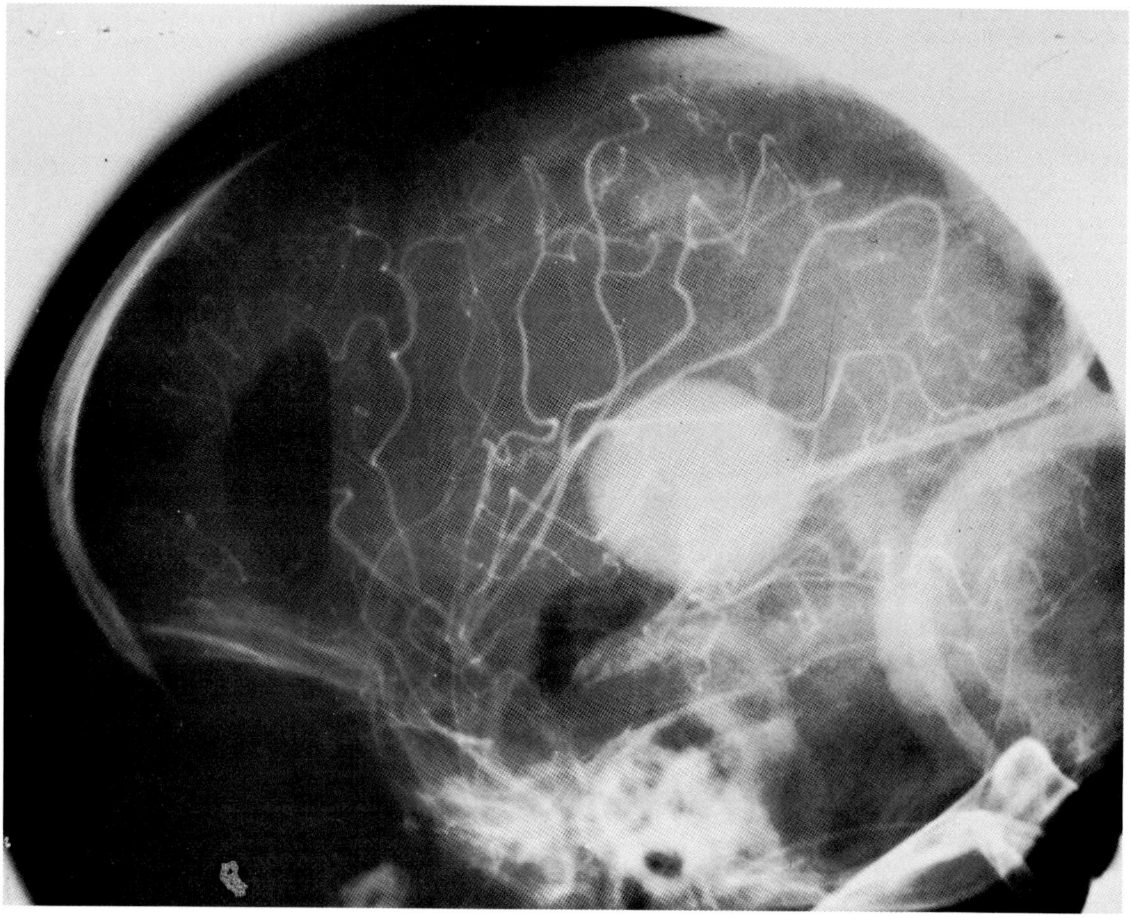

Fig. 55. Lateral view of carotid arteriogram demonstrates a markedly dilated vein of Galen. (Note air in dilated lateral ventricle from previous pneumoencephalogram.)

HEMISPHERIC MALFORMATION. This malformation involving branches of the internal carotid artery is most frequently found over the convexity of the brain in the territory of the middle cerebral artery. The lesion consists of an enlarged feeding artery and a mass of dilated, tortuous veins. The onset of clinical manifestations is most commonly in late childhood or in adolescence. The child may complain of periodic migrainoid headaches for many years, but diagnosis is frequently not made until the acute onset of subarachnoid hemorrhage. The child with a hemispheric malformation may complain of and localize a pulsatile sound in the head, and a pathologic bruit may be heard on auscultation. The cardinal clinical manifestations are related to the site of the malformation. Involvement of branches of the middle cerebral artery is characterized by clinical manifestations referable to the motor cortex with focal, motor or sensory, and generalized seizures followed by transient postictal paralysis which gradually becomes a permanent lateralizing sign. Parietal lobe involvement is suggested by contralateral sensory seizures and hemisensory deficit involving position, stereognosis, discrimination, and localization of tactile stimuli and body image. Posterior fossa malformations produce signs of cerebellar dysfunction and evidence of increased intracranial pressure.

Routine laboratory studies are often unrewarding, as skull x-rays, electroencephalogram, and cerebrospinal fluid analysis are often normal. Special studies are usually required. Visual fields may demonstrate a homonymous hemianopia. Radioactive isotope studies may show an abnormal uptake. The diagnosis can be confirmed only by cerebral angiography.

Traumatic Arteriovenous Fistula

This fistula can occur only in the region of the cavernous sinus where artery and vein are in juxtaposition. Following trauma there develops a highly characteristic clinical picture with pulsating exophthalmos, intracranial bruit, and involvement of the first two branches of the trigeminal nerve (facial sensory loss and diminished corneal reflex) and the oculomotor, trochlear, and abducens nerves (dilated and fixed pupil, diplopia, and extraocular muscle palsies).

Carotid angiogram is diagnostic, with demonstration of the cavernous sinus during the arterial phase.

Intracranial Aneurysm

Ruptured saccular aneurysms are a rare cause of subarachnoid hemorrhage in children. Many cases go unrecognized because the aneurysm commonly involves the bifurcation of the smaller peripherally placed arteries.

Clinical manifestations are due to direct pressure of the aneurysm on surrounding structures or to hemorrhage from rupture. The onset is often dramatic without warning, and death may result from massive bleeding. Hemorrhage into the subarachnoid space results in signs and symptoms of meningeal irritation and increased intracranial pressure. Intracortical hemorrhage may give rise to focal neurologic signs dependent on the areas involved. Unless the aneurysm is occluded by a thrombus, its presence can often be demonstrated by cerebral angiography. Early angiography is indicated except in the presence of coma with fluctuating vital signs.

Diagnosis of Cerebrovascular Diseases

Differential diagnosis must distinguish among the various types of cerebrovascular conditions and other conditions involving the central nervous system, such as brain tumors, abscess, trauma, epilepsy, and meningitis.

Treatment of Cerebrovascular Diseases

A rational therapeutic program must consist of a complete understanding of the pathologic process and its resultant alteration of function. For a given disease there are both nonspecific and specific therapeutic measures.

Nonspecific therapy consists of fluids to prevent dehydration and maintain circulation, antibiotics to combat infection, anticonvulsants to control seizures, and anticoagulants when indicated to prevent extension of the thrombus. Increased intracranial pressure secondary to cerebral edema may be managed by the introduction of light hypothermia and the use of corticosteroids and/or urea.

Venous and dural sinus thromboses are managed by strict control of fluids and electrolytes and, when indicated, antibiotics and anticonvulsants. Mastoidectomy with decompression of the lateral sinus is indicated when this dural sinus is involved. Repeated and often daily lumbar punctures may be necessary to reduce the pressure, but if ineffective a lumboperitoneal shunt may be required to preserve vision.

Arterial thromboses are treated symptomatically. Anticoagulation is contraindicated. The only indication for vascular surgery is thrombosis of the extracranial portion of the internal carotid artery.

The management of arterial emboli is mainly symptomatic, including skillful nursing care. Anticoagulation may be used to prevent the formation of future emboli.

The treatment of arteriovenous malformations is both medical and surgical. Medical therapy includes treatment of cardiac decompensation, phlebotomy to control blood volume, and the careful management of fluids and electrolytes. Surgery is hazardous but offers the only possibility for a cure. It may be indicated if the vascular lesion is accessible and neither involves the dominant hemisphere nor supplies vital structures.

References

GENERAL

A classification and outline of cerebrovascular diseases. Neurology, 8:395, 1958.

Poser, C. M., and Taveras, J. M. Clinical aspects of cerebral angiography in children. Pediatrics, 16:73, 1955.

CEREBRAL VENOUS AND DURAL SINUS THROMBOSIS

Byers, R. K., and Hass, G. M. Thrombosis of the dural venous sinuses in infancy and in childhood. Amer. J. Dis. Child., 45:1161, 1933.

Greer, M., and Schotland, D. Abnormal hemoglobin as a cause of neurologic disease. Neurology, 12:114, 1962.

——— and Berk, M. S. Lateral sinus obstruction and mastoiditis. Pediatrics, 31:840, 1963.

Symonds, C. P. Otitic hydrocephalus. Neurology, 6:681, 1956.

CEREBRAL ARTERIAL THROMBOSIS

Banker, B. Q. Cerebral vascular disease in infancy and childhood: 1. Occlusive vascular diseases. J. Neuropath. Exp. Neurol., 20:127, 1961.

Bax, M., and Mitchell, R., eds. Acute Hemiplegia in Childhood. London, William Heineman, Ltd. (Little Club Clinics in Developmental Medicine, No. 6), 1962.

Bickerstaff, E. R. Aetiology of acute hemiplegia in childhood. Brit. Med. J., 2:82, 1964.

Byers, R. K., and McLean, W. T. Etiology and course of certain hemiplegias with aphasia in childhood. Pediatrics, 29:376, 1962.

Carter, S., and Gold, A. P. Acute hemiplegia in infancy and childhood. Pediat. Clin. N. Amer., 14:851, 1967.

Davie, J. C., and Coxe, W. Occlusive disease of the carotid artery in children. Arch. Neurol., 17:313, 1967.
Dyke, C. G., Davidoff, L. M., and Masson, C. B. Cerebral hemiatrophy with homolateral hypertrophy of the skull and sinuses. Surg. Gynec. Obstet., 57:588, 1933.
Freeman, J. M., and Gold, A. P. Porencephaly simulating subdural hematoma in childhood. Amer. J. Dis. Child., 107:327, 1964.
Gold, A. P., and Yahr, M. D. Childhood lupus erythematosus: a clinical and pathological study of the neurological manifestations. Trans. Amer. Neurol. Ass., 1960, p. 96.
Gross, R. E. Arterial embolism and thrombosis in infancy. Amer. J. Dis. Child., 70:61, 1945.
Hilal, S. K., Solomon, G. E., Gold, A. P., and Carter S. Primary cerebral arterial occlusive disease in children. Part I: Acute acquired hemiplegia. Radiology, 99:71, 1971.
——— Primary cerebral arterial occlusive disease in children. Part II: Neurocutaneous syndromes. Radiology, 99:87, 1971.
Ouvrier, R. A., and Hopkins, I. J. Occlusive disease of the vertebro-basilar arterial system in childhood. Develop. Med. Child. Neurol., 12:186, 1970.
Pitner, S. E. Carotid thrombosis due to intraoral trauma. New Eng. J. Med., 274:764, 1966.
Shillito, J., Jr. Carotid arteritis: a cause of hemiplegia in childhood. J. Neurosurg., 21:540, 1964.
Solomon, G. E., Hilal, S. K., Gold, A. P., and Carter, S. Natural history of acute hemiplegia of childhood. Brain, 93:107, 1970.
Tyler, H. R., and Clark, D. B. Incidence of neurological complications in congenital heart disease. A.M.A. Arch. Neurol. Psychiat., 77:17, 1957.
——— and Clark, D. B. Cerebrovascular accidents in patients with congenital heart disease. A.M.A. Arch. Neurol. Psychiat., 77:483, 1957.
Wisoff, H. S., and Rothballer, A. B. Cerebral arterial thrombosis in children: Review of literature and addition of two cases in apparently healthy children. Arch. Neurol., 4:258, 1961.
Wolman, L. Cerebral dissecting aneurysms. Brain, 82: 276, 1959.

CEREBRAL EMBOLISM

Clark, R. M., and Linell, E. A. Case report: Prenatal occlusion of the internal carotid artery. J. Neurol. Neurosurg. Psychiat., 17:295, 1954.
Cohen, A. C. et al. Air embolism. Ann. Intern. Med., 35:779, 1952.
Schneider, R. C. Fat embolism: A problem in the differential diagnosis of craniocerebral trauma. J. Neurosurg., 9:1, 1952.
Wells, C. E. Cerebral embolism: The natural history, prognostic signs, and effects of anticoagulation. A.M.A. Arch. Neurol. Psychiat., 81:667, 1959.

INTRACRANIAL HEMORRHAGE

Chalgreen, W. S. Neurologic complications of the hemorrhagic diseases. Neurology, 3:126, 1953.
Gold, A. P., Ransohoff, J., and Carter, S. Vein of Galen malformation. Acta Neurol. Scand. (Suppl. I), p. 40, 1964.
Groch, S. N., Sayre, G. P., and Heck, F. J. Cerebral hemorrhage in leukemia. A.M.A. Arch. Neurol. Psychiat., 2:439, 1960.
Levine, O. R., Jameson, A. G., Nellhaus, G., and Gold, A. P. Cardiac complication of cerebral arteriovenous fistulas. Pediatrics, 30:563, 1962.
Lewis, I. C., and Philpott, M. G. Neurological complications of Schönlein-Henoch syndrome. Arch. Dis. Child., 31:369, 1956.
Silverstein, A. Intracranial bleeding in hemophilia. A.M.A. Arch. Neurol. Psychiat., 3:141, 1960.
Sullivan, M. P. Intracranial complications in leukemia in children. Pediatrics, 20:757, 1957.

Chapter 8
TRAUMA TO THE NERVOUS SYSTEM

JAMES F. HAMMILL

Trauma results in the death of 15,000 children per year and 100,000 individuals of all ages. The number of deaths in this country due to trauma in the age group from birth to 14 years exceeds the combined fatalities from infectious disease, malignancy, and cardiovascular-renal syndromes.

Forty percent of all traumatic cases in childhood involve head injuries either alone or combined with other injuries. The peak age incidence is in the second year of life, with males outnumbering females 2:1. Peak seasonal incidence is in the spring and summer months during the late afternoon and early evening hours.

In spite of this magnitude of serious injury the mortality rate is in the range of only 0.5 percent, indicating three million childhood injuries per year with over 90 percent not requiring hospitalization.

Head injuries may affect the scalp, skull, or the nervous system; they may occur alone or in combination. Most injuries involving the nervous system represent simple concussion or mild contusion, and there is complete recovery without complications. Some, however, may be more serious or even life-threatening and require careful analysis and management.

Scalp Injuries

Lacerations

Scalp injury is most often due to blunt trauma; however, the resulting wound is usually a smooth linear cut due to the unyielding surface of the bone over which the blow occurs. Wounds of the skin layer are separated only minimally owing to fixation by the underlying fibrous tissue septa. When the galea is involved the wound will gape, particularly if it is in a transverse direction. Bleeding is quite marked because of the rich anastomatic blood supply of the

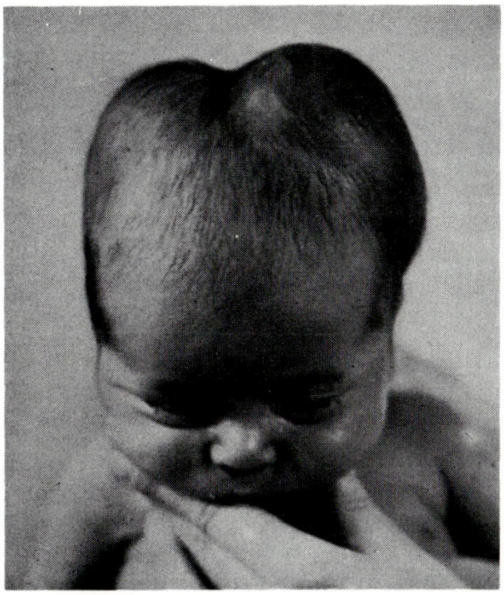

Fig. 56. Cephalohematoma involving both parietal bones in an infant 13 days old.

scalp and the limited contraction-retraction ability of the vessels firmly anchored in the dense connective tissue layer. Consequently, large lacerations heal quite well, and infection rarely occurs unless there is gross contamination or tissue destruction. However, the potential hazards of infection of the skull and intracranial contents are of considerable importance because of the magnitude of the problem when it does occur. Infectious complications are invariably the result of poor initial handling.

If the child's general condition prohibits immediate definitive wound care, and if hemorrhage is not excessive, a sterile pressure dressing may be applied. Where necessary, primary closure may be delayed for 8 to 12 hours without any significant increase in the incidence of infection. In the majority of cases the wound may be treated at once.

Hematoma and Cephalohematoma

Hematomas resulting from bleeding into an area of injury within the dense connective tissue layer of the scalp are common, but because of the density of the tissue they are generally not very large and absorb within two or three days. Galeal laceration permits bleeding from above to permeate the subgaleal loose connective tissue layer and may result in an extensive, rapidly appearing swelling that can assume enormous proportions, as there is no limiting membrane to prevent its spread.

Bleeding beneath the pericranium is most common in, but not restricted to, the incompletely ossified and highly vascular skull characteristic of the first two years of life. These collections are restricted by the pericranial suture line attachment, occur most often in the parietal area, and are the swellings for which the term cephalohematoma is usually reserved (Fig. 56). Both subgaleal and subpericranial hematomas present findings on palpation that may be confused with an underlying depressed fracture. Subgaleal collections of partially clotted blood may develop a soft center surrounded by an indurated ring which may be mistaken for a rim of bone about an area of skull depression. The pericranial fibrous suture attachment demarcating cephalohematomas is also commonly confused with a depressed skull fracture. Fracture sites, depressed or linear, underlying hematomas require radiographic examination to clarify the diagnosis.

The larger hematomas are absorbed in 2 to 4 weeks. When cephalohematomas persist, pericranial proliferation occurs with the production of bony callus; ultimately a thin layer of bone may be formed in the involved area. Only rarely is there calcification of an entire nonabsorbed hemorrhagic area. Aspiration or open evacuation of hematomas is contraindicated as the partially clotted blood is difficult to aspirate and the risk of infection is great. In the infant, cephalohematomas may be of such size as to play a significant role in the development of anemia, and their breakdown products are commonly responsible for varied degrees of jaundice. A scalp swelling associated with an underlying linear fracture, meningeal tear, and leakage of cerebrospinal fluid into the subgaleal space may be noted. Collections of this type are termed subgaleal or subepicranial hydromas and are not uncommon over linear skull fractures in children. They are usually less extensive and softer than hematomas and have a less well-defined ring of induration. When the fluid is not mixed with blood, transillumination is greater than in the case of hematomas, and the mass may be noted to fluctuate with coughing and straining. These collections subside spontaneously with healing of the underlying dural tear. If they are large or if they persist beyond 4 to 7 days, the swelling may be reduced by lumbar puncture. This procedure may also be used as a differential diagnostic test to determine the type of fluid present. Pressure dressings do not hasten absorption of hematoma or hydroma and may contribute to skin breakdown and infection.

Craniocerebral Trauma

PATHOPHYSIOLOGY. The human head may withstand tremendous force and yet maintain both skull and cerebral integrity. The position of the head at impact, suture patency, and degree of movement at the craniospinal junction are important variables. Blood pressure may increase to 150 percent or more above normal to compensate for increased intracranial pressure in an attempt to maintain cerebral circulation.

Shock rarely occurs on a purely neural basis and is usually due to blood loss from associated extracerebral injuries. It may be noted terminally where it is an ominous prognostic sign correlated with extensive and irreversible cerebral damage. Adequate respiration and oxygenation are essential to blood pressure maintenance. Hypoxia may result in an increased blood pressure due to chemoreceptor effect in the absence of increased intracranial pressure but will soon result in hypotension due to cardiac hypoxia.

Experimental cerebral injury in the acute postconcussive phase shows marked circulatory slowing associated with the onset of cerebral edema. Within minutes brain volume may increase over 5 percent.

The mass movement of the intracranial contents following injury results in varied contusion patterns both at the point of impact and at a distance from it both ipsilaterally and contralaterally. Disruption of the blood-brain barrier results in laceration and subarachnoid and intracerebral bleeding. Marked movement may tear blood vessels between the brain and meninges and result in subdural collections. This vascular damage most commonly involves the cortical bridging veins entering the dural-encased superior longitudinal sinus, but may occur at any point. Disruption of extradural vessels, either venous or arterial, will result in extradural hematoma.

Transient unconsciousness after injury reflects a sudden physiologic block at the brainstem level. The brainstem reticular formation has an alerting function, mediating sensory input to higher centers. Following trauma, this formation may enter an absolutely refractory state, recovery from which directly correlates with return to consciousness. This mechanism is the commonest cause of the transient concussion picture and is due to increased cervicocranial mobility after impact permitting transmission of increased angular acceleration and shear strains to the entire brain but particularly the brainstem. Animals with the head relatively fixed can routinely sustain a head injury force double that usually resulting in concussion.

Skull Fractures

CLINICAL MANIFESTATION. Skull fractures may involve the vault or base and may be of the simple linear type, diastatic (abnormal suture separation occurring at the time of impact), simple depressed, comminuted, or the ping-pong or pond variety. They may occur as an isolated manifestation of head trauma but more often are associated with underlying cerebral injury. Simple linear fractures and diastatic fractures resulting in suture separation are of little immediate significance other than to indicate the force of the blow and the point of maximal impact. Over 80 percent of all skull fractures are of the simple linear type and the parietal area is involved five times more commonly than other regions of the skull. Diastatic fractures have the same medicolegal significance as a fracture line and most often involve the lamboidal suture. A lamboidal suture separation wider than 1.5 mm, particularly at several points in its course, is usually considered abnormal, as is a coronal suture spread of greater than 2 mm (Fig. 57).

Children less than one year of age have significantly less calcification of the vault than do older children, and there is greater elasticity of both its inner and outer tables. This explains the fact that fractures occur in the neonatal period, and occasionally later, in which both outer and inner skull tables are displaced inward but without an actual break in either. These have been termed ping-pong or pond fractures.

Fractures of the base of the skull may be indicated by bilateral orbital ecchymoses in anterior fossa lesions (Fig. 58) and by retroauricular ecchymosis (Battle's sign) with tympanic membrane discoloration in involvement of the petrous bone in the middle fossa (Fig. 59). Otorrhea and rhinorrhea imply basilar skull fracture and are potentially of more serious consideration because of the risk of infection. The posttraumatic collection of intracranial air in any of the meningeal spaces (aerocele) or the ventricular system (pneumoencephalocele) implies fractures through the paranasal sinuses.

LABORATORY DATA AND DIAGNOSIS. Skull x-rays are the essential aid to diagnosis. There is seldom an indication for emergency films, as they rarely add to management of the immediate problem and are best delayed until the child's condition permits optimal radiographic study both of the skull and of all suspected areas of trauma. A skeletal survey to detect areas of multiple osseous injury is essential in infants and very young children; beyond these ages it becomes a matter of clinical judgment. Questionable drainage from the nose may be differentiated by collecting a specimen of the discharge and analyzing for glucose, which is present in negligible amounts in nasal secretions compared to cerebrospinal fluid. This may be done chemically or by the use of a glucose reacting test tape.

TREATMENT. Simple linear fractures without underlying damage do not require treatment other than analgesics for headache and irritability. It is important to emphasize to the parents that a simple fracture of the skull is of itself little to be concerned about. Its mere demonstration in an otherwise intact child should not cause alarm, limit usual activities, or be considered ominous as regards prognosis. It is good practice to secure repeat skull films 3 months after the injury to demonstrate a uniting fracture line. In the absence of union, further films should be obtained at 2- to 4-month intervals to detect such complications as a leptomeningeal cyst. Fractures in children generally heal in 6 to 12 months.

Pond or ping-pong fractures of infancy usually do not require surgical elevation. In extremely rare instances an underlying defect of cerebral cortex may result in a lack of brain growth and failure of the skull depression to elevate; a 3-month period of ob-

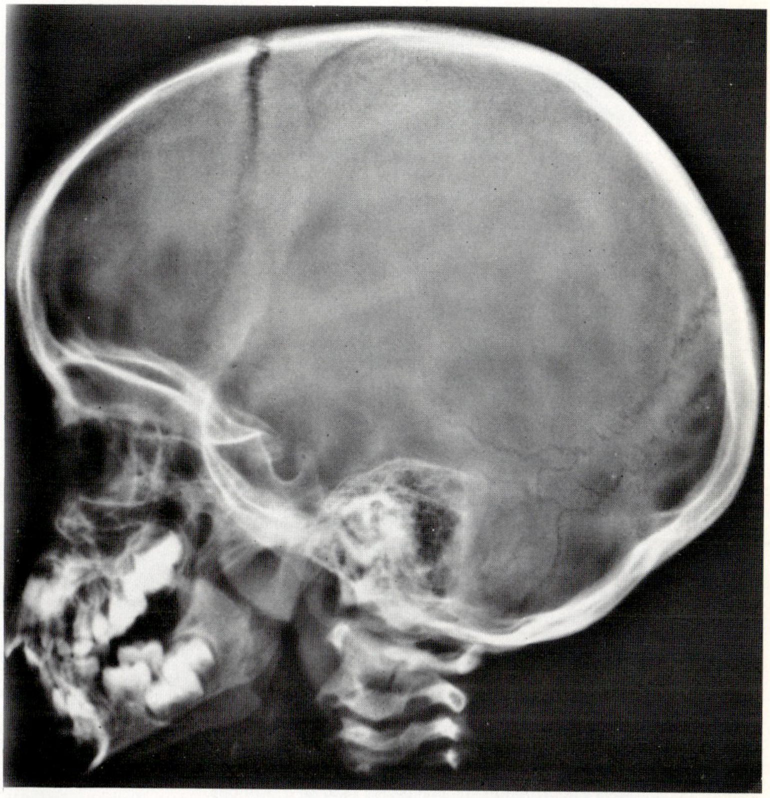

Fig. 57. Lateral skull film of a 4-year-old child with diastatic coronal suture separation.

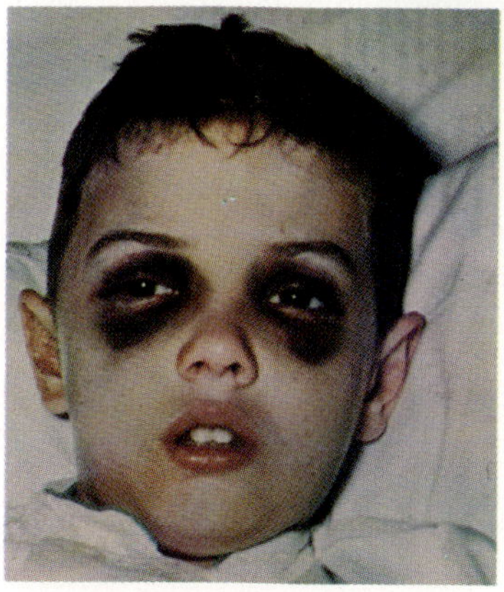

Fig. 58. Five-year-old child with bilateral orbital ecchymoses secondary to an anterior fossa basilar fracture.

servation will decide this. Early surgical intervention is rarely warranted regardless of the location or size of the depression (Fig. 60).

Fractures depressed more than 0.5 cm should be elevated to avoid the formation of undesirable cerebromeningeal cicatrices with the attendant danger of focal neurologic defect and seizures. Early surgery is indicated, as it is in all compound and comminuted skull fractures.

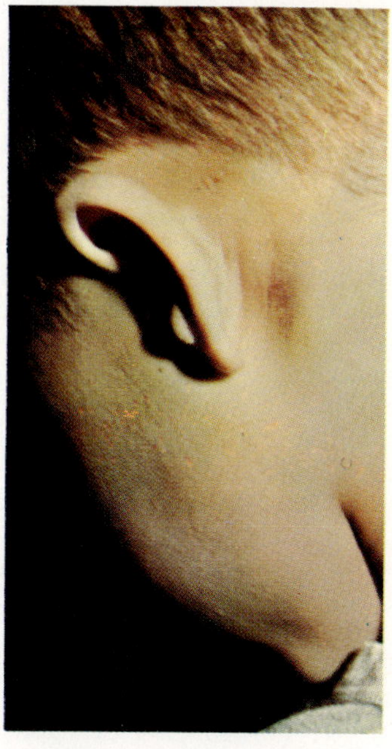

Fig. 59. Same child as Figure 58. Retroauricular ecchymosis (Battle's sign) due to fracture of the petrous bone in the middle fossa.

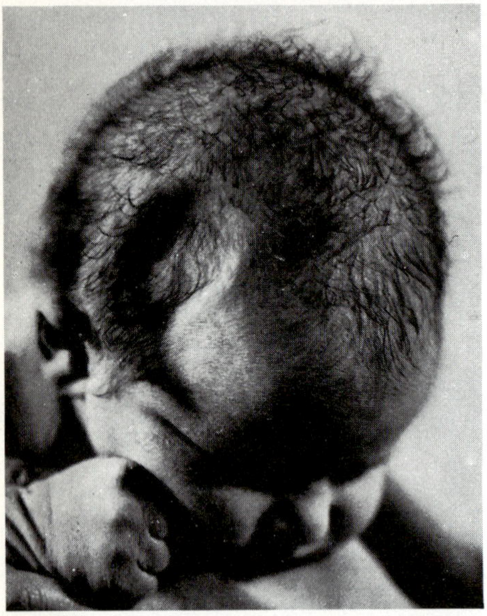

Fig. 60. Depressed fracture of skull from birth injury. Infant delivered by version and extraction with application of forceps to aftercoming head. Depressed fracture of right parietal bone, said to be related to abnormality of mother's pelvis. Difficulty in resuscitation and cyanosis during the first few hours. Right internal strabismus. No signs of increased intracranial pressure. Patient made a complete recovery without operation. Physically and mentally normal at age of 5½ years.

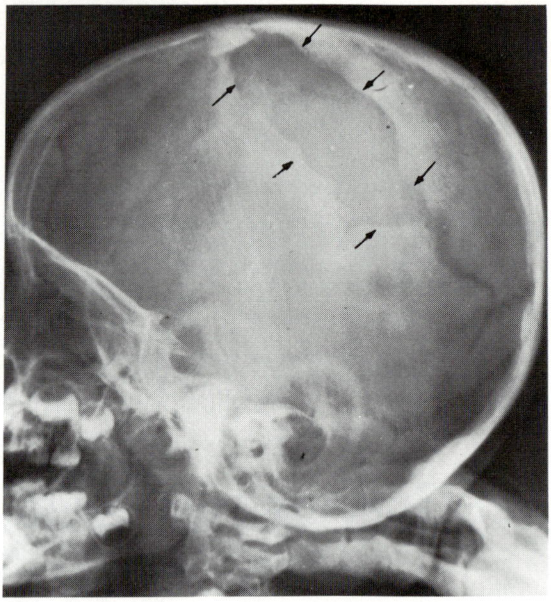

Fig. 61. Leptomeningeal cyst showing large area of parietal skull erosion eight months after a simple linear fracture.

Basal skull fractures resulting in rhinorrhea or otorrhea require hospitalization. The child is maintained in a semiupright bed position, and plugging or irrigation of the involved orifices is contraindicated. The use of prophylactic antibiotics and chemotherapy is controversial; however, in the presence of a demonstrated cerebrospinal fluid leak, therapy is comparable to that for undiagnosed bacterial meningitis. Spontaneous cessation of cerebrospinal fluid drainage may occur. If flow persists beyond a week, surgical repair should be considered, as the danger of meningitis is overwhelming. This hazard remains as long as fistulous patency exists and may result in repeated infections, diffuse arachnoiditis, and secondary hydrocephalus.

Traumatic aerocele, if persistent, is also an indication for operative intervention. Intracranial air tends to be rapidly absorbed. If x-rays at 48- to 72-hour intervals show persistence of air or an increased collection, surgery should not be delayed.

In cases of rhinorrhea, coughing and sneezing may produce increased drainage and actually permit air to enter the intracranial cavity. Accentuation of headache under these circumstances may be the result of delayed intracranial air collection and be documented by repeat x-rays. Suppression of coughing and sneezing is indicated in all patients with posttraumatic otorrhea or rhinorrhea.

A late sequela of a linear fracture in young children is a leptomeningeal cyst, or more accurately, a growing skull fracture. This results from dural laceration, projection of the arachnoid membrane into the fracture site and brain herniation producing bone erosion of the overlying skull over a period of months to years. The late onset of focal seizures, increased intracranial pressure, focal neurologic signs, and occasionally visible and palpable skull deformity should alert one to this posttraumatic complication. Skull x-rays are diagnostic (Fig. 61), revealing an area of erosion over a prior fracture site. Growing skull fractures are usually in the parietal area and should be suspected when the initial fracture line is wide or has been associated with a subepicranial hydroma.

Extradural Hematoma

Extradural hematoma refers to bleeding between the skull and dura usually from a tear in the middle meningeal artery due to a temporal bone fracture. Laceration of the dural sinuses or other branches of the extradural vascular complex may also result in hemorrhage into the extradural space. As the skull matures, vessels in this location are firmly imbedded in bony grooves and are more vulnerable to damage by fractures that involve these channels. Children less than 2 years of age rarely sustain extradural hemorrhage, as these vessels are less adherent to the calvarium. Because of the greater elasticity of the young skull, damage of this type may exist without any radiographic demonstration of fracture.

The typical clinical syndrome is apparent during the first 12 to 24 hours after initial injury. The child may be rendered briefly unconscious by the original trauma, regain awareness, and after a period of several hours lapse into coma with signs of increased intracranial pressure, hemiplegia, and at times focal seizures. An equal number present without a lucid interval; these children progressively merge from a moderate initial lethargy or stupor into a state of profound coma.

There is no mechanism for the absorption of an extradural hemorrhage, and its increasing mass rapidly raises intracranial pressure with a progressive rise in systolic blood pressure and slowing of the pulse. The eventual result is a decreased irregular respiratory rate with terminal hypotension and tachycardia. The relatively sudden elevation in intracranial pressure is responsible for subhyaloid retinal hemorrhages and early third nerve compression on the affected side, resulting in a fixed, dilated pupil. Subhyaloid hemorrhages are globular extravasations of blood onto the retina, rather than into it. They may change shape and position with head movement, being a mobile fluid collection between the retina and the subhyaloid membrane overlying it. In young children a fracture line may be absent, or not visible, suture diastasis may be the only evidence of trauma, and the lucid interval may be absent. The syndrome usually runs a course of 6 to 12 hours in adults but may extend from 24 to 96 hours in children because of the greater incidence of venous versus arterial bleeding. Either type is more commonly associated with anemia than in comparable adult injuries.

Extradural hemorrhage represents the most lethal complication of head injury, with a mortality rate in untreated cases of 100 percent and in operatively treated cases of almost 50 percent. It is one of the few medical emergencies requiring immediate operative intervention. Untreated cases seldom survive more than 2 to 3 days, although occasional instances with a course of 1 week or more have been noted.

Treatment demands immediate diagnosis via plain skull x-rays, echoencephalography, and arteriography, where feasible, followed by definitive surgery. Local conditions or the patient's status may preclude detailed evaluation and necessitate immediate surgery on clinical grounds. Prognosis for survival and neurologic integrity is directly proportional to the patient's preoperative status and duration of unconsciousness. Under optimal conditions complete recovery without residua may be expected.

Subdural Hematoma

In contrast to the infrequent occurrence of extradural hematomas in children and their relative rarity in patients less than 2 years of age, subdural hematomas are common, with approximately 85 percent occurring in children 1 year of age or less. The syndrome may present as an acute problem (within 3 days), subacutely (within 4 to 20 days), or chronically (greater than 20 days) as dated from the time of presumed trauma.

TABLE 22. *Frequency of Signs and Symptoms of Subdural Hematomas*

	Percent
Anemia	70
Seizures	65
Vomiting	50
X-ray signs of increased pressure	50
Enlarged head	40
History of trauma	40
Retinal hemorrhages	40
Hyperirritability	35
Bulging fontanel	35
Focal neurologic defect	35
Slowed development	20
Skull fracture	20

Hemorrhage in this instance is venous, the blood collecting in the potential space between dura and arachnoid. It arises from laceration veins bridging the area from the cortex to the superior longitudinal sinus or less often from venous bleeding associated with cerebral laceration or an actual venous sinus tear. Such collections in children are bilateral in 80 percent of the cases. These hemorrhages seldom absorb and tend to become encapsulated by dural proliferation.

In infancy the clinical picture differs from that in the older child and often consists of a gradually increasing intracranial pressure syndrome with an enlarging head, bulging fontanel, anemia, seizures, irritability, vomiting, and failure to thrive. The relative frequency of signs and symptoms is indicated in Table 22.

In young children the syndrome of subdural hematoma may be further delineated by subdural puncture through the lateral recess of a patent anterior fontanel. This must be performed bilaterally. When the diagnosis has been established, repeated daily aspirations of 50 ml or more of subdural fluid from alternate sides, within the limits of patient tolerance and ease of flow, may be made. This technique attempts to empty the subdural space and permit cortical reexpansion to obliterate it. If after 10 to 14 days this regimen has not been effective, it is unlikely that further attempts will be successful. Inability to tap the subdural space "dry" may be due to absolute enlargement of the cranial cavity by the hematoma to such a degree that the brain cannot reexpand to fill it, failure of expansion due to membrane formation about a chronic hematoma, secondary cerebral atrophy, a fistula from the subarachnoid into the subdural space, or continued bleeding. Surgical drainage, craniotomy with membrane removal, or a shunting procedure will be necessary. Careful attention must be directed to preventing or correcting

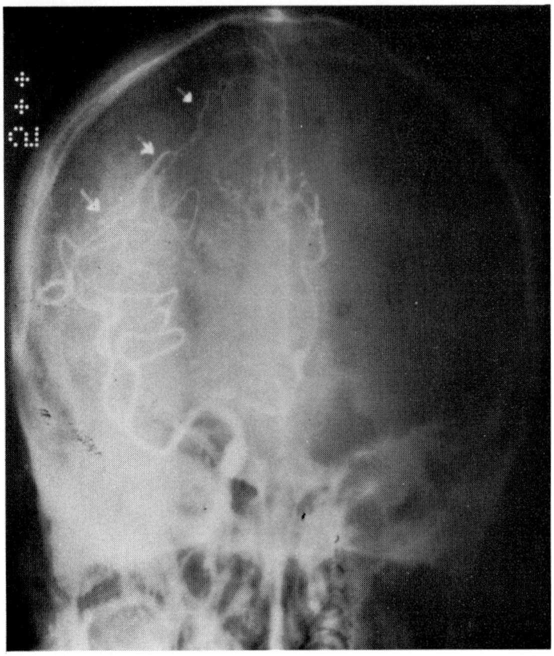

Fig. 62. Carotid arteriogram anteroposterior view, showing a subdural hematoma (arrows) displacing surface vessels and brain from the inner table of the skull.

anemia, hypoproteinemia, and electrolyte abnormalities during the period of therapy.

Subdural hematomas in older children require surgical drainage and seldom reaccumulate after operation.

Negative findings from subdural punctures do not absolutely rule out subdural collections. The exploring needle may not enter the fluid lake, or viscous, compartmented liquid may preclude withdrawal. Evidence of increasing intracranial pressure, focal seizures, and deterioration in general neurologic status and level of consciousness should alert one to the problem. Electroencephalography may reveal marked unilateral or bilateral cortical depression over subdural collections but is often normal or nonspecific. There is no absolute clinical picture that indicates the presence of a subdural hematoma. Cerebral angiography is the best diagnostic test to indicate the presence and extent of subdural collections and should be considered whenever the patient's course and findings are suggestive of this complication (Fig. 62).

Treatment is usually successful when the diagnosis is made early before cerebral atrophy and a fixed neurologic deficit have occurred.

Posttraumatic lacerations of the arachnoid membrane resulting in cerebrospinal fluid collections in the subdural space, termed subdural hygromas, present the same general clinical picture and problems as subdural hematomas.

Concussion

Closed head injuries make up the largest group of cases of craniocerebral trauma. The term implies no injury to the underlying bone beyond that of a linear fracture.

The simplest type of head trauma is cerebral concussion. This refers to the situation following a sudden head blow in which transient loss of consciousness occurs but is followed by full recovery without sequelae. More prolonged unconsciousness often associated with some evidence of focal neurologic defect and varying degrees of amnesia implies a cerebral contusion or laceration.

Children with either category of injury often vomit and later are pale, apathetic, or quite irritable. Overwhelming cerebral stimuli of any type may result in convulsive phenomena. In young children this is particularly true following head injury, and such an episode, occurring usually within a matter of minutes after impact, does not necessarily imply a severe degree of trauma, an abnormality of seizure threshold, or significant increase in the possibility of future convulsive episodes.

The physician's problem is how extensively to evaluate the injury and how to manage the patient in the period immediately postinjury. In cases of simple concussion or mild contusion the child should be examined carefully with attention to gross evidence of skull fracture and associated damage to viscera and bones. Observation until full recovery of consciousness is mandatory, as is the recording of vital signs. In most cases the child will have partially recovered by the time he is seen and, other than pallor, irritability, and bruises, will have few signs on examination. These children are best managed at home, provided intelligent, not overly distraught parents can cooperate in noting the youngster's pupillary equality, level of responsiveness, and general motor power. Arousal of the patient every 2 hours to determine the level of awareness and other signs is advisable for 12 to 24 hours postinjury.

Cerebral Contusion and Laceration

Most severe degrees of head injury or prolonged unconsciousness require hospitalization with more detailed evaluation and management to delineate the extent of injury and the need for specific therapy. Immediate attention must first be given to airway maintenance, the treatment of shock, fractures, the alleviation of hemorrhage, the prevention of fat embolization, or the care of splenic rupture, lung perforation, aspiration, atelectasis, or other emergency.

Primary or subsequent evaluations of the head injury will require some details of history and time sequence of events related to the injury and an accurate record of the initial status and findings. Examination should include precise evaluation of the individual's level of consciousness with regard to lethargy, stupor, or coma and content of his verbalizations and performance. Is the child irritable, agitated, confused, disoriented, confabulatory, amnesic, or completely unresponsive? Is there a response to sound and pain stimuli? Is it appropriate or purposeless?

The reason for hospitalization is to assess the course of postinjury and intelligently anticipate and treat complications. All pertinent items must therefore be clearly recorded to afford any examiner or consultant the comparative analysis that is the essential feature in the management of head injury patients. Pupillary size and reaction, observed extraocular movements, findings from examination of the fundi, symmetry of facial movement (either spontaneous or with pain stimulus), corneal responses, gag reflex, spontaneous or induced limb movements, tonus, deep tendon reflexes, and response to plantar stimulation should be listed in addition to the vital signs, evidence of meningeal irritation, a description of the external discharge from ears or nose, and a careful examination of the scalp and skull.

Cerebrospinal fluid studies are of limited value in cases of head injury, and their routine use cannot be justified. On the other hand, when there is suspicion of concurrent meningitis, a lumbar puncture is clearly indicated. In the acute posttraumatic period a spinal tap has little differential value, since intracortical, subdural, or extradural hematomas may be characterized by either clear or bloody fluid. An elevated cerebrospinal fluid pressure is usual after any significant degree of cerebral contusion, whether or not there has been a posttraumatic subarachnoid hemorrhage. In the latter instance, headache and meningeal discomfort may be relieved by the withdrawal of cerebrospinal fluid after the patient's general condition has been stabilized for 72 hours or more.

The meningeal signs of subarachnoid hemorrhage are often delayed, not appearing until 8 to 24 hours after bleeding. Posttraumatic hemorrhage of this type is common. It is seldom a significant complicating factor other than in its production of discomfort and prolonging convalescence. Rarely, obstruction to the cerebrospinal fluid pathway may develop secondary to blood in the subarachnoid space by obstruction at the incisura. This situation is often temporary, but posttraumatic hydrocephalus on this basis, necessitating a shunting procedure, must be borne in mind. Depending on the degree of cerebral damage, the child may not regain full consciousness for a period of hours to several weeks. During this time supportive care may be complicated by problems involving nutrition and electrolyte balance, restlessness, seizures, respiration, fever, bladder care, and otorrhea or rhinorrhea.

Patients remaining unconscious for any significant period of time may present a problem in fluid balance secondary to posttraumatic diabetes insipidus, paradoxic antidiuretic hormone excretion, and varied degrees of hyponatremia or hypernatremia. Fluid intake and urinary output should be recorded in conjunction with weight and serum electrolyte determinations until intake and output return to normal. Restlessness, increasing stupor, and seizures may result from gross electrolyte imbalance, usually on the basis of failing to recognize an increased thirst or by iatrogenic water intoxication. As soon as feasible, nutrition and fluid balance should progress from intravenous to nasogastric feedings and finally to normal oral feeding. Posttraumatic diabetes insipidus is usually transient but may require a period of Pitressin therapy, either by injection or as snuff. A number of children have a brief vasodepressor shocklike reaction to Pitressin tannate in oil and initially are best treated with an aqueous Pitressin preparation.

An agitated, lethargic-stuporous state characterizes many injured patients. Depressant drugs of the barbiturate or phenothiazine groups are best avoided in the acute period after injury. Valium, 2 to 4 mg intramuscularly or orally every 4 to 6 hours as needed, is safe as is paraldehyde 2 to 4 ml via the same routes. Bladder drainage, adequate hydration, loose restraints about wrist and ankles, boxing gloves for older children, and a well-padded crib or bed rails may be necessary to calm and protect the disturbed patient.

Convulsions, other than at the time of the initial impact episode, demand suppressant therapy. This usually implies an initial phenobarbital or paraldehyde regimen in conjunction with Dilantin therapy. Dosages, routes of administration, and the management of convulsive status are described in detail elsewhere (p. 147). The appearance of generalized or focal seizure phenomena may reflect the presence of a subdural or intracortical hematoma; however, convulsions are seldom the only manifestations in such cases and most often reflect underlying cortical contusion and laceration rather than a specific vascular complication.

Maintenance of a clear respiratory passage by proper positioning, suction, oropharyngeal airway, or tracheostomy is essential. Tracheostomy should be an elective procedure and preferably performed on a previously inserted endotracheal tube. In cases of severe brain damage with impaired gag and cough mechanisms, tracheostomy is an initial step in management to prevent aspiration, atelectasis, and pneumonia. In the young child requiring respiratory aid a properly positioned high tracheostomy with a tube of maximal caliber is essential.

Significant temperature elevations in the absence of infection occur after head injury. However, even in cases with posttraumatic subarachnoid hemorrhage, the temperature rarely exceeds 102° F unless there is severe cortical and brainstem involvement. The latter patient is usually in profound coma and may demonstrate marked temperature variations with elevations to 105° F or more. In these cases, if the patient is unresponsive to aspirin and sponging, the use of hypothermia may be considered with the temperature maintained at 92° to 96° F in an effort to decrease cerebral and general metabolic requirements in a situation of probable hypothalamic damage.

Urinary care may become a problem either because of continued soiling with skin irritation and breakdown or periodic retention. The usual diaper, urinary collection bag, or catheter techniques may be utilized. Should an indwelling catheter be necessary, prophylactic Gantrisin or similar drugs are not effective in preventing infection in the absence of scrupulous aseptic catheter technique and bladder irrigation.

Varying degrees of cerebral edema occur after head injury. It may be restricted to the contused, lacerated area or become generalized and present a picture not unlike that of acute lead encephalopathy with markedly increased intracranial pressure, focal neurologic signs, and seizures. Differentiation from hematoma formation or active intracranial bleeding is often impossible. The diagnosis is most frequently made retrospectively after clot or hemorrhage has been ruled out. General supportive care is all that is usually needed, but in critical situations efforts to decrease brain bulk and metabolism by intravenous urea and/or hypothermia may be of value. Osmotic loading substances, such as urea, produce a marked diuresis and decrease in cerebral bulk by dehydration. Rebound swelling does occur, and therapy may be needed over a period of days. Urea is given intravenously 1 g per kilogram of body weight each 8 to 12 hours with an indwelling bladder catheter in place and careful attention to electrolyte balance. Dosages of urea given in conjunction with hypothermia should be on a basis of 0.5 g per kilogram of body weight, as reduced elimination of urea occurs with lowered body temperature. Substances of this type always present danger when bleeding is present or a clot is developing. A more effective means of treating cerebral edema is with the use of steroids. Dexamethasone (Decadron) 4 to 16 mg daily for 3 days and gradually decreasing thereafter is the drug of choice in the treatment of cerebral edema. Therapy of this type is best accomplished in specialized treatment units where the necessary equipment and nursing personnel are available.

Intracortical hematomas are most often small; large solitary posttraumatic collections are uncommon. Surgically significant hematomas are usually clinically indistinguishable from extradural or subdural collections. Increasing intracranial pressure and progressive focal neurologic signs may result from an intracerebral clot in the absence of the more common hematomas. Diagnosis here reflects the same principles as in other intracranial collections, with detection being a function of ancillary studies. Many resolve without the need for surgical intervention; however, with increasing neurologic deficit and intracranial pressure and with angiographic and echoencephalographic evidence of progressive displacement, surgery should be considered.

Sequelae of Craniocerebral Trauma

Combinations of fixed neurologic defects may exist after brain injury but are usually self-evident. The less predictable sequelae are seizures, organic mental changes, and the posttraumatic syndrome.

SEIZURES. Posttraumatic seizures are most often generalized rather than focal but may be of any type other than petit mal. The incidence of persistent convulsive phenomena after head injury is unknown and extremely difficult to determine. The severity of the injury, the duration of unconsciousness, the occurrence of early seizures other than at the time of impact, and serial electroencephalographic patterns are of some value in analyzing the problem.

Penetrating depressed fractures have a residual seizure incidence of 30 to 60 percent, particularly if associated with periods of unconsciousness greater than 24 hours and the presence of convulsions during the acute phase. Children surviving subdural, extradural, or intracortical hematomas have a similar late seizure potential. A normal electroencephalogram with absence of paroxysmal or focal abnormalities 3 months after injury tends to make posttraumatic epilepsy less likely than when such discharges exist. A progressively worsening tracing is quite suspect; however, a delay of months to a year or more in the development of any electrical abnormality may be seen in patients who have or will subsequently develop seizures. Gross irregularity of the electroencephalogram may be present after head trauma in a perfectly normal child, and at times the tracing may appear relatively normal in the presence of frank focal neurologic defect. Nevertheless, a tracing should be obtained after significant head trauma as a base line in cases with or without seizures concomitant with acute episode. Unfortunately, the electroencephalogram is often of little help, or actually misleading, in predicting the chances of epilepsy developing after any given injury.

In closed head injuries, late epilepsy occurs in less than 5 percent of cases. The seizures may present in 3 months to 4 or more years after injury, the peak incidence occurring between 6 to 18 months. Previously controlled seizure states in known epileptics may be exacerbated after head injury, although analysis of such groups has revealed no consistent pattern.

Convulsive phenomena during the acute episode will usually result in the patient being placed on anticonvulsant therapy, which should be maintained for at least a 2-year period of freedom from seizures before gradual withdrawal of the drug. The appearance of the electroencephalogram at this time bears little relationship to the occurrence of subsequent convulsions, either with or without medication. Some authorities feel a paroxysmal or focally abnormal electroencephalogram after injury is in itself an indication for prolonged anticonvulsant drug therapy. This remains a controversial point.

ORGANIC MENTAL SYNDROMES. Self-limited memory defects and minor personality changes may be noted after head injury. Persistent frank organic dementia is uncommon in children, as is intellectual defect, although with extremely severe and extensive injuries, particularly in infancy, psychomotor retardation is seen.

POSTTRAUMATIC SYNDROME. The problem of general sequelae following head injury, the posttraumatic syndrome, is less common in children than in adults; however, it does occur. The symptoms tend to vary somewhat from those in the adult (headache, irritability, and postural vertigo). They are more commonly in the realm of enuresis, disturbances of sleep pattern, episodically aggressive behavior, and decline in school performance. How much is due to organic rather than primarily psychologic factors is difficult to state. Symptomatic management with sedatives, tranquilizers, and sometimes psychotherapy may be needed. Investigation as to the presence of typical or fragmentary convulsive phenomena may be profitable, and improvement may be noted after the institution of anticonvulsant therapy.

A commonsense attitude toward general care during the acute phase is extremely important. Overhospitalization, unfounded gratuitous remarks about possible future brain damage, and prolonged litigation correlate highly with the incidence of posttraumatic behavioral dysfunction. The physician must maintain an attitude of expectancy for return to normal function both with the parents and with the child. The avoidance of oversolicitous, unnecessary limitation of school, play, and social activities will reduce a common factor in the etiology of the posttraumatic reaction syndrome.

Group statistical studies would tend to indicate that children with behavioral and mental defects are more prone to head injury and more prone to display sequelae than mentally stable individuals.

Injuries to the Spinal Cord

ETIOLOGY AND PATHOGENESIS. Trauma to the vertebral column and spinal cord constitutes less than 5 percent of childhood injuries. The enclosure of the spinal cord in a bony canal is of great protective value; however, the mobility of the cervical spine and enlargement of the spinal cord at this level make it the single most common area of spinal injury at all ages. Dislocation may occur without fracture and result in a neural defect well beyond what might be inferred from the seemingly minimal osseous-ligamentous disturbance. The additional support given the thoracic vertebrae by the trunk and the smaller size of the spinal cord in this area are further protective factors which can only be overcome by excessive force. The pelvis gives additional support to the lumbar spine; however, as the spinal cord ends at the second lumbar vertebra in the older child, there is somewhat less protection of the lower thoracic–upper lumbar area.

In infancy, birth injury is the commonest cause of spinal cord trauma. Forceful breech extraction with spinal hyperextension is the situation in which this is most likely to occur. Birth injuries of this type may also be seen with cephalic presentation or complications necessitating version maneuvers, cephalocervical angulation, and unusual traction. The majority of these injuries result in cord transection in the midcervical to upper thoracic area. Those resulting in high cervical lesions involve the cervicomedullary junction and are seldom compatible with life.

In older children, trauma may be indirect, as in whiplash injuries, where the spine is either hyperextended or flexed beyond its normal range. Direct trauma resulting in crush injuries to the spine and its contents is less common and most often due to impact secondary to falls from a considerable height. The general pathology of spinal cord injury varies from complete severance through contusion and compression.

DIAGNOSIS. Cord injuries in the newborn period may be suspected in any case of difficult extraction necessitating considerable force. Resuscitation may be difficult with intercostal paralysis, a retracted thorax, prominent abdomen, diaphragmatic respiration, and a weak cry. The child is noted to have flaccid, abducted, and motionless lower extremities. Sensory evaluation is difficult, but a level of decreased response may be detected compatible with the usual midcervical–upper thoracic area of pathology. Because of the site of injury, only upper extremity movements are noted, with shoulder and forearm motions but little else. In this areflexic spinal shock stage, respiratory, urinary, and skin infection is common and often fatal. Hyperreflexia may occur subsequently with mass reflex upon stimulation resulting in a total flexion in the involved areas that may be misinterpreted as functional return.

If there is survival, the late picture depends upon the site and severity of the spinal cord lesion. Whether or not the patient's paraplegia assumes a position of flexion, extension, flaccidity, or spasticity depends upon the completeness and extent of the spinal cord defect. A sharply demarcated level is uncommon, as the defect is more often of such longitudinal extent as to cover many segments and preclude the development of spasticity. Intercurrent infection, whether acute or chronic, will delay the development of spasticity or decrease its extent. Early bladder function tends to manifest itself as an overflow with constant dribbling, while later automatic function occurs with reflex emptying upon distension to a moderate volume.

Laboratory evaluation should include spinal x-rays, which are usually normal, although fracture or subluxation may be detected. A number of normal variations of the cervical spine in childhood (pseudodislocation, hypermobility, etc.) often make radiologic interpretation difficult and are causes of interpretive error. The cerebrospinal fluid is usually bloody and has an increased protein content.

The diagnosis is often self-evident but may at times be confused with neonatal asphyxia, intracranial injury, congenital defects, or progressive infantile spinal muscular atrophy.

MANAGEMENT. The newborn requires immediate airway attention, oxygenation, suction, and meticulous skin, bladder, and bowel care. Antibiotics may be of value if long-term catheterization is required and should be given early with evidence of any acute infection. Myelography and surgery are not indicated; they decrease survival potential and in no way enhance recovery.

Survivors are expected to have normal intelligence; they can use their upper extremities fairly well but rarely ambulate or even sit without support. Early in life urinary and rectal sphincter control may be adequate. However, as the child grows older, surgery may be required to maintain adequacy of function. Surgical procedures may also be indicated for the orthopedic problems.

Trauma to the spinal cord of older children presents many similar problems; however, immediate management tends to be more definitive, the initial goal being safe, rapid transportation of the patient to where he will receive definitive care. Injury in this group is more likely to be complicated by damage to the vertebral column. It is of paramount importance that the patient be handled so that additional injury to the cord is not produced by improper posture or undue mobility of the vertebrae at the level of injury. Other bodily injuries may also have occurred, and judgment must be exercised for their proper care in keeping with the demands of the spinal cord injury.

The patient must be so placed on the litter as to maintain the normal cervical and lumbar lordosis and to prevent movement which might cause additional injury. Intravenous fluids, intranasal oxygen, and catheterization are often invaluable adjuncts in the initial management of spinal cord injuries. During the early stages, the patient must not be given anything by mouth nor strong sedatives or any drugs which would mask neurologic changes.

Open injuries must be treated surgically. Closed cord injuries may require either surgical or nonsurgical treatment. Unwise surgery in patients with cervical injury may be fatal and indications for surgery must be appraised with great care.

The cervical spinal cord is typically injured by a fracture, a dislocation, or a fracture-dislocation of one or more vertebrae. Severe injury above the level of the fifth cervical cord segment is rarely compatible with life. The radiograms may show marked crushing of the bodies, fragmentation of the pedicles, laminae, and spines, and such dislocation that facets are locked entirely out of position. Under no condition whatsoever must the grave error be made of trying to reduce such dislocation anywhere in the cervical spine by closed manipulation. In most severe lesions of the vertebrae there will be a complete transverse physiologic loss of cord function, often at one or more segments above the uppermost visible vertebral injury. In other instances, the vertebral lesions demonstrated roentgenologically will be minimal in comparison with the marked neurologic loss. There are no means of knowing whether an early spinal cord injury is due to contusion, with physiologic interruption and anatomic preservation, or whether the lesion is one of frank anatomic discontinuity. Closed injuries to the cervical cord with evidence of vertebral dislocation are best treated by placing the patient on a firm mattress or special frame and applying continual traction to the slightly extended head. The vertebrae will in most instances relocate in almost normal alignment within 24 to 36 hours. Serial lateral bedside portable x-ray pictures will demonstrate progress of the restitution. Occasional spinal puncture may also be done to follow the manometric effect of the closed decompression. Traction is maintained for at least 6 weeks.

Immediate decompressive laminectomy for the injured cervical cord is attended by severe morbidity and high mortality, but there are two instances when it is proper to operate early: (1) if the state of the patient was initially one of incomplete loss of cord function and hours or days later increasing loss of function appears; and (2) if at any time after the injury, immediately or days later, good radiograms show clearly that a bone fragment rests upon the cord in such a way that traction could not or has not relieved its pressure. The possibility of a mass of centrally extruded intervertebral disk substance as a result of injury must not be overlooked.

The thoracic segments of the vertebral column form a relatively rigid mass. The thoracic vertebral canal is the narrowest of all parts of the canal, and the spinal cord throughout its thoracic extent has a somewhat less rich blood supply than at either the cervical or lumbar levels. Spinal cord injury at this level is usually the result of direct severe trauma and carries a poor prognosis. All these factors must be considered in the early care of closed injuries to this area. Cord compression will almost invariably reveal total block of the flow of cerebrospinal fluid. The value of surgical decompression is highly variable.

As with injury at the thoracic level, dislocation of one lumbar vertebral body under another, wedging of a body with kyphosis, or fracture of the posterior arches calls for immediate decompressive laminectomy. Injury of the conus medullaris (T_{12}-L_1 vertebral levels) is of grave significance. Below that level the delicate filaments of the cauda equina may be badly torn and attenuated, the injury being associated with considerable subarachnoid hemorrhage.

The long-term care and rehabilitation of patients with spinal injuries is a challenge that is often best met in a special center or unit geared to this type of care. Extensive efforts to reestablish bowel and bladder function will be needed as well as attention to skin integrity, to nutrition, and to late syndromes of pain, spasms, autonomic dysfunction, genitourinary complications, psychiatric problems, and programs of education and training.

Peripheral Nerve Injuries

Injuries to the peripheral nervous system are not common in childhood. Those seen early in life are usually due to damage of the brachial plexus or sciatic nerves.

The spinal roots of the fifth cervical through the first thoracic nerves form the brachial plexus. These roots are poorly stabilized at birth, and traction damage is rarely transmitted to the spinal cord. Injuries to infants result in almost pure root syndromes in comparison to the more distally involved and diffuse damage seen with injuries in older children and adults. Recovery is better in children than in adults as regards both spontaneous resolution and surgical results.

Etiologically any force changing the normal relationship of arm, shoulder, and neck may result in plexus injury. Birth trauma is the commonest cause. The plexus has points of fascial fixation to the first rib medially and the coracoid process of the scapula laterally. Abduction of the arm stretches the nerves under and against the coracoid, resulting in stretch, avulsion, or compression of the lower plexus. Lateral deviation of the head and shoulder depression stretch the nerves over and against the first ribs, resulting in similar damage to the upper plexus. Traction injuries of these types may occur with breech or cephalic deliveries.

Upper plexus root injuries, Erb-Duchenne type, are commonest. The shoulder sags, the arm hangs limp in internal rotation, and the wrist is pronated reflecting paralysis of spinati, deltoid, biceps, brachioradialis, and extensor carpi radialis muscles and often rhomboids, serratus, and levator scapulae as well. The deep tendon reflexes of the involved extremity are usually lost, but it is unusual to be able to demonstrate a sensory defect. Treatment requires the deformity be overcome to prevent posterior subluxation of the humeral head from the glenoid fossa. The arm is placed in abduction and external rotation by a brace or by pinning a towel over the wrist and fixing it to the mattress in the desired position. A full range of motion of the shoulder by passive exercises is performed daily. Well over 80 percent of these patients will have complete recovery in 3 months or less. Anomalous plexus configuration may include the fourth cervical root, or trauma may be transmitted to this level resulting in phrenic nerve damage and ipsilateral diaphragmatic paralysis, which is rarely a problem unless significant bilateral injury has occurred.

Lower plexus root injuries, Klumpke-Dejerine type, show more sensory and vasomotor involvement with paralysis of the flexors and extensors of the forearm and the intrinsic muscles of the hand. Marked involvement of the first thoracic root results in cervical sympathetic damage and a Horner's syndrome, often with delay of normal pigmentation of the ipsilateral iris. The deep tendon reflexes are usually intact, with a poor grasp response. Sensory changes involve the ulnar side of the hand and forearm. Dependent edema and cyanosis are common. Treatment involves splinting the forearm and wrist in a neutral position and passive range of motion exercises. The majority of cases completely recover within 3 to 6 months, although the overall prognosis is not as favorable as in the upper plexus lesions (Fig. 63).

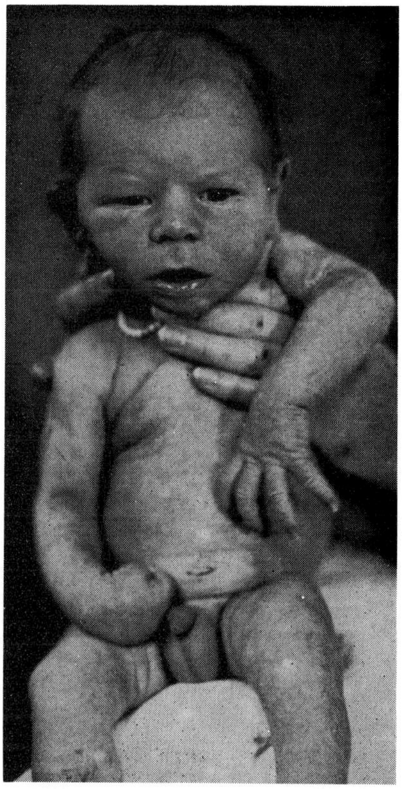

Fig. 63. Brachial plexus injury to an infant 12 days old. Involvement of the upper, middle, and lower trunks of the right brachial plexus, combined with right enophthalmos, a component of Horner's syndrome.

Injuries to the brachial plexus in older children are usually of mixed upper and lower plexus types. If due to traction and hyperabduction, the prognosis may be good, although at this age the usual cause is severe trauma which often results in root avulsion or a degree of hemorrhage and scarring that precludes functional recovery.

Direct plexus surgery is consistently unprofitable. In cases with persistent defects, orthopedic procedures to stabilize joints in favorable positions and tendon transplantation, where feasible, are the only available treatments.

The peripheral nerves in the upper extremity may be involved alone or in varied combinations, due usually to direct laceration trauma or severe injuries with combined osseous-vascular-neural damage. Compression neuropathies are uncommon in childhood.

Serratus anterior palsy due to involvement of the long thoracic nerve (nerve of Bell) is usually a result of pressure on the shoulder or excessive forceful activity with the arms elevated. It is most frequently seen in prepuberal athletic boys in association with baseball pitching, weight-lifting, or carrying heavy loads. The scapula "wings" with horizontal forward pressure of the arms and there is weakness in lifting and arm elevation due to impaired scapula fixation. Treatment is expectant with full functional recovery anticipated, although some residual scapular winging may persist. Activities possibly associated with the lesion should be discontinued. During the first week the weight of the shoulder may be removed from the scapula by a simple arm sling, which is often not necessary unless the paralysis is total or there is considerable discomfort. Range of motion exercises, then more active shoulder strengthening maneuvers, are the only measures indicated.

The axillary or circumflex nerve that innervates the deltoid and teres minor muscles is usually injured only in association with anterior dislocations of the shoulder, particularly when associated with fractures of the greater tuberosity of the humerus. The axillary nerve winds around the surgical neck of the humerus and may be injured by fractures in this location. Injury to the nerve is detected by inability to abduct the arm to the horizontal position and a zone of hypesthesia of the lower posterior deltoid area. Therapy is that of the primary injury, and with rare exceptions full neural recovery can be anticipated.

Radial nerve injury is most commonly a result of fracture through the middle third of the humerus with neural stretch or contusion. The triceps muscle may not be involved, but there is marked weakness of the brachioradialis and the extensors of the wrist and fingers (wristdrop). Sensory loss in an area between index finger and thumb on the dorsum of the hand. In the acute state it is impossible to tell whether or not the nerve has been lacerated or severed. Therefore, where feasible, open reduction of the fracture and nerve repair are reasonable considerations. Later, electrical testing will give information as to whether or not there is anatomic continuity of the nerve. Where permanent residua exist in spite of all efforts, tendon transplantation gives quite effective wrist, finger, and thumb extension.

The ulnar nerve may be lacerated along its course in the forearm near the wrist or in conjunction with fractures as it passes behind the medial epicondyle of the humerus at the elbow. The epiphysis of the medial epicondyle does not fuse to the humerus until late adolescence and is particularly prone to avulsion. The ulnar nerve may be contused at the time of injury or compressed later by scar formation. Sensory loss involves the fifth digit and ulnar half of the fourth and extends along the medial side of the palm to the lower forearm. Weakness may involve the interossei, lumbicales, hypothernar muscles, adductor pollicis, the flexor carpi ulnaris, the deep flexor of the fourth and fifth digits, resulting in a defect in spreading the fingers, adducting the thumb, flexing the fourth and fifth digits at the distal interphalangeal joints, and poor opposition of the fifth finger.

Treatment is that of the primary injury. Surgical intervention depends upon the intactness of the nerve as determined by clinical and electrical studies and can consist of suturing or grafting the involved nerve.

The median nerve may be damaged similarly to the ulnar and is often injured with it. In addition to the more common laceration injury, there may be damage in anterior dislocation fractures at the elbow or wrist. Sensory loss is on the palmar surface of the hand and involves thumb, index, middle and radial half of the ring fingers, and the radial surface of the palm. Weakness of the pronators of the forearm, long flexors of the fingers, and short adductor and opponens of the thumb is the major motor defect. Therapeutic considerations are similar to cases of ulnar palsy.

Peripheral nerve injuries involving the lower extremities are almost exclusively of the sciatic nerve and its branches. It is the largest nerve in the body and at the knee divides into the tibial and common peroneal nerves. Iatrogenic trauma secondary to intramuscular injections is the leading cause of sciatic neuropathy in infancy. Lesions of this type are also seen in older children and adults. The "normal course" of the sciatic nerve in the hollow midway between the ischial tuberosity and the greater trochanter under cover of the gluteus maximus muscle varies greatly. This fact, taken together with the small size of the infant gluteal mass and the potential neurotoxicity of many antibiotics, makes it unwise to utilize this area for intramuscular injections. Intragluteal injections are contraindicated in infancy and should be used in older children with extreme caution. The anterolateral compartment of the thigh and deltoid areas is safer and always preferable.

Complete sciatic lesions produce total foot paralysis and loss of leg flexion. There is a flail footdrop, absent ankle jerk, and a sensory loss below the knee involving the entire leg except for its medial aspect.

The tragedy of nerve injury in infancy is accentuated by residua of short, small extremities due to lack of stimulation of muscular-tendon movement essential to bone growth. All cases of sciatic palsy must be carefully evaluated with a view toward surgery, although high lesions of this type rarely show complete recovery and are usually associated with a marked permanent disability.

The peroneal nerve is vulnerable to pressure neuropathy as well as other injury. It descends from the popliteal fossa to a superficial position on the lateral aspect of the leg passing posterior to the head of the fibula. Injury here results in sensory loss over the dorsum of the foot and anterolateral surface of the leg with weakness of the dorsiflexors and evertors of the foot and toes.

The tibial nerve descends deep in the calf, rounds the posterior aspect of the medial malleolus, and enters the foot. It innervates muscles controlling plantar flexion of the foot and toes and the intrinsic muscles of the foot. Sensory loss is usually confined to the sole.

Combined peroneal and tibial nerve injuries often occur. Treatment is similar to that described for ulnar nerve injuries.

Cranial Nerve Injuries

Trauma to the cranial nerves is seldom an isolated occurrence and usually reflects more diffuse craniocerebral injury.

The olfactory nerve is frequently torn as its filaments pass from the subfrontal area of the brain through the cribriform plate. The defect is rarely complete and usually asymptomatic. If severe anosmia persists, distortion of taste is the presenting complaint.

Trauma to the optic nerve occurs in association with orbital fracture but may be seen with cerebral contusion and hemorrhage into the nerve sheath. Injury to the chiasmal area is uncommon. The hypothalamus and brainstem usually receive the brunt of injury in this region with resulting fatality.

The commonest cranial nerve injuries are those involving the third, fourth, sixth, seventh, and eighth nerves.

Laceration of the carotid artery in its cavernous sinus position due to fractures or transmitted trauma may result in a carotid-cavernous fistula. Complications of this type are less common in children than in adults but may occur. Either immediately or within several days of injury the patient may become aware of a bruit. Subsequently third, fourth, and sixth cranial nerve paresis may occur with associated exophthalmos, periorbital engorgement, and diminished sensation in the first two divisions of the fifth cranial nerve. The bruit is strikingly prominent over the involved side and far more pronounced than the nonspecific cephalic bruits of childhood. It is obliterated or considerably reduced by ipsilateral carotid compression. Spontaneous occlusion of the fistula rarely occurs. Carotid ligation in the neck and often intracranially above the cavernous sinus is necessary.

Damage to the oculomotor nerves is more common, and permanent or transient dysfunction of the extraocular muscles occur more frequently in the pediatric age group than in the adult.

Fractures through the petrous portion of the temporal bone may damage the facial nerve. Paralysis may be immediate or delayed. Neonatal facial paralysis may follow forceps extraction or reflect unusual in utero positions. Immediate treatment is directed to corneal protection. Damage to the nerve distal to the geniculate ganglion may be associated with blood behind the tympanic membrane and a conductive hearing loss. Injury central to the ganglion tends to be associated with labyrinthine dysfunction and a pattern of sensorineural hearing loss, implying a level of injury that is not amenable to direct therapy. In all other instances evaluation and management are aimed at the functional state of the nerve. Electrodiagnostic tests to follow and determine the degree of degeneration and estimate anatomic continuity of the nerve are not infallible; however, when there is evidence of neural degeneration, careful evaluation and consideration should be given to operative intervention.

Surgical decompression and/or nerve graft, where feasible, give the best results. Hypoglossal facial anastomosis and plastic procedures to enhance facial symmetry are less satisfactory but are at times the only possible approach to the problem.

Fractures through the base of the skull, direct blows on or near the ear, or the extravasation of blood from subarachnoid hemorrhage may affect both vestibular and auditory components of the eighth cranial nerve as well as causing direct damage to the labyrinth, cochlea, or middle ear. Posttraumatic neural deafness has a relatively poor prognosis for full recovery. Labyrinthine dysfunction as evidenced by postural vertigo and increased sensitivity to motion is usually transient.

References

Boshes, B. Trauma to the Spinal Cord. *In* Baker, A. B., ed., Clinical Neurology, 2nd ed. New York, Paul B. Hoeber, Inc., 1962, Vol. 3, Chap. 36, pp. 1639-1678.

Campbell, E. D. R., Hickey, R. P., Nixon, K. H., and Richardson, A. J. Value of nerve-excitability measurements in prognosis of facial palsy. Brit. Med. J., 2:7, 1962.

Caverness, W. E., and Walker, A. E., eds. Head Injury Conference Proceedings. Philadelphia, J. B. Lippincott Co., 1966.

Cloward, R. B. Single suture scalp closure. J. Neurosurg., 21:142, 1964.

Dillon, H., and Leopold, R. L. Children and the postconcussion syndrome. J.A.M.A., 172:86, 1961.

Drake, C. G., and Jory, T. A. Hypothermia in the treatment of critical head injury. Canad. Med. Ass. J., 87: 887, 1962.

Epstein, J. A., Epstein, B. S., and Small, M. Subepicranial hydroma. J. Pediat., 59:562, 1961.

Gil, D. G. Physical abuse of children; findings and implications of a nationwide survey. Pediatrics, 44:857, 1969.

Gilles, F. H., and Shilli, T. O., Jr. Infantile hydrocephalus: retrocerebellar subdural hematoma. J. Pediat., 76:529, 1970.
Gurdjian, E. S., Lissner, J. R., and Patrick, L. M. Protection of the head and neck in sports. J.A.M.A., 182: 509, 1962.
Hanson, D. J. Intramuscular injection injuries and complications. Practitioner, 27:109, 1963.
Hawkes, C. O., and Ogle, W. S. Atypical features of epidural hematoma in infants, children and adolescents. J. Neurosurg., 19:971, 1962.
Haymaker, W., and Woodhall, B. Peripheral Nerve Injuries, 2nd ed. Philadelphia, W. B. Saunders Co., 1953.
Hjern, B., and Nylander, I. Acute head injuries in children. Acta Pediat. (Suppl.), 152, 1964.
Jacobziner, H., and Culbert, R. W. Non-fatal accidents in the school age child. Clin. Pediat., 2:484, 1963.
Jennett, W. B. Epilepsy After Blunt Head Injuries. Springfield, Ill., Charles C Thomas, Publ., 1962.
Kempe, C. H., Silverman, F. N., Steele, B. F., Droegemueller, W., and Silver, H. K. The battered child syndrome. J.A.M.A., 181:17, 1962.
Kozmin, P. J., Ritz, N. D., Moss, A. H., and Kaufman, A. Massive hemorrhage—Scalps of newborn infants. Amer. J. Dis. Child., 108:413, 1964.
Lende, R. A., and Erickson, T. C. Growing skull fractures of childhood. J. Neurosurg., 18:479, 1961.
Leventhal, H. R. Birth injuries to the spinal cord. J. Pediat., 56:447, 1960.
Lindsay, W. K., Walker, F. G., and Farmer, A. W. Traumatic peripheral nerve injuries in children: results of repair. Plast. Reconstr. Surg., 30:462, 1962.
Low, N. L., and Correll, J. W. Head pain due to leptomeningeal cysts. Brit. J. Surg., 53:971, 1966.
McLaughlin, H. L. Trauma. Philadelphia, W. B. Saunders Co., 1959.
McLaurin, R. L., King, L. R., Elam, E. B., and Budde, R. B. Metabolic responses to craniocerebral trauma. Surg. Gynec. Obstet., 110:282, 1960.
Mealey, J., Jr. Pediatric Head Injuries. Springfield, Ill., Charles C Thomas, Publ., 1968.
Monthly Vital Statistics Report. The U.S. Dept. Health, Education and Welfare, Vol. 19, No. 5, 1970.
Ommaya, A. K., Rockoff, S. D., and Baldwin, M. Experimental concussion—a first report. J. Neurosurg., 21: 249, 1964.
Rasmussen, J., and Gulati, D. R. Cortisone in the therapy of post-operative cerebral edema. J. Neurosurg., 19:535, 1962.
Rickham, P. P. Head injury in childhood. Helv. Chir. Acta, 28:560, 1961.
Selby, I. Skull fractures in infants. Acta Chir. Scand., 122:30, 1961.
Shulman, K., and Ransohoff, J. Subdural hematoma in children; the fate of children with retained membranes. J. Neurosurg., 18:175, 1961.
Tenner, M. S., and Stein, B. M. Cerebral herniation in the growing fracture of the skull. Radiology, 94:351, 1970.
Watkins, E. S., Stubbs, J. D., and Lewin, W. Urea in the management of head injuries. Lancet, 1:358, 1961.
Zimmerman, B. Effects of injury on electrolyte metabolism. J. Trauma, 3:141, 1963.
Zollinger, R. W., Creedon, P. J., and Sanguily, J., Jr. Trauma in children in a general hospital. Amer. J. Surg., 104:855, 1962.

Chapter 9
PAROXYSMAL DISORDERS

DORA CHAO

Epilepsy

Epilepsy is as old as the human race. The early Greeks and then the Romans looked upon epilepsy as a sacred disease, a curse by some capricious gods. Although disputed by no less an authority than Hippocrates about 400 B.C., this misconception has persisted through the ages. Even today many epileptics and their families still suffer from social prejudices and feel the shame of a stigma. The period of scientific inquiry and social enlightenment began in the middle of the nineteenth century. The astute observations of Hughlings Jackson led him to theorize that fits were caused by occasional, excessive, and disorderly discharge in the cerebral gray matter. It was upon this fundamental premise that scientific studies have subsequently flourished in many directions, leading to the present-day understanding. The major advances have been:

1. The development of modern neurology, neuroanatomy, neuropathology, neuroradiology, especially knowledge of the functional anatomy of the brain.
2. The development of electroencephalography and its fruitful applications in clinical and experimental investigations.
3. The advance of drug therapy.
4. The development of surgical treatment of focal epilepsy and the knowledge gained therefrom.
5. The more recent development of neurochemistry, electron microscopy and electroneurophysiology have brought research on seizure mechanism to the cellular level.

While these developments opened up new vistas of knowledge, the clinician still has the age-old problem of adequate care and treatment of epileptic patients.

There is no accurate census of the incidence of epilepsy in the United States. One recent estimate places epilepsy at the head of a list of chronic disorders with 17 million active cases, or approximately 1 in every 100 individuals in the United States. In pediatric practice the problem of seizures is indeed a major one. About 5 in 100 children have had a seizure at one time or another in their lives, if only in association with fever; and the prevalence of bona fide epilepsy has been estimated to be 0.5 percent.

There is a brighter side of the picture, however. Overall, medical therapy of epilepsy with today's drugs and available service is about 50 to 60 percent effective. Increased understanding and acceptance by the public have also brought improvement in the social and economic outlook to the epileptic patient and his family. On this happy note the student of today may look forward to gratifying experiences in facing the challenge of the problems of the epileptic child.

DEFINITIONS. ***Epilepsy.*** The word *epilepsy* has its origin in Greek and means "to lay on" or "to seize." A *seizure* (an *attack,* a *fit,* a *spell*) is an episode of cerebral dysfunction produced by abnormal, excessive, neuronal discharge occurring in the brain which may be caused by a great variety of conditions. A seizure is therefore a symptom and not a disease. Its manifestations depend upon the location of the discharge and its spread. Thus, a seizure may manifest as a change in the state of consciousness, an abnormal sensory experience, disordered motor activities (tonic or clonic contractions), or disturbance of vegetative, intellectual, and behavioral functions. When seizures become recurrent, the condition is termed *epilepsy.*

Gibbs and Lennox defined epilepsy as a "paroxysmal cerebral dysrhythmia." They emphasized not only the abnormal rhythms but also their paroxysmal occurrence as the essential features of the epileptic dysfunction.

Convulsion. Convulsion implies generalized or widespread abnormal motor activity as a prominent component in an epileptic attack. Not all convulsions are epileptic in nature, and many types of epilepsy are without a convulsive element.

Prodrome. The prodrome consists of symptoms that appear hours or days before the onset of the actual seizure. For example, on the basis of past experience the family might recognize that the coming of a seizure is habitually heralded by the child becoming whiny, anorexic, and irritable.

Aura. Aura is the name given to the subjective sensations or experiences which habitually precede an epileptic attack and which are frequently recognized by the patient as immediate warning of an impending seizure. Physiologically, an aura is the beginning of the abnormal neuronal discharge and hence may be a helpful sign for localization of the epileptogenic focus.

Ictal. Ictus is derived from Latin and means a sudden attack. The adjective *ictal* means pertaining to an attack. *Preictal* and *postictal* refer to the time immediately before and shortly after a seizure; *interictal* refers to the interim period between attacks.

Classification

Until recently, four systems of classification were in general use: clinical, anatomic, electroencephalographic, and etiologic. This is inevitable because epilepsy is only a symptom of many disease conditions of diverse functional disturbances. It is recognized that by using them all in a given case, a broader understanding of the patient's ailment may be gained. Indeed, it was based upon this viewpoint that a new classification combining clinical seizure type, electroencephalographic expression, anatomic substrate, etiology, and age was proposed by the Vienna Congress, International League Against Epilepsy. The reader should consult the original publication for complete information; the reference is given in the bibliography.

TABLE 23. *Clinical Classification of Seizures*

Generalized convulsions (major motor)
- Tonic-clonic (grand mal)
- Tonic

Focal seizures
- Focal motor
- Focal sensory
- Frontal adversive
- Occipital
- Inhibitory
- Temporal lobe

Petit mal

Minor Motor
- Akinetic
- Myoclonic
- Infantile spasms

Psychomotor epilepsy

Autonomic epilepsy (convulsive equivalent seizures)

Miscellaneous

1. CLINICAL CLASSIFICATION. This oldest and most widely used system is purely descriptive of the clinical features of the seizures. Some of the terms are apt because the pattern of attack is simple, for example, lapse or absence, akinetic or drop seizure, and massive myoclonic (jackknife) spasms. Some other terms are more ambiguous and require further definition because the seizure patterns are complex and cannot be characterized by a simple descriptive term or phrase; for example, minor motor seizure is a misnomer because the adjective "minor" gives a false implication in relation to the severity of the symptoms and the usually grave prognosis. These criticisms notwithstanding, classification by seizure pattern is meaningful and useful when used in correlation with other systems of classification. The major seizure types are listed in Table 23.

2. ANATOMIC CLASSIFICATION. Hughlings Jackson was the first epileptologist to attempt an anatomic classification when he used such terms as "uncinate fits" and "rhinencephalis seizures." This concept of focal origination of seizure discharge has led to extensive studies of functional anatomy of the brain. The advent of electroencephalography including cortical and depth electrography and the advancement of surgical treatment of focal epilepsies have extended such anatomic studies directly to the epileptogenic human brain in the modern operating theater. To the neurosurgeons it is not only logical and desirable but absolutely necessary to classify seizure symptoms on an anatomic basis. Inevitably the anatomic terms have become more or less identified with certain clinical epilepsies, for example:

Centrencephalic seizures:	Grand mal epilepsy Petit mal epilepsy
Diencephalic epilepsy (thalamic-hypothalamic):	Convulsive equivalent syndrome (autonomic epilepsy)
Focal cortical seizures	
Temporal lobe epilepsy:	Psychomotor epilepsy
Frontal lobe epilepsy:	Adversive seizures, Jacksonian epilepsy
Parietal lobe epilepsy:	Focal sensory seizures
Occipital lobe epilepsy:	Visual sensations

It should be noted that the anatomic system is still far from perfect or complete, and some anatomic designations, e.g., "temporal lobe," require additional definition (see psychomotor epilepsy). To the clinician the anatomic classification is an essential element in diagnosis.

3. ELECTROENCEPHALOGRAPHIC CLASSIFICATION. The electroencephalogram provides a pictorial record of cerebral activity reflected at the cortex in electrical terms. In the course of its clinical application many specific patterns have been found to correlate with various clinical types of epilepsy with varying degrees of concordance. Some of the well-known examples of electroencephalographic patterns follow.

a. *Three per second spike and wave dysrhythmia* is the classic electroencephalographic abnormality found in genetic epilepsy of the pure lapse or petit mal attack. However, it also occurs in patients who may have grand mal attacks only, or both types of attack (Fig. 64).

b. *Paroxysmal polyspike and wave dysrhythmia* is closely correlated with myoclonic jerks (Fig. 65).

c. *Paroxysmal or continuous slow spike and slow wave dysrhythmia* is generally associated with diffuse encephalopathy of known or unknown etiology. The seizures are chiefly akinetic or myoclonic with or without generalized convulsion. The EEG pattern was referred to as "petit mal variant" by Lennox and the clinical picture has borne such names as minor motor seizures, atypical petit mal, myokinetic epilepsy, and the Lennox syndrome (Fig. 66).

d. *Hypsarhythmia* is a continuously abnormal electroencephalographic pattern characterized by high-voltage, poorly organized, slow and sharp wave activity mixed with bursts of irregular spikes and polyspikes and wave activity showing poor interhemispheric correlation. It is found in 90 percent of children with massive myoclonic spasms (Fig. 67).

e. *The 14 and 6 per second positive spike dysrhythmia* (Fig. 68) occurring in drowse or light sleep was believed to arise from diencephalic nuclei and/or limbic system, and is often found in children with seizure equivalent. More recently several investigators have observed it in 15 to 55 percent of apparently "normal school children" with a peak age incidence at 12 years. Although these observations appear to suggest an age and maturation dependence, and to have raised doubt regarding its pathologic significance, its frequent concordance (with or without other EEG abnormalities) with vegetative dysfunctions, posttraumatic, postbreath-holding, choreic and migraine syndromes remains an intriguing finding.

f. *Focal (or multifocal) discharges* may arise from epileptogenic focus (or foci) in the cerebral cortex or subcortical centers. The clinical seizure symptoms are dependent upon the functional attributes at the site of discharge and the manner of spread. Focal seizures may escalate into generalized convulsions. The so-called temporal lobe is the most common site of epileptogenic discharge (Fig. 69). Sometimes a primary lesion located elsewhere may remotely activate the temporal regions. The concordance between temporal lobe focus and psychomotor epilepsy is about 60 percent.

On the basis of correlative studies, certain electroencephalographic terms have frequently been used interchangeably with clinical terminology. This practice is not justified because the correlation is rarely perfect. For the clinician, the electroencephalogram is an invaluable tool in diagnosis, but it is unwise to dogmatically equate a certain electrographic pattern with a specific clinical seizure type.

4. ETIOLOGIC CLASSIFICATION. The epilepsies may be divided into two general etiologic groups: genetic and symptomatic. The genetic epilepsies are characterized by the absence of a demonstrable structural lesion of the brain, the tendency to spontaneous cerebral dysrhythmia being genetically inherited. In contrast, the symptomatic epilepsies are associated with metabolic disorders or organic pathology of the brain acquired through developmental error, injury, or disease. In some cases symptomatic and genetic epilepsy may occur concomitantly.

a. Genetic Epilepsy. The etiologic role of heredity, first implicated by Hippocrates, has been established by extensive studies of epileptic families and relatives. Both Conrad and Lennox found that when epilepsy occurred in monozygous twins, both twins were affected in about 85 percent, whereas in dizygous twins, both were affected in only 3 percent and 15.9 percent of their cases, respectively. EEG studies of the epileptic families led Lennox and Gibbs to suggest that cerebral dysrhythmia underlying epileptic diathesis was inherited as a mendelian dominant factor. These observations were confirmed by the studies of Metrakos and Metrakos, who demonstrated further that the EEG trait and the clinical seizure of genetic epilepsy manifest themselves with greatest frequency between the ages of 5 and 12 years. The seizure manifestation is either generalized convulsion, pure petit mal, or a combination of the two, often with myoclonic components. In 4 to 8 percent of epileptics a hereditary factor seems involved. Even when there is no overt epilepsy, a low

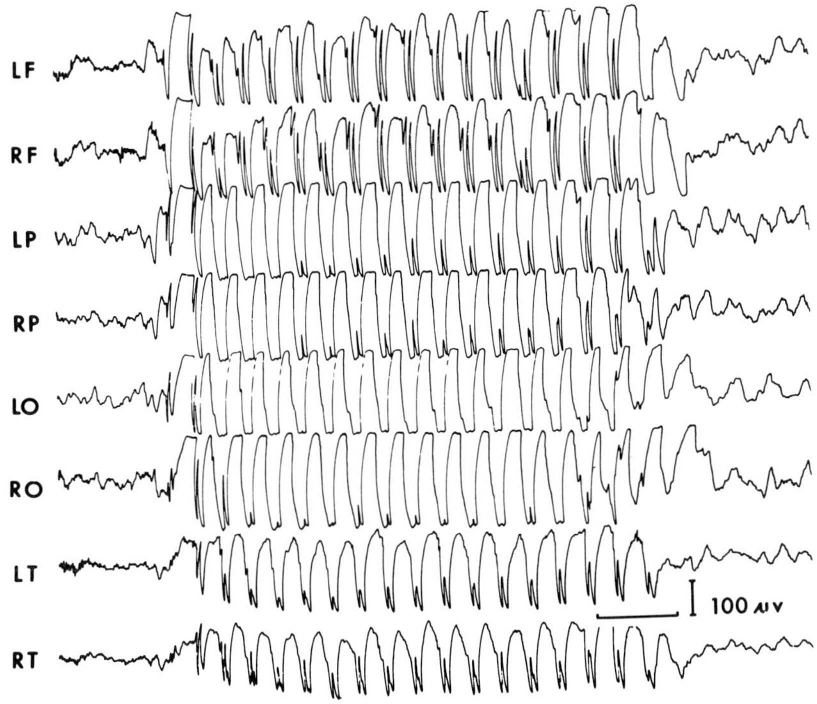

Fig. 64. Three per second spike and wave dysrhythmia.

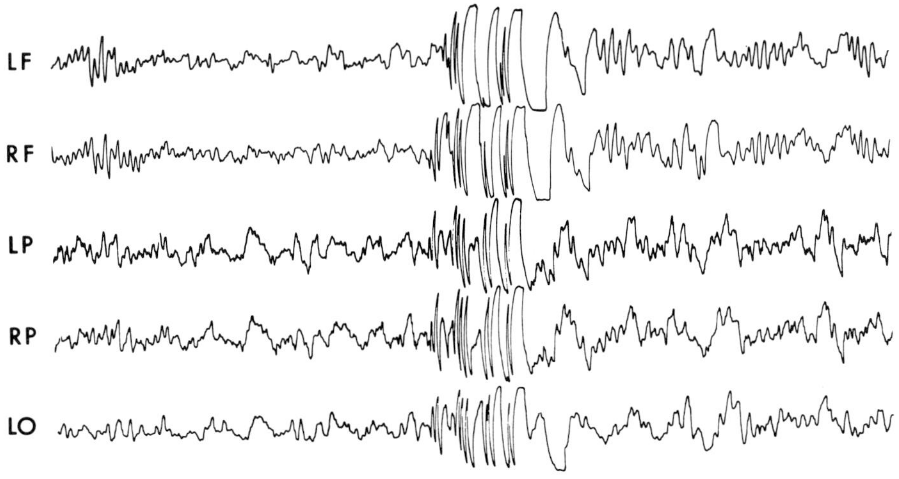

Fig. 65. Paroxysmal polyspike and wave dysrhythmia.

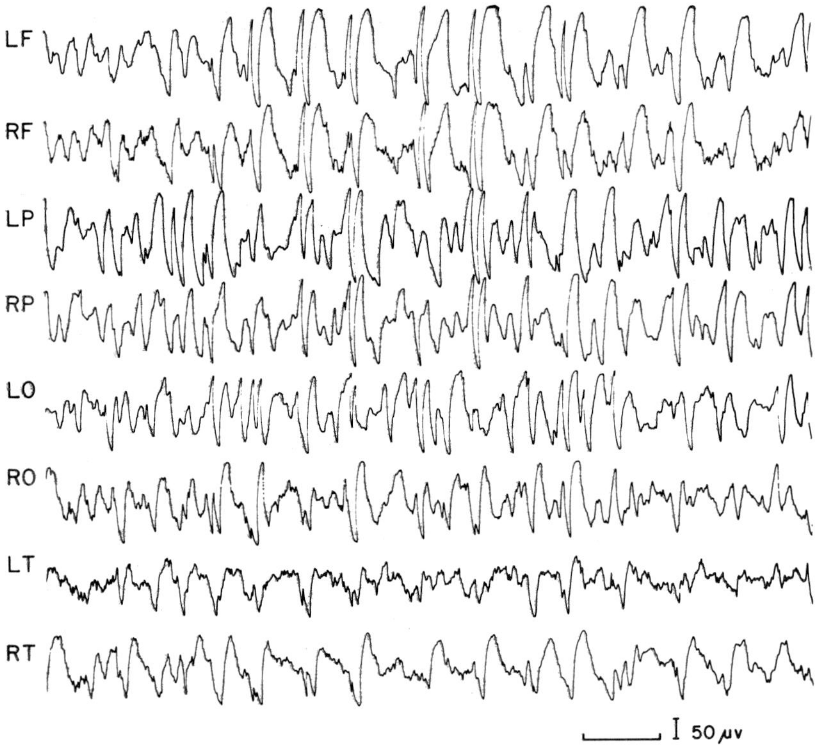

Fig. 66. Generalized slow spike and wave dysrhythmia.

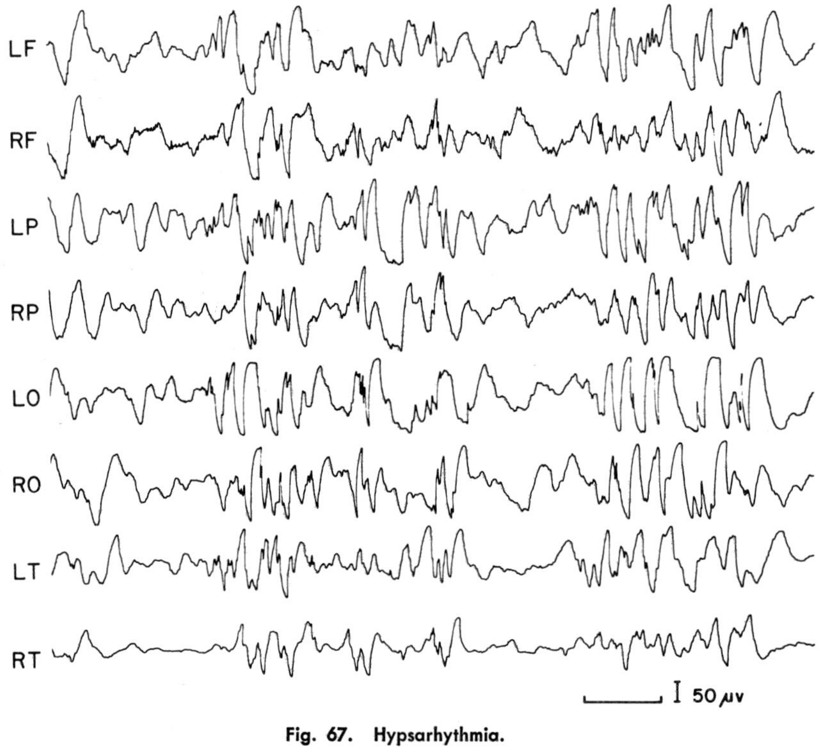

Fig. 67. Hypsarhythmia.

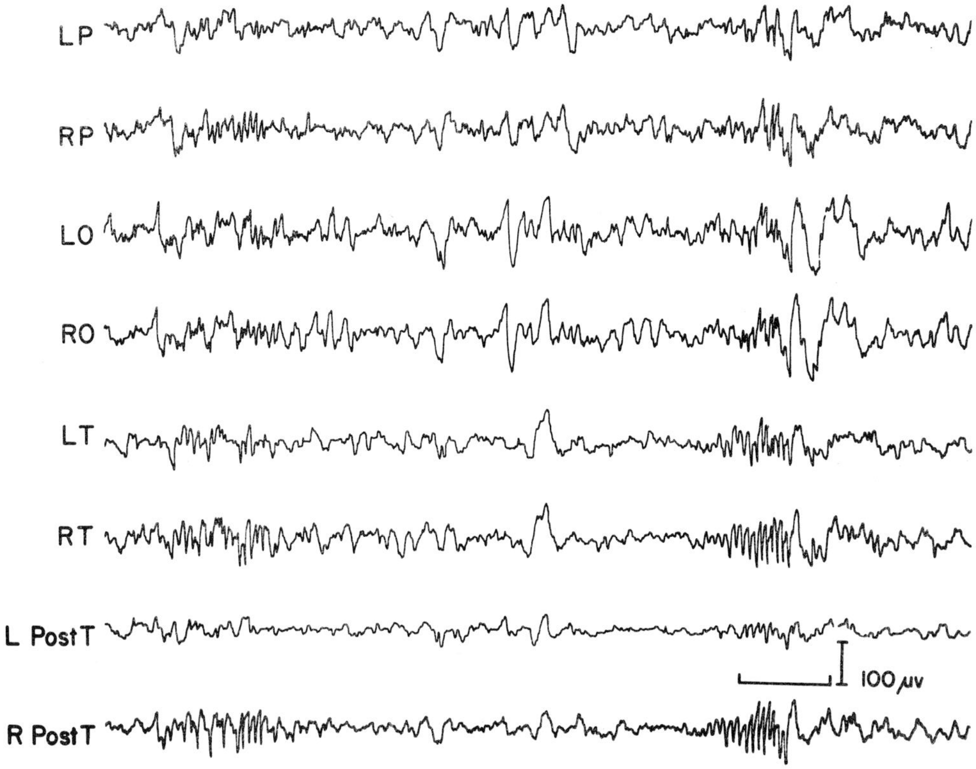

Fig. 68. Fourteen and six per second positive spike dysrhythmia.

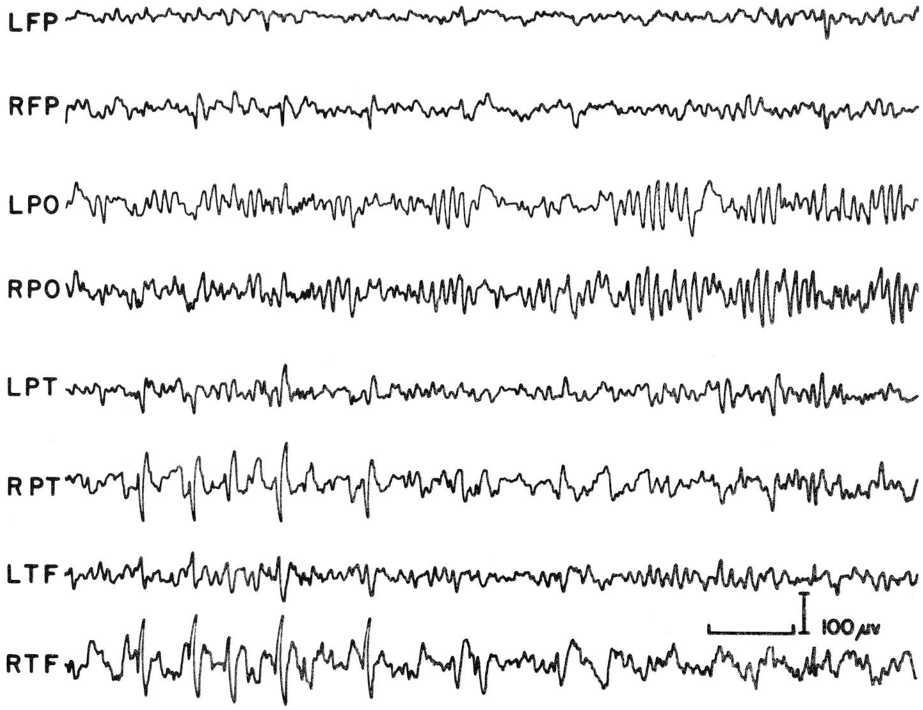

Fig. 69. Temporal spike focus.

TABLE 24. *Etiologic Factors Associated with Epilepsy*

Prenatal Factors
- Genetic
  - Genetic epilepsy
  - Inborn errors of metabolism
    - Carbohydrate: glycogen storage disease, hypoglycemia
    - Protein: phenylketonuria, maple syrup urine disease
    - Fat: cerebral lipidoses, leucodystrophies
  - Heredofamilial diseases: myoclonus epilepsy
- Congenital structural anomalies
  - Porencephaly
  - Vascular malformations
  - Neurocutaneous syndrome
  - Developmental defects of the brain
- Fetal infections
  - Viral encephalopathy: rubella, cytomegalic inclusion disease
  - Protozoan meningoencephalitis: toxoplasmosis
- Maternal diseases
  - Toxemia of pregnancy
  - Chronic renal disease
  - Diabetes mellitus
  - Radiation during pregnancy
  - Drug usage and drug intoxication
  - Trauma

Perinatal Factors
- Trauma
- Hypoxia
- Jaundice
- Infection
- Prematurity
- Drug withdrawal

Postnatal Factors
- Primary infection of central nervous system
- Infectious diseases of childhood with encephalopathy (e.g., measles, mumps)
- Head trauma
- Circulatory diseases
  - Vascular anomalies
  - Occlusive diseases: arterial, venous
  - Hemorrhage
  - Hypertensive encephalopathy
- Toxic encephalopathy
  - Thallium
  - Lead
  - Convulsogenic drugs: INH, steroids
- Allergic encephalopathy
  - Immunization reactions
  - Drug reactions
- Physical and metabolic encephalopathies
  - Fever and febrile convulsions
  - Anoxia and hypoxia
  - Prolonged convulsions with cyanosis
  - Electrolyte disturbance
  - Acute porphyria
  - Hypoglycemia
  - Hypocalcemia
  - Hypomagnesemia
  - Hypo- and hypernatremia and others
  - Pyridoxin deficiency or dependency
- Degenerative diseases of the brain
- Tumors

seizure threshold may be evidenced by paroxysmal spike-and-waves or polyspike-and-waves occurring spontaneously or by activation of sleep, intermittent photic stimulation, or hyperventilation. The risk of producing epileptic offspring is about 2 to 4 percent.

b. Symptomatic or Acquired Epilepsy. The causes of symptomatic epilepsies are very diverse; but the end results are similar: a structural or metabolic cerebral lesion develops and serves as the focus of epileptogenesis. This process may be localized or diffuse, static or progressive, traumatic or inflammatory, neoplastic or degenerative, vascular or allergic. Some of the more common etiologic factors are listed in Table 24.

Pathogenesis

The common denominator in the pathology of epileptogenic diseases is a structural or a metabolic disturbance in the brain giving rise to seizure discharge.

A typical epileptogenic cortical scar consists of a central zone, in which no nerve cells survive, and an intermediate zone, in which the surviving cells are diminished in number and undergoing different phases of degeneration. An intermediate zone also intervenes between a tumor or other structural lesion and the normal surrounding tissue. In either case the blood supply to the intermediate zone is compromised, and the degenerating cells are more excitable. It is these unstable cells which constitute the epileptogenic focus.

Regardless of etiology and pathology of the cerebral lesions, the pathophysiology of seizure discharge may be identical. The basic mechanism appears to be prolonged depolarization with consequent hyperactive and hypersynchronous discharge from abnormal neurons. Such epileptic discharge may be circumscribed or may spread, and thus activate distant neurons, causing them to become secondarily or in some instances independently epileptogenic.

The biochemical basis of epileptic discharge remains incompletely understood. Experimental studies with epileptogenic cortex from animals and human patients suggest that the production and maintenance of such discharge involves (1) an accumulation of excess acetylcholine or other excitatory substance, (2) increased membrane permeability with increase in intracellular sodium ions, and (3) depletion of intracellular potassium ions. Systemic metabolic disturbances, such as hypoglycemia, hypocalcemia, anoxia, hypocapnia, and pyridoxin deficiency, are believed to exert their influence upon these basic factors and may become secondarily responsible for initiation of the epileptogenic discharge.

TRIGGERING MECHANISM. By and large epileptic attacks appear suddenly and fortuitously without any apparent immediate cause. On the other hand, many seizures do seem to occur under the influence of a triggering factor. The onset of these seizures may be cyclic and thus suggest a periodically recurring triggering mechanism, or provoked in an erratic manner. In the cyclic group the hormonal factors related to menstrual period, menarche, and menopause are conspicuous examples. In the induced seizures the provoking agents encompass a diversity of factors and mechanisms. These may be divided into nonsensory and sensory. Among the nonsensory group are hyperthermia, hyperventilation, metabolic disorders, physical stress, sleep deprivation, emotional disturbances, and so forth. The sensory triggers may be visual (e.g., photogenic, television, reading), auditory (musicogenic), vegetative, tactile, and proprioceptive; they may be spontaneous normal sensory stimuli of daily life or unexpected sensory experiences (startle reaction), and at times self-induced. Of the last group, the so-called startle epilepsy in brain-damaged children with or without cerebral palsy is an example. In these children hyperexcitable brainstem structures provide the pathologic substrate for escalation of normal startle reactions to epileptic seizures.

AGE FACTOR. Age and epilepsy are related in many ways. It is well known that epilepsy is much more common in children than in adults. In genetic epilepsy the appearance and disappearance of the clinical seizures and the electrical dysrhythmia are age dependent. Thus, pure petit mal attacks and the 3 per second EEG pattern have a peak incidence between 4 and 10 years and tend to disappear by the end of adolescence.

Seizures that occur before 2 years of age suggest a metabolic disorder or an underlying structural defect of the brain. Newborn infants are more likely to have poorly organized movements, such as twitching, trembling, or shaking, rather than a bona fide tonic-clonic convulsion. They often have apneic or blue spells, limp or stiff spells, vasomotor changes with flushing, pallor, and clamminess. Such seizure discharges probably originate mostly in subcortical structures; as the cortex develops, more differentiated types of seizure patterns become evident.

Seventy-five percent of structural growth of the brain occurs in the first 2 years of life. Generally speaking, the younger the child and the more immature the brain, the more susceptible it is to injury, and the more far-reaching the resultant functional disorganization.

Seizure Types

GENERALIZED CONVULSIONS. Generalized convulsions constitute the most common type of seizure in childhood. In the genetic type of epilepsy the seizure discharge is believed to originate in centrencephalic structures and to spread rapidly to both cerebral hemispheres with immediate loss of consciousness and generalized convulsions. As a rule, there is no aura preceding the onset and no localizing neurologic sign following the attack. In contrast, the symptomatic type may be associated with an aura and/or a postictal phenomenon that suggest a focal origin of the generalized seizure. With the rapid spread of the seizure discharge from the epileptogenic focus, the memory of the aura may be obscured. This is especially true in children.

The classical grand mal attack is usually precipitous in onset. Typically, the eyes roll up or to one side, the pupils dilate, and the face becomes flushed or pale. Consciousness is quickly lost, and the entire body is seized by a tonic spasm. There is often a sharp cry, and if standing, the child falls heavily to the ground. With the tonic spasm respiration is arrested and the child becomes cyanotic. After a period of 10 to 30 seconds, the tonic phase gives way to generalized clonic jerking lasting from 1 to 5 minutes or longer. Breathing is resumed but labored. There may be profuse perspiration and salivation, involuntary bladder and bowel evacuation, and the tongue may be bitten. Gradually the attack diminishes in severity; the muscle contractions become less violent and finally cease. If the duration of the attack is short, the child may recover his senses quickly and show little or no after effect. More commonly, however, he remains stuporous and sinks into postictal sleep lasting an hour or more. When he awakens, he may have headache, generalized fatigue, and restlessness for a variable duration. Postictally, transient neurologic deficits may be present, and these sometimes may be of significance in the diagnosis of a focal lesion.

Status Epilepticus. Grand mal seizures may occur in series without consciousness being regained between attacks. This condition is known as "status epilepticus." It may be induced by sudden withdrawal of anticonvulsant medication, incident to intercurrent infection, or without known cause. If not treated promptly and effectively, the status may persist for many hours or days with development of serious sequelae or even death. Transient postictal signs and symptoms include aphasia, ataxia, and mental sluggishness. Persistent symptoms and signs may develop indicating that irreversible brain damage has occurred as a result of prolonged cellular hypoxia. Status epilepticus should therefore be treated as a medical emergency.

Tonic Seizures. This is a type of seizure in which the patient's body stiffens, with increased tonicity of the entire musculature, and consciousness is lost. Such attacks arise when the midbrain is primarily involved in the seizure discharge.

FOCAL SEIZURES. When the initial event of a seizure consistently indicates a local origin in some part of the brain, it is focal epilepsy. The epileptic discharge may originate at any level of the nervous system. It may remain localized or spread across the midline to the opposite side and become generalized. Focal discharging lesions may be transient in young children. The significance of focal seizures in the young child is not the same as in older children or adults. Not infrequently the focal attack may vary from side to side, giving rise to multifocal epilepsy.

Focal Motor Seizures. These may manifest as involvement of one entire side of the body simultaneously (hemiconvulsion), or be limited to one extremity and/or the face. Jacksonian epilepsy is one which originates in one part of the motor cortex and spreads to involve the rest of the motor strip. The common points of onset are the thumb, the face, and the toe—structures having relatively large cortical representation. The orderly spread of the electrical discharge is reflected in the classical "march" which was described by Jackson 100 years ago. Jacksonian seizures frequently escalate into grand mal attacks. Following a seizure there may be transient paresis or paralysis lasting minutes or hours. This phenomenon, known as Todd's paralysis, is believed to result from a localized neuronal exhaustion. When Todd's paralysis becomes progressively longer in duration, or when the weakness persists during the interictal periods, one should suspect a progressive lesion. *Epilepsia partialis continua* refers to local convulsive movements of a continuous type, when a discharge maintains itself at a certain point continually.

Focal Sensory Seizures (somatic sensory seizures). Numbness and tingling are the usual sensations in seizures arising from the sensory cortex. The abnormal sensations may also proceed in a "march" and at times spread to the motor area with resultant motor seizures.

Focal Adversive Seizures. These attacks consist of turning of the head, eyes, and trunk away from the side of the cerebral lesion, with loss of consciousness. The seizure discharge is generally located in the prefrontal area, but other areas such as the occipital and temporal cortex may give rise to such attacks.

Occipital Seizures. Seizure discharges in the visual cortical areas produce simple visual impressions, such as dimness of vision, seeing shadows and clouds in front of the eyes, or a transient blindness.

Inhibitory Seizures (ictal paralysis). The epileptic discharge, even from the motor areas may produce inactivation or paralysis instead of excitation or motor activity. Such attacks are called inhibitory seizures.

Temporal Lobe (Psychomotor) Epilepsy and Diencephalic (Convulsive Equivalent) Epilepsy. These are the most common types of seizures of focal origin in childhood. They will be discussed separately.

PETIT MAL. In its "pure" form, absence or lapse attacks are characterized by episodes of abrupt, momentary loss of consciousness accompanied by cessation of voluntary activities. The child has a blank expression and stares into space (Fig. 70). The duration of each attack rarely exceeds 5 to 15 seconds. Just as abruptly, the child recovers his senses and resumes his activity as if no interruption had occurred. Typically, there is no aura and no postictal disturbance.

In 60 to 70 percent of patients, myoclonic jerks may occur. The common forms are slow rhythmic blinking of the eyes and rhythmic jerking of the head, arms, or trunk. The child rarely falls or loses bladder control. While having a petit mal attack, some children may perform semipurposeful motor acts such as snapping of the fingers, patting movement, or walking around or in circles. These have been termed *"petit mal automatism."*

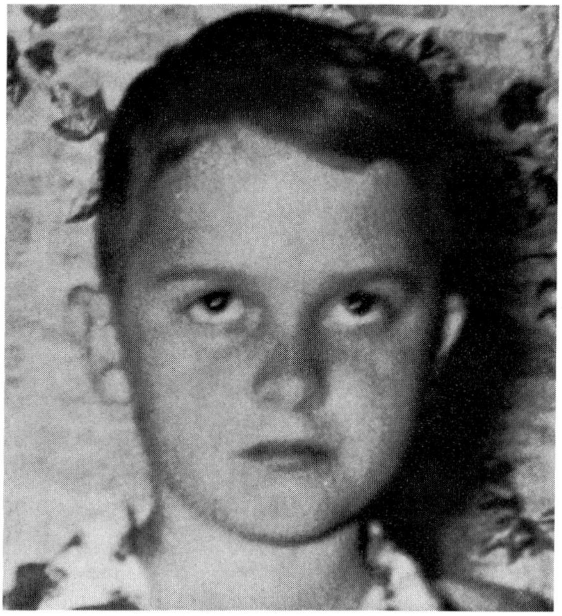

Fig. 70. A 10-year-old having an absence attack.

The frequency of absence attacks varies widely, from occasional to hundreds a day. Attentiveness in work or play diminishes the number of attacks; idleness, fatigue, excessive hydration, emotional stress, menstruation, overventilation, and photic stimulation tend to increase the frequency.

When attacks occur in close succession for a prolonged period of time, mental function is continually impaired and the child remains dazed and confused. The sudden obtunding of mental function may lead to a false impression of degenerative or toxic encephalopathy. This is known as *"petit mal status"* (Fig. 71). It may be ushered in by a febrile illness, an emotional upset, menstrual period, or occur without obvious cause. The occurrence of petit mal status seldom affects the ultimate prognosis.

The age of onset of pure petit mal epilepsy is usually between 4 and 10 years. The incidence is slightly higher in girls than in boys (6:4). The child's physical and mental development is usually unaffected, and the neurologic findings are entirely normal. The attacks tend to decrease with time and approximately 50 percent completely disappear in the late teens; they may however, persist into adult life.

About one-third to one-half of patients with petit mal may develop grand mal seizures. In these, the petit mal seizures usually make their appearance first.

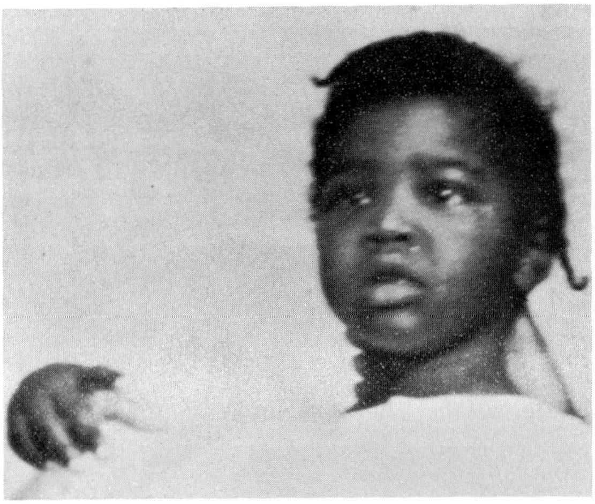

Fig. 71. A 4-year-old in petit mal status. Note obtund appearance and myoclonic jerk of hand.

The EEG abnormality of absence attacks is characteristic. Bursts of generalized bilaterally synchronous 3 per second spike and wave complexes appear, usually against a background of normal activity. Short bursts of such activity may not be accompanied by an overt clinical seizure, but may be associated with subtle impairment of mental efficiency. Bursts lasting longer than 5 seconds are often accompanied by clinical attacks.

MINOR MOTOR SEIZURES. ***Akinetic Attacks.*** Akinetic attacks are also known as drop fits. Postural tone is controlled by a balanced discharge of facilitatory and inhibitory impulses from the reticular formation in the upper brainstem. Drop seizures are believed to result from a sudden increase of inhibitory discharges which transiently overwhelms the influence of the facilitatory center and leads to sudden loss of postural tone.

The muscles involved may be limited to the neck, giving rise to head bobbing, or more generally resulting in collapse of the body. The attacks are so abrupt and unexpected that the patient and parents are caught unprepared, and significant injury may result.

Although akinetic attacks have been seen in genetic petit mal epilepsy, the majority of such attacks occur in patients with symptomatic epilepsy.

Akinetic attacks of symptomatic origin are by far the more common type. The children affected are much younger than the genetic group. The nodding seizures appear when the infant is able to assume sitting position, and the drop seizures occur when the child is able to get about. The frequency may be as high as several hundred seizures a day. Severe physical injuries are common, and there is a constant danger to life. The cause is frequently unknown; but in many cases the history may strongly implicate diffuse encephalopathy incident to past infections due to measles, other viral agents, immunization antigens, toxins, residua from tuberculous meningitis or tuberous sclerosis.

The EEG may show continuous runs of generalized slow spike and 1½ to 2 per second slow waves.

Various degrees of brain damage as evidenced by mental retardation and neurologic abnormalities —such as a Babinski sign, unequal deep tendon reflexes, abnormal muscle tone, apraxia, and incoordination—are frequently present.

As a rule the course is protracted, the seizures subsiding slowly and the EEG reverting gradually to a slow dysrhythmia. The child may become a slow learner or frankly retarded.

Myoclonic Epilepsies. Myoclonus is a phenomenon of clonic spasms of an isolated muscle or groups of muscles. Neither term necessarily implies epilepsy, although in some epileptic disorders myoclonus is a prominent symptom. Physiologically, myoclonus is believed to occur because of sudden release from inhibitory control of motor centers in the midbrain, the brainstem, or the spinal cord. The "uninhibited" discharge from these centers may spread to high structures, which may influence the myoclonus but are not essential in its occurrence. A variety of pathologic conditions may produce myoclonus, particularly those with diffuse involvement of the brain.

Clinically, *myoclonic seizures* may occur in genetic epilepsies in association with petit mal or grand mal attacks. More severe myoclonic seizures are not uncommon in symptomatic epilepsies incident to nonprogressive and progressive diffuse encephalopathies. That these myoclonic phenomena are epileptic in nature is attested to by the presence of cerebral dysrhythmia. The various types are:

1. *Myoclonic Seizures in Genetic Epilepsies.* Slow rhythmic jerks of the eyelids, the neck, or the arms are seen in 60 to 70 percent of children with absence attacks. These jerks do not alter the course or prognosis of the pure petit mal epilepsy. The EEG is that of the absence pattern.

Some patients with genetic epilepsy may have mixed seizures of myoclonic and grand mal attacks. The myoclonic seizures usually antedate the grand mal attacks by months or years. They tend to come on in the morning, causing the child to fall or to drop things without alteration of consciousness. Sometimes the parents may mistake these episodes for mere carelessness or teen-age clumsiness, only to realize their true nature when a long train of myoclonic jerks merges into grand mal attacks. The EEG may reveal paroxysmal multiple spike, slow wave, with normal background activity.

2. *Myoclonic Seizures in Nonprogressive Diffuse Encephalopathies.* The incidence in this group is highest between 2 and 6 years. Although the cause is often unknown, symptoms and signs of brain damage are almost always present, and a past history of undiagnosed infection or reaction to immunization may be obtained. Sometimes a history of childhood

infectious disease among the siblings may be a significant clue that the patient might have had a subclinical infection by the same etiologic agent. The myoclonus may occur alone or in association with akinetic attacks or grand mal seizures. In some cases the myoclonus may be no more than a shudder or quick jerks of the eyes, which may be unnoticed by the parents. In other cases the myoclonus may be more gross and more widespread. The jerks are usually arrhythmic. The EEG frequently shows generalized multiple spike and slow wave dysrhythmia. The course may be protracted with gradual improvement and subsidence of seizures in two or more years. Some degree of mental subnormality and residual neurologic deficit is quite common.

3. *Myoclonic Seizures in Progressive Diffuse Encephalopathies.* Severe or moderate myoclonus is a prominent feature in the middle stages of subacute sclerosing panencephalitis (inclusion body encephalitis, Dawson) and in neuronal storage diseases. The myoclonic attacks are usually diffuse in nature. The EEG may show periodic succession of high-voltage complexes which are synchronous in all leads with the myoclonic jerks. Treatment is ineffective. The underlying disease runs a protracted course with uniformly bad prognosis.

4. *Familial Myoclonus Epilepsy of Unverricht.* This is a relatively rare heredofamilial degenerative disease first described by Unverricht in 1891 and later by Lundborg. The onset occurs in childhood or at puberty and is marked by increasingly severe, arrhythmic myoclonic attacks involving chiefly the trunk and limb muscles. As the disease progresses, dementia, ataxia, and spasticity appear, and the myoclonus tends to diminish and disappear with the onset of generalized rigidity. Bulbar palsy and deepening stupor lead to death in 10 to 20 years. Pathologically, Lafora bodies having acid mucopolysaccharide reaction have been demonstrated in the ganglion cells of cerebellar and subcortical nuclei in many reported cases.

Massive Myoclonic Spasms. Massive myoclonic spasms (infantile spasms, massive spasms, lightning seizure, jackknife seizures) are types of seizures peculiar to infants and occur in diffuse encephalopathies of disparate causes. The seizures may first occur in apparently normal infants or in infants obviously defective since birth. The cause is unknown in about one-half of the cases. In the remainder, a history of cerebral insult occurring during gestation, birth, or infancy may be obtained. The nature of the cerebral insult may be a developmental anomaly, intrauterine factors of placental and maternal origin, birth trauma, anoxia, phenylketonuria, tuberous sclerosis, postnatal head injury, meningoencephalitis of bacterial or viral origin, and toxic or allergic encephalopathies. More recently there has been a growing belief that the basic disturbance responsible for epileptogenesis may be biochemical rather than structural, although its exact nature remains to be elucidated.

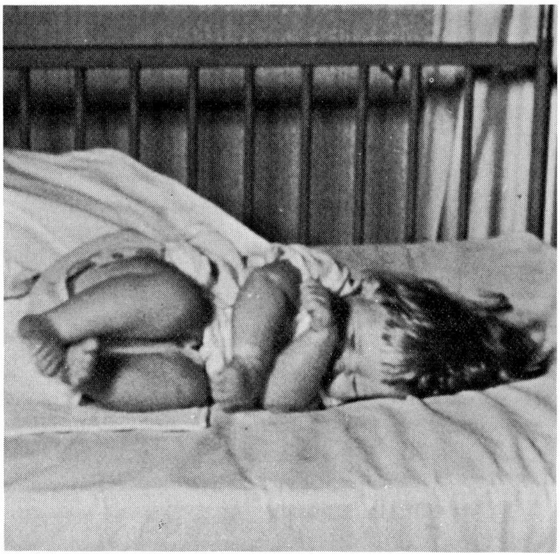

Fig. 72. A 6-month-old infant having a jackknife or flexor type of massive myoclonic spasms.

Massive myoclonic spasms are not an uncommon infantile epilepsy, second in incidence only to grand mal seizures. The peak incidence is between 3 and 6 months, although it has appeared as early as one day after birth; onset after the age of 2 years is uncommon. There is no significant difference in sex incidence.

The attacks may occur singly, but more often in series of successive episodes. Each attack is characterized by sudden, forceful myoclonic contractions involving the musculature of the trunk, the neck, and the extremities. In the flexor type, the patient adducts and flexes his limbs, drops his head, and doubles upon himself, much like closing a jackknife (Fig. 72). In the extensor type, the neck is extended, the arms spread out, and the body is bent backward in a manner aptly described as spreadeagle. A cry or grunt may accompany the more severe attacks. The infant may grimace or laugh, or appear fearful during or after the attack.

Individual attacks are momentary in duration, never exceeding one minute. The frequency varies from a few attacks to hundreds a day.

In 90 percent of the cases, the EEG shows a characteristic pattern known as hypsarhythmia; the severity of the electrical disturbance generally correlates with the severity of the clinical seizures.

The natural course of massive myoclonic spasms is protracted. After a period of months or years, the spasms may gradually diminish in frequency and severity and then cease. Occasionally they give way to focal seizures, grand mal seizures, or minor motor seizures. The sequelae of brain damage are permanent. With the onset of the seizures, development is arrested or regresses. As the attacks persist, mentality and motor functions continue to deteriorate. Ultimately 10 to 15 percent of the children succumb; of the surviving, more than 90 percent are mentally retarded.

PSYCHOMOTOR EPILEPSY. Psychomotor epilepsy is common in childhood; the incidence is highest between 3 and 6 years and becomes much lower after the age of 12 years. There is a slight preponderance of boys over girls. The seizure discharge usually originates in the "temporal lobe," which comprises the gray matter of the Sylvian fissure, the insula, the uncus, the amygdala, and the hippocampus, in addition to the three lateral temporal convultions. In the author's series of 250 cases, a temporal EEG focus was found in 60 percent in routine studies. Atrophic lesions due to birth injury, postnatal trauma, febrile convulsions in infancy, and thrombotic and infectious meningoencephalopathies are far more common than expanding lesions.

Prodromal symptoms of irritability or gastric upset may precede the onset of a seizure by hours or days. Sleep is a common precipitant. An aura of fear, gastric sensation, buzzing in the ear, or bad odor may usher in the attack. An infant who cannot express himself may hold up his hands to his ears or to the epigastrium with a facial expression of fear, pain, or alarm. The seizures are characteristically of brief duration, lasting from half a minute to 5 to 10 minutes. Consciousness is often impaired but rarely completely lost. The most common motor symptoms are drawing or jerking of the mouth and face, usually opposite to the side of the discharge. Aphasia or dysphasia may be present if the discharge originates from the dominant side. The eyes may stare in a searching manner. There may be tonic posturing or a desire to urinate. Coordinated but inappropriate movements may be performed repeatedly in a stereotyped manner (automatism), common examples being clutching, fumbling, kicking, walking or running in circles, swallowing, smacking, chewing, licking, and spitting. Pill-rolling, athetoid, or flinging movements are less common. Inhibitory seizures with loss of tone (limpness) or arrest of motion (freezing) may occur. Affective expressions such as laughing or crying are not unusual. Psychical symptoms such as forced thinking, rage, illusions, or hallucinations are rare in children. Chronic behavior disorder may be present. When the attack is over, there may or may not be postictal sluggishness or sleep. Amnesia of the attack is the rule.

AUTONOMIC EPILEPSY OR SEIZURE EQUIVALENT SYNDROME. This syndrome may be defined as an entity of epilepsy characterized by paroxysmal attacks of autonomic disturbances with or without associated seizures of other types and with or without disorders of other cerebral functions. The syndrome occurs in children of all ages with peak incidence at 6 to 7 years. Boys predominate by a 2:1 ratio. A history of birth injury, postnatal head trauma, encephalopathies, or prenatal injury, in the order named, may be elicited in 40 to 50 percent of the children. A family history of epilepsy is present in 20 to 30 percent of the patients.

The most common symptoms are headache and abdominal pain. The headache may be severe or mild, diffuse or ill-defined, and almost never hemicranial. The abdominal pain, which also varies in severity and may be accompanied by nausea, vomiting, and other visceral symptoms, has been diagnosed as an acute surgical emergency, leading to unnecessary laparotomy. Unexplained diarrhea may suddenly appear. Profuse salivation, thermal disturbances, and various vasomotor symptoms may be observed. Unexplained fits of rage or uncontrollable laughter have been reported. Syncopal episodes and sudden collapse with complete limpness may alarm the parents. The seizures generally last for minutes and rarely hours.

Not all of the above symptoms are observed in all the patients, but more than three symptoms should be present in recurrent attacks before such a diagnosis can be considered. Overexertion, anxiety, and sleep are the usual precipitants.

Nearly half of the children may have other types of epilepsy; psychomotor seizures, grand mal, and limp attacks are the commonest. Penfield described attacks of the above symptoms in a patient with a tumor in the third ventricle and suggested the term diencephalic autonomic epilepsy. Gibbs described the 14 and 6 per second positive spikes in sleep and suggested their thalamic-hypothalamic origin. It is probable that these seizure discharges originate in or near the hypothalamus. The correlation of convulsive equivalent with 14 and 6 EEG pattern is about 50 percent in our experience. Autonomic symptoms may also be produced by discharge from the insular and the orbitofrontal regions.

OTHER NONEPILEPTIC ICTAL PHENOMENA. The EEG may sometimes reveal abnormal activities in children with no overt seizures but with behavior or personality disorders. Besides focal abnormalities, generalized bilateral synchronous paroxysmal activity may be present. Similar findings may be recorded in children with aphasia, learning problems, and sleep disturbances. That an ictal discharge plays an important role in the mechanism of the disorder in such cases is supported by the fact that a good response to anticonvulsant therapy is sometimes obtained.

Diagnostic Evaluation

The first step in the study of a child who has a convulsion is to document its occurrence. Although anxious parents are, as a rule, poor witnesses, every effort should be made to obtain a description of the seizure, particularly premonitory symptoms, loss of consciousness, convulsive movements, duration of the attack, and the state of the patient following the attack. Breath-holding spells in infants may simulate convulsive seizures. In breath-holding spells there is always a precipitating factor, usually a slight injury or some emotional disturbance which results in violent crying, ending suddenly in respiratory apnea.

The cyanosis in such attacks appears before loss of consciousness and convulsive movements.

The second step is to determine whether the seizure is associated with some organic lesion of the central nervous system or with some metabolic disturbance. Every child who has had a convulsion should be subjected to thorough study, including a complete history, general physical and neurologic examinations, x-rays of the skull, electroencephalogram, and contents of the blood.

HISTORY TAKING. Frequently a good history in itself provides the essential evidence for the diagnosis. Besides a description of the seizure per se, certain other details are of relevance: The *frequency* of attacks may increase with passage of time in untreated cases of petit mal, but remain stationary in psychomotor and convulsive equivalent seizures. The *duration* of the attack is pertinent. Absence attacks seldom exceed 30 seconds in duration, whereas psychomotor seizures often last for several minutes. Any prolonged convulsion accompanied by cyanosis may be detrimental to the brain. The *time* of occurrence may be of value in diagnosis. Early morning attacks or episodes recurring after a meal may suggest the possibility of hypoglycemia.

Factors tending to *precipitate* seizures, such as bright light, television, flickering light, loud noise, overbreathing, emotional disturbance, physical fatigue, hunger, menstruation, and fever, should be ascertained so that appropriate measures may be taken to diminish their influence.

Maternal history of illnesses, operations, medication during pregnancy, and miscarriage may be of importance. The events of *birth* must be recalled in detail. Precipitous delivery is as significant as prolonged labor. Induction of labor, instrumentation, operative procedures, and other obstetric complications are relevant. The condition of the *placenta,* if known to the mother or available in the hospital record, should be noted.

The *status* of the infant at birth and as a neonate is of utmost importance. His vitality, vigor, color, and activities (feeding, sleep, crying) are clues to future development.

In *infancy* and *childhood,* head injury, untoward reaction to immunizations, and infections are significant. Febrile convulsions are also important. The milestones in early childhood and school records are informative data of the patient's mental and motor development.

Headache, abdominal pain, restless sleep, and behavior disorders are frequent *"side"* symptoms, worthy of note. Their persistence after commencement of epilepsy treatment may indicate that medication is not sufficient. Symptoms referable to speech, vision, fine skills, and higher mental functions are also of relevance; their progressive deterioration is often a bad omen.

The type, dosage, duration of *previous medication,* and the patient's response are important data helpful in planning treatment.

FAMILY HISTORY. Inasmuch as epilepsy continues to be regarded as a stigma, a positive history of epilepsy in the family may not be obtained on the first round of inquiry. As it is of some importance in diagnosis, prognosis, classification, and epidemiology, renewed efforts should be made to conclusively establish the answer. A different approach in the inquiry or use of such terms as "fever spasms" or "fainting spells" in the place of epilepsy may sometimes be rewarding.

ORDER OF EXAMINATION. The examination begins with the interview. Much information may be gained by observing the child. His general behavior and affect, his response to the environment and to questions and commands constitute an impression and provide clues as to how he could best be examined later. He may be given a puzzle to work, pictures to color, or building blocks. His activities should tell something about his motor skills and his mental development. He may show subtle seizure activity that is not evident to the parents.

The sequence of examination should be flexible, and the most difficult parts, for instance, fundoscopy, should be reserved for the last. Often the parents may be asked to leave and the child be observed unobtrusively by the examiner alone.

NEUROLOGIC EXAMINATION. The head size should be measured. Before 2 years of age the head and chest circumference coincide. An abnormally large head may suggest congenital hydrocephalus, subdural hematoma, intracranial mass, cerebral neurofibromatosis, or Tay-Sachs disease. An abnormally small head may indicate brain damage with cerebral atrophy or congenital dysplasia. The fontanel and sutures should be noted for early closure or evidence of separation. Dilated venous channels on the scalp suggest increased intracranial pressure. Clusters of venous patches suggest arteriovenous malformation. Auscultation of the skull should be done with the child recumbent; a localized loud bruit suggests a vascular abnormality. Transillumination of the skull is useful in young infants. Asymmetry or other abnormality in the configuration of the skull must be explained. The spinal axis should be examined for dimples, sinus tracts, tufts of hair, or lipomatous deposits. Certain skin lesions are clues of cerebral anomalies, since the skin and nervous system have a common embryologic origin from ectoderm. Port-wine nevus flammeus of trigeminal distribution is a clue for Sturge-Weber-Dimitri disease; adenoma sebaceum and cutaneous depigmentation suggest tuberous sclerosis; and café-au-lait spots and nodular masses over peripheral nerve distribution signify neurofibromatosis. All three conditions may be associated with epilepsy.

The retina, an extension of the brain, is a rewarding structure to examine carefully. In early infancy, choreoretinitis may be due to toxoplasmosis or cytomegalic inclusion disease. Cherry-red spot or pigmentary changes in the macular area point to cerebral lipidosis. Other retinal changes such as hemorrhage, exudate, papilledema, and optic atrophy also provide important clues to various other diagnoses which may be associated with the epilepsies. The eyes should be examined for cataracts; their presence suggests the possibility of prenatal viral infection or an inborn error of metabolism. Apart from the above, a complete neurologic examination as described elsewhere in this section should be followed. The presence of focal signs, however minimal, may contribute importantly to the total evaluation of the child. A brief psychologic evaluation should always be included, even though accurate psychometric tests may be left to the experts.

GENERAL PHYSICAL EXAMINATION. The findings of high blood pressure or evidence of congenital heart disease is of importance because hypertensive encephalopathy and cerebral anoxia may cause convulsions. The existence of multiple dysplastic features (e.g., hypertelorism, low-set ears, simian line, receding chin, yellow skin, silky skin) suggests the possibility of cerebral dysplasia being the cause of epilepsy. Hepatic and splenic enlargement may be indications of glycogen storage disease, Gaucher's disease, or Niemann-Pick disease.

If the history suggests petit mal absence seizures, hyperventilation for three minutes (approximately 100 deep breaths) may induce an attack and help confirm the diagnosis; a negative result should not be considered to rule out this possibility.

LABORATORY EXAMINATION. The diagnostic impression derived from the history and physical examination should determine the indication for laboratory studies and which tests should be performed.

Electroencephalography. Of the various labotory tests, the electroencephalogram is the most informative and least painful procedure. It frequently provides the only objective evidence of cerebral disorder in seizure patients. It is also helpful in differentiating diffuse encephalopathies from localized lesions. With serial studies, it may provide evidence as to whether the lesion is static or progressive. However, the electroencephalogram should not be considered as a means of obtaining a "penny in the slot" diagnosis. As has been discussed in the section on classification, although certain specific electroencephalographic patterns have been shown to correlate closely with certain seizures, it is not safe or wise to adopt without question a diagnosis suggested by the electroencephalogram contrary to that indicated by clinical evidence.

Electrocorticography and depth electrode recordings are highly specialized procedures to be carried out only when precise localization of an epileptogenic lesion is required prior to surgical exploration.

Radiographic Studies. Radiographic examination of the skull occasionally provides unique information. Asymmetry of the cranium with unilateral thickening of the vault, elevation of the sphenoid and petrous ridges, and increased development of the sinus cells are indicative of a cerebral hemiatrophy. Asymmetry associated with localized thinning and bulging of the vault may suggest an underlying expanding lesion such as porencephalic cyst. Increased intracranial pressure may be reflected by sellar changes and separation of sutures. Abnormal calcifications may help localize and provide a clue to the nature of the cerebral lesion.

More specific procedures such as cerebral angiography and air studies are indicated when there is a possibility of a vascular or neoplastic lesion. Ventriculography is the procedure of choice where there is evidence of increased intracranial pressure. Echoencephalography and brain scan may also be helpful.

Other Tests. Lumbar puncture and examination of the cerebrospinal fluid are of particular value when cerebral tumor or progressive degenerative or inflammatory disease is suspected.

A complete blood count and urinalysis should be routine tests; these data are useful as a base line for future reference, especially in case of drug toxicity. In a Negro child, a sickle-cell preparation should be done. The urinary amino acid screening test may be considered in epileptics whose etiologic factor is unknown. The urinary sediment should be examined for cytomegalic inclusion bodies and metachromatic bodies when indicated. The test for porphobilinogen in the urine is indicated in children with acute abdominal pain and convulsions and may result in the rare diagnosis of porphyria. A phenylpyruvic acid test of the urine should be routine, as 25 percent of PKU patients have epilepsy. Serum calcium and phosphorus determinations as well as a fasting blood sugar should be routinely performed to rule out a metabolic basis for the seizures.

Differential Diagnosis

The child with episodic disturbances in the state of consciousness may have a seizure disorder, syncope, migraine, or a functional disorder. In the epileptic patient it is essential to determine whether the attacks are associated with an underlying organic or metabolic disorder (symptomatic), are of undetermined cause (unknown), or are hereditary (genetic).

A. Diagnostic Criteria of Genetic Epilepsy:
   1. Age: grand mal—onset between 2 to 16 years
      petit mal—onset between 4 to 16 years
      mixed seizures—petit mal usually precedes grand mal
   2. Seizure pattern: absence, generalized tonic clonic, myoclonic, (rarely) akinetic seizures with no focal features
   3. Family history: family incidence of similar seizures or febrile convulsions
   4. Normal neurologic and physical findings. Usually normal intelligence
   5. Characteristic EEG pattern: bilaterally synchronous 3 per second spike wave or bilaterally synchronous paroxysmal slow dysrhythmia

B. Diagnosis of Symptomatic Epilepsy:

1. Space-occupying lesions should always be considered with focal seizures and focal EEG abnormalities. There is no need, however, to perform all kinds of investigations at the beginning. If the seizures are refractory to drug therapy or if the child develops progressive symptoms or signs, more definitive diagnostic studies may be necessary. Temporal lobe neoplastic lesions may be very slow growing and simulate genetic epilepsy.
2. Degenerative and infectious encephalopathies: Epilepsies are common in many types of chronic disease of the central nervous system. The presence of other manifestations of cerebral dysfunction is suggestive. These include regression of mentation and speech, change in personality or sleeping habits, visual complaints, headache, general or specific incoordination and clumsiness. Progressive EEG changes often accompany these manifestations. Subacute sclerosing panencephalitis, cerebral lipidosis, and some of the leucodystrophies are examples of this group.

Epilepsy must be distinguished from other paroxysmal phenomena including the following:

1. *Syncope.* These attacks are always provoked, not spontaneous. Careful history will reveal the precipitating factor. In infants, two types of syncope occur: the more common type is the breath-holding spell. Less frequently, fainting spells may follow trivial but unexpected trauma to the head; the infant may or may not cry before passing out. Older children may faint upon painful stimulation, fear, or strong emotional upset. In all these conditions, there is usually a positive family history of a similar disorder. In breath-holding attacks and syncope in older children, the mechanism is cardioinhibitory or Valsalva-like effect. In the infant who passes out following head trauma, a reflex mechanism involving the medullary centers appears responsible. In all types the tendency for this hyperparasympathetic activity is believed to be hereditary. In adolescents, particularly females, hyperventilation may precipitate a syncopal episode.

2. *Hysteria.* Older children from 6 to 16 years, may have episodes which stimulate epileptic attacks because of anxiety or other psychologic causes. Neurologic examination and EEG in such children show no evidence of abnormality.

3. *Migraine.* (p. 154).

Course and Prognosis

Epilepsy is, by definition, a chronic disorder with recurrent paroxysmal symptoms. The course and prognosis vary with the nature and severity of the underlying disease. Medication is continued for 3 to 4 years after the attacks are arrested. In case of relapse, which is more frequent around puberty, drug therapy has to be reinitiated and a full course maintained for another 2 or 3 years.

The prognosis of genetic epilepsies is generally good. Pure petit mal attacks tend to diminish in frequency with age and by adolescence disappear in approximately 50 percent of patients. Favorable outcome is seen even in cases with petit mal status. Grand mal seizures of genetic type are often nocturnal and generally respond to medical therapy but they tend to disappear after age 20. Mixed grand mal and petit mal seizure pattern is more difficult to control.

Of the symptomatic epilepsies posttraumatic and focal epilepsies have a favorable prognosis. About one-half to one-third of psychomotor seizures are difficult to control. A time factor seems important in the treatment of psychomotor seizures. All efforts should be made to gain seizure control at the earliest possible time. Delay in initiating appropriate treatment may result in discrete EEG focus giving way to mirror foci and subsequently more diffuse abnormalities. In such cases the seizures may be more complex, protracted, and refractory to anticonvulsants. As a consequence the patient's intellect may be adversely affected. Other acquired epilepsies including massive myoclonic, minor motor, and mixed types are difficult to treat but the end result is not all unrewarding. In addition to the seizures, most children in this category may have other manifestations of brain dysfunction. In a small number of cases the physician would have to prepare the parents for the possibility of institutional care and help them in the painful process of making this decison.

Age factor is not as important as the pathologic nature of the cerebral lesion and the type of seizures produced. The *duration of seizure history,* however, is important. The prospect of successful treatment is diminished if symptoms are of long standing.

Serial EEG's are helpful as general guide in prognosis. The prognosis is better if EEG shows progressive improvement and finally normalizes. Generally the EEG reverts to normal before seizures arrest. In some cases the EEG abnormality persists for a long time but the child remains well. One should not attempt to "treat" the EEG. Progressive worsening of EEG calls for reevaluation.

Conditions which tend to *precipitate attacks* are important factors in prognosis; ways and means to eliminate or minimize these will be helpful. Sometimes surgical extirpation of a sensitized and accessible area of the brain may eliminate seizure build-up completely.

The *attitude of the family,* relatives, school authorities, and schoolmates may exert intangible but important influence upon the child's own reaction toward his illness. The physician can play an important role in obviating these influences by thoughtful counseling. The possibility of brain damage or even sudden death from seizures per se are common fears besetting the parents. Severe convulsions with prolonged anoxia may be fatal but this seldom occurs.

Convulsions with cyanosis lasting over 30 minutes may cause brain damage. The child who develops periodic bouts of status epilepticus generally has a poor prognosis.

Management

The management of the epileptic child should be considered in three aspects, namely, (1) the specific therapy of the seizure, (2) the overall management of the child as a person, and (3) the counseling of the parents. The emphasis may vary with individual patient and family; all should receive full attention of the physician.

PARENT COUNSELING. It must be realized that all parents need counseling and reassurance. They may be prejudiced about their child's "unspeakable affliction," have a sense of guilt or shame, and be worried, anxious, fearful, or even hostile. They may have "shopped around" without a clear idea of what the real trouble is or what the future holds for the child. The strain on their emotional and economic resources may threaten the welfare of the entire family. Clearly it is the obligation of the physician to enlighten, to reassure, to answer questions, and to help solve secondary problems. After a thorough work-up, in which the parents have participated in history taking, they should be apprised of the diagnosis, treatment plan, and prognosis as nearly as is known or presumed. The result is often surprising and gratifying. Most parents can become reconciled to even the worst diagnosis or the poorest prognosis if they are kept informed. As they learn to understand what it is and what to expect, they will be in a much better position to carry on the care of their child without unduly dislocating their family life. The importance of this to the total welfare of the epileptic child cannot be overestimated. Wisely carried out, parent counseling is a small investment in terms of time and effort on the part of the physician, with huge dividends to the family as their fears of uncertainty are allayed by understanding the definitive diagnosis and plans of treatment.

MANAGEMENT OF THE CHILD AS A PERSON. The epileptic child should be treated as a "person," not a "case." It should be reemphasized that epilepsy is only a symptom of an underlying disease which may exhibit other symptoms of equal or more serious import. The child may have emotional problems, either because of his seizures or because of poor schoolwork secondary to cerebral dysfunction. In addition, as the child grows into adolescence and young adulthood, educational, social, and economic problems arise and demand solution. The physician should provide suggestions and direction.

Generally speaking, the epileptic child should be encouraged to live as normal a life as is consistent with safety. If the seizures are under good control, such physical exercises as riding a bicycle, jumping rope, roller skating, and swimming (under supervision) may be permitted; and if the child is able, certain competitive sports may be also allowed. Other than the ketogenic diet, dietary and fluid restrictions play no role in the management of epilepsy.

TABLE 25. *The Drugs of Choice for the Various Seizure Types (in order of preference)*

Generalized (major motor), focal, psychomotor, and convulsive-equivalent epilepsy
- Dilantin
- Phenobarbital or Mebaral
- Mysoline
- Mesantoin
- Celontin
- Phenurone
- Bromides

Petit mal
- Zarontin
- Tridione
- Valium
- Diamox
- Milontin
- Aralen

Minor Motor
- ACTH or adrenal corticosteroids
- Mogadon
- Ketogenic diet
- Zarontin, Tridione, Valium, and Celontin
- Dexedrine
- Meprobamate
- Gemonil

Status epilepticus
- Valium (iv)
- Sodium Nembutal (iv)
- Sodium phenobarbital (iv or im)
- Paraldehyde (iv, im, or rectal)
- Volatile anesthetics

Although petit mal seldom affects the intellect, the same assurance may not be given for all genetic epilepsies expecially when the seizures are prolonged and numerous. Many types of symptomatic seizures are associated with brain damage. In addition to their seizures, these children usually have mental, motor, or speech deficits as well. These difficulties may in turn lead to secondary emotional disorders, and such children should receive special assistance to overcome their handicaps. They may need to attend special classes at school and require special vocational and social guidance.

DRUG THERAPY. Drugs are the principal weapons in the treatment of the epilepsies. With proper choice and dosage of drugs appropriate to the seizure type, about 60 percent of all epileptic attacks can be satisfactorily controlled.

Phenobarbital was introduced in 1912 and remains the best anticonvulsant among the barbiturates. The discovery of diphenylhydantoin (Dilantin) in 1936 marked the beginning of modern drug therapy for epilepsy. Eight years later, trimethadione (Tridione) was tested, and quickly proved its specific usefulness in the petit mal group. Since then a large number of new drugs have been added. Several barbituric acid derivatives with less sedative action have

TABLE 26. *Anticonvulsants for Childhood Epilepsy*

	Indications	Dosage				Toxicity
		0-1 Year	5 Years	12 Years and Up	mg/kg/day	
Aralen (chloroquine)	Petit mal*	60 mg, 1-2 times per day	200 mg per day	400 mg per day	15-20	Bleaching of hair, blurring vision
Bromides	Same as Dilantin	250-500 mg daily	500 mg, 2-3 times daily	500 mg, 4-6 times daily	50-100	Drowsiness, skin rash, mental dullness, toxic psychosis
Celontin (methsuximide)	Psychomotor* Minor motor†	75 mg, 2-3 times daily	150 mg, 3 times daily	300 mg, 2-3 times daily	15-20	Drowsiness, ataxia, skin rash, rare aplastic anemia
Dexedrine (dextroam-phetamine)	Petit mal	1.25 mg, 2-3 times daily	5 mg, 2 times daily	10 mg, 2-3 times daily	0.25-0.75	Restlessness, irritability, sleeplessness
Diamox (acetazolamide)	Petit mal* All types†	125 mg, 3 times daily	250 mg, 3 times daily	250 mg, 4 times daily	15-30	Anorexia, paresthesia, drowsiness, polyuria, hyperpnea, headache
Dilantin (diphenyl-hydantoin)	Generalized Psychomotor Focal	20 mg, 3-4 times daily	50 mg, 3 times daily	100 mg, 3-4 times daily	3-8	Gum hypertrophy, ataxia, diplopia, nystagmus, rash, fever, nausea, vomiting, hirsutism
Gemonil (metharbital)	Minor motor*	25 mg, 4-6 times daily	50 mg, 4-6 times daily	100 mg, 3-4 times daily	5-15	Rare drowsiness
Librium (chlordiazepoxide)	Same as Phenobarbital	15 mg, 4-5 times daily	32 mg, 3-4 times daily	100 mg, 3-4 times daily	2-8	Drowsiness, irritability, rash
Mebaral (mephobarbital)	Minor motor	—	—	30-150 mg per day		Nausea, lethargy, dizziness
Meprobamate (Equanil, Miltown; methylpropyl pro-panediol dicarbamate)	Petit mal* Minor motor†	200 mg, 2-3 times daily	200 mg, 3-5 times daily	400 mg, 2-3 times daily	20-40	Drowsiness, hyperactivity

Mesantoin (methylphenylethyl hydantoin)	Same as Dilantin	25 mg, 3-4 times daily	50 mg, 3-4 times daily	100 mg, 4-6 times daily	4-10	Rash and fever, leucopenia and agranulocytosis, ataxia
Milontin (phensuximide)	Petit mal* Minor motor†	50 mg, 4-5 times daily	250 mg, 3-4 times daily	500 mg, 3-6 times daily	20-40	Nephrotoxic (slightly)
Mogadon (nitrazepam)	(not available in U.S.A.)					
Mysoline (primidone)	Same as Dilantin	50 mg, 3-4 times daily	125 mg, 2-3 times daily	250 mg, 4-6 times daily	12-25	Drowsiness, ataxia, skin rash
Paradione (paramethadione)	Same as Tridione					
Paraldehyde (paracetaldehyde)	Status epilepticus	1 ml, im or iv; 2 ml, rectally	3 ml, im or iv; 6 ml, rectally	3-6 ml, iv; 8 ml, im		Unpleasant odor, drowsiness
Peganone (ethyl phenyl hydantoin)	Same as Dilantin		500 mg, 2-4 times daily	1,000 mg, 3-4 times daily		Same as Dilantin except for hirsutism and gum hypertrophy
Phenobarbital (ethyl phenyl-barbituric acid)	Same as Dilantin* Minor motor†	15 mg, 3-4 times daily	30 mg, 2-3 times daily	60 mg, 2-3 times daily	1-5	Drowsiness, skin rash, and fever, hyperirritability in infants
Phenurone (phenacemide)	Psychomotor	125 mg, 3-4 times daily	250 mg, 4-6 times daily	500 mg, 4 times daily	20-35	Hepatotoxic, leucopenia, agranulocytosis, rash, irritability, and mental derangement
Tridione (trimethadione)	Petit mal* Minor motor†	25 mg, 4-6 times daily	150 mg, 4-6 times daily	300 mg, 4-6 times daily	20-50	Rash, leucopenia and agranulocytosis, nephrosis, photophobia, irritability
Valium (diazepam)	Status epilepticus*	1-2 mg, iv	5 mg, iv	10 mg, iv	Slow injection, 1-2 mg/ minute	Drowsiness, ataxia
	Minor motor Petit mal	1 mg, 1-3 times daily	2 mg, 1-3 times daily	5 mg, 1-3 times daily		
Zarontin (ethosuximide)	Petit mal* Minor motor†		250 mg, 2-3 times daily	250 mg, 3-4 times daily	20-50	Drowsiness, skin rash, gastric upset, rare aplastic anemia

*Primary indication.
†Secondary indication.

become available: Mebaral (Mephobarbital), Gemonil (Metharbital), Mysoline (Primidone).

To the hydantoin family the following have been added: Mesatoin (methylphenylethyl hydantoin) and Pegonone (ethotoin) in the 1940's.

The suxinimides (Milontin, Celontin, Zarontin) have been found valuable in petit mal and psychomotor seizures. Meanwhile, a host of other drugs, not primarily anticonvulsant in action, have proved useful. Among these is acetazolamide (Diamox), whose effect is related to its inhibitory action on brain carbonic anhydrase.

Some tranquilizing agents have antiseizure properties: Librium is a weak antiepileptic agent but two of its analogs have been found more effective: Valium (diazepam) has become the drug of choice for all types of status epilepticus; Mogadon (nitrazepam) is widely used with success for minor motor seizures in Europe and South America but is not available in this country.

Tegretol (carbamazepine), chemically related to Tofranil (imipramine hydrochloride), a drug for trigeminal neuralgia, has been used in major motor and psychomotor epilepsies.

The amphetamines and the antimalarials also have their places in the antiepileptic armamentarium.

Finally, the adrenal steroids and ACTH preparations have produced some dramatic results in massive myoclonic and minor motor seizures.

For the indications, dosage, and toxic reactions, reference may be made to the drug tables (Tables 25 and 26).

General Principles of Drug Therapy. Of the large number of tested drugs, some are wide-spectrum (Dilantin, phenobarbital, Diamox) and others more specific (Tridione, Celontin, Zarontin) in their antiepileptic activity. The selection of the most effective drug or drugs for each individual patient requires judgment and experience. Some general guidelines are therefore of fundamental importance:

1. A prime factor in successful therapy lies in the choice of the most effective drug, which depends upon correct identification of the clinical seizure type and the associated EEG pattern of the epilepsy in question. Except for emergencies, therapy can be withheld until the clinical and laboratory studies have been completed and a diagnosis has been established.

2. Use one drug at a time. Give it a fair trial before discarding it as ineffective. Increase dosage to tolerance and give it for a reasonable period of time. A combination of two or more drugs may be required, especially for mixed seizures. Give each addition or deletion thoughtful consideration until a satisfactory regimen is found.

3. Give adequate dosage. Young children can tolerate comparatively large doses of anticonvulsants. They are also consistently outgrowing their dosage, requiring adjustment from time to time.

4. Duration of therapy should be prolonged; early termination of medication may be followed by relapse. A safe rule is to continue the medication for at least three or four years after the *last* attack.

5. Weaning from medication should always be gradual, with stepwise reduction of dosage and withdrawal of one drug at a time.

6. One hundred percent control of symptoms may not be achieved in every patient. It is better to have a functional child with satisfactory control than complete control at the expense of a drug-toxic child.

7. Sometimes a drug, or a combination of drugs, may activate instead of suppress the seizure activity. Be ready to review the problem and revise the treatment from a different approach.

8. Factors which trigger or aggravate seizures should be prevented or controlled; these include fever, constipation, allergic states, emotional upset, frustration, physical exhaustion, and premenstrual edema.

Specific Anticonvulsant Therapy. *Grand mal.* Most grand mal seizures, regardless of cause, respond well to Dilantin or phenobarbital, or both. It is wise to use only one drug at the beginning. Dilantin is the first choice because phenobarbital may cause hyperactivity and irritability in young children and sluggishness in children of school age. Mebaral (mephobarbital) is also an effective barbiturate and is usually well tolerated by children. Mebaral is metabolized to phenobarbital, and in equivalent doses its effect is half that of phenobarbital. The individual effective dose is therefore twice that of phenobarbital. Mesantoin (methylphenylethyl-hydantoin) may be used in place of Dilantin.

All these drugs may cause toxic symptoms from overdosage or idiosyncrasy. Fever, morbilliform rash, even exfoliative dermatitis may develop, and the drug should be discontinued. Sometimes, after the symptoms clear, another trial with smaller dosage may be tolerated. Other common toxic reactions from Dilantin overdosage are cerebellar signs (usually reversible), nausea, vomiting, and irritability (more common in infants). The more subtle symptoms of headache, dizziness, mental depression are often not recognized as idiosyncrasy or mild toxicity to Dilantin and may mislead to suspicion of disease of CNS, psychoneurosis, or even brain tumor. Most of these symptoms are reversible. More severe forms of idiosyncrasy to Dilantin may result in the development of Stevens-Johnson syndrome, lupus erythematosus, lymphadenopathy simulating lymphoma. These are urgent indications to stop Dilantin therapy immediately. Recent reports indicated that Dilantin, Mysoline, and phenobarbital, alone or combined, may cause subnormal serum folate values. Whether or not megaloblastic anemia reversible by folic acid therapy occurs in children and how prevalent needs further investigation. Gum hypertrophy occurs in about 50 percent of children on Dilantin therapy. This is not a contraindication to the use of Dilantin. Firm massage of the gums may alleviate this side effect. Excessive hair growth is also common in young children but this is generally reversible after the drug is discontinued. Mesantoin is more toxic than Dilantin and may produce neutropenia or aplastic anemia; periodic blood counts are indicated when this agent is used.

Mysoline (Primidone) is a satisfactory anticonvulsant drug. The desired dosage should be built up gradually, lest the child become oversedated. Mysoline may cause irritability, anorexia, and lethargy but is generally well tolerated by the majority of children.

Gemonil (Metharbital), a weaker anticonvulsant, is almost devoid of side effects and can be used as an adjunctive drug.

Individual Seizure Management. If the initial seizure, febrile or nonfebrile, is witnessed and found to be unduly prolonged (10 minutes or more), it should be controlled by the use of intravenous sodium phenobarbital. In such circumstances an infant under the age of 1 year may require 0.06 to 0.1 g; a child between the ages of 2 and 5, 0.12 to 0.2 g; and the older child, up to 0.3 g.

Status epilepticus. This condition is a medical emergency requiring immediate treatment. The mortality rate is 5 to 10 percent. The airway must be open, and oxygen is administered if cyanosis is present. The convulsions must be stopped and recurrence prevented by effective medication.

The specific anticonvulsants should always be given by the intravenous route and in amounts large enough to stop seizure activity quickly. A common error is the frequent use of small aliquots of anticonvulsants with resultant toxicity but continued status. In recent years diazepam (Valium) has superseded the barbiturates and paraldehyde as the drug of choice for the treatment of status epilepticus. The drug is given by slow intravenous injection at a rate of not exceeding 1 mg per minute. For infants the optimal single dose is 1 to 2 mg, for young children 2 to 5 mg, and for older children 5 to 10 mg. The response of the patient to intravenous therapy with diazepam may be monitored by EEG if available and the injection may be stopped promptly as electrical and clinical arrest of the seizure becomes evident. The majority of cases will respond favorably with prompt termination of seizure discharge and subsidence of clinical symptoms. In most instances one injection is sufficient. But if symptoms should recur, a second or even third injection may be required at 20 to 30 minute intervals. Diazepam has been found to be safe and less toxic than barbiturates or paraldehyde with respect to respiratory and cardiovascular depression. It should be borne in mind that Valium potentiates barbiturates. This form of therapy has also been used for petit mal status and epilepsy partialis continua. The focus of depressive action is believed to be in the brainstem reticular system. The next drug of choice is sodium nembutal administered intravenously because of its fast action. The dosage is 0.1 to 0.4 g depending on age. If respiration is depressed, it is preferable to use paraldehyde, another highly effective agent, to be given as a dilute solution of 4 ml in 100 ml of 0.25 N saline in 5 percent glucose in water solution. Untoward side effects of paralydehyde are respiratory distress and acute cardiac failure. If used judiciously in a diluted solution, these complications are rarely seen. It can also be given rectally with a wide margin of safety. Volatile anesthetic agents including vinyl ether or chloroform may be useful in controlling status, especially when it is difficult to give medications by the intravenous route. Concomitant with the acute emergency therapy, long-acting drugs, preferably phenobarbital or Dilantin should be initiated by the intramuscular route.

Focal cortical epilepsy. Focal seizures respond favorably to the same drugs used in grand mal attacks. Multifocal seizures are less easy to conrtol.

Psychomotor seizures. Among focal cortical epilepsies, psychomotor epilepsy is the most common. Dilantin is the drug of choice and may be combined with phenobarbital. Celontin (methsuximide) is useful in some children, and its side effects include drowsiness, anorexia, skin rash, fever, and occasionally neutropenia. In some instances Celontin has proved to be more effective than Dilantin.

Because of the possible toxic action on the liver and bone marrow, Phenurone (phenacemide) has not attained popularity in the treatment of psychomotor epilepsy.

"Pure" petit mal absence. Zarontin (ethosuximide) is the drug of choice in the treatment of petit mal attacks. Untoward reactions include anorexia, abdominal pain, drowsiness, and occasional skin rash. Aplastic anemia has been rarely reported. Tridione (trimethadione) is also a relatively specific anti petit mal drug. A common cause of failure is timidity in dosage. Monthly blood count should forewarn the possibility of neutropenia. As the neutrophil count approaches the level of $1600/mm^3$, reduction of dosage or change of medication should receive serious consideration. Skin rash with fever is an indication to stop the drug or decrease the dosage. Lupus erythematosus is an uncommon complication of both Tridione and Zarontin therapy. Other less important side effects are photophobia, drowsiness, and eosinophilia. Diamox (acetazolamide), either alone or combined with Tridione, is effective. In a rare patient in whom none of the foregoing drugs brings relief, an antimalarial agent, Aralen (chloroquine), has proved useful. The side effects are visual disturbances (lacrimation, blurred vision, ptosis, and strabismus), skin sensitivity, and occasional peripheral neuropathy. These symptoms are reversible except the retinopathy. Periodic examination of the visual field is mandatory since visual field defects precede the onset of retinitis and at this stage the eye lesions are still reversible.

Myoclonic epilepsy. This seizure type is more difficult to manage than pure petit mal attacks. The drug of choice is Celontin, whose effect may also be dramatic. Next choices are Valium, Tridione, Diamox, and Meprobamate. Corticosteroids or corticotropins may be effective in some resistant cases.

The myoclonic epilepsy seen in degenerative diseases is resistant to drugs.

Minor motor seizures. Akinetic Seizures. These seizures are almost always associated with organic brain disorders and are notoriously difficult to control. In a small percentage of patients beneficial results may be obtained from Valium, Celontin, Tridione, Zarontin, or Diamox. In some cases a trial of ACTH therapy is highly recommended (for dosage schedule, see massive spasms). With severe drop seizures, children often sustain bruises of face and eyes or even fractures of teeth or skull. Wearing a padded football helmet may prevent or minimize such injuries. The ketogenic diet may be the most effective form of treatment for this type of seizure but this requires the full cooperation of the child and the family.

Massive Myoclonic Spasms. This type of spasm is very resistant to the usual anticonvulsants. ACTH is the drug of choice. The efficacy of ACTH or steroid therapy appears to depend upon the underlying cause of the spasms and the promptness and intensity of the medication. The earlier and the more intensive the therapy, the better the response. In 50 percent of the cases the seizures may be controlled or improved. The attendant mental impairment, however, is much less affected by steroid or any type of therapy. The dosage and duration of treatment have varied at different clinics. The following schedule for Acthar gel by intramuscular injection in two divided doses is recommended:

1st week—40 IU/day
2nd week—40 IU/day
3rd week—30 IU/day
4th week—20 IU/day
5th week—20 IU for 3 days and
10 IU/day for 3 days

Proper precautions of steroid therapy should be closely followed. The sleeplessness and irritability which are often seen during the second or third week of therapy may be counteracted by oral or rectal chlorpromazine. Moon facies and acne are not uncommon. Significant electrolyte imbalance and hypertension are rarely observed.

Convulsive Equivalent (Autonomic Epilepsy). The majority of these patients can be successfully treated with anticonvulsant drugs. Dilantin, alone or in conjunction with Diamox, is most satisfactory. Diamox alone may sometimes be effective. Meprobamate, Mebaral, and Tridione may also be useful.

DIETARY TREATMENT. The value of starvation in the control of epileptic seizures has been recognized for centuries. However, it was not known that the effect was due to ketosis until shortly before the ketogenic diet was introduced as a form of antiepileptic treatment by Wilder in 1921. Since the advent of modern anticonvulsant drugs in ever increasing variety and effectiveness, the need of dietary therapy has become limited to selected patients in whom drugs have utterly failed or have to be discontinued because of intolerance or idiosyncrasy. The diet is most effective in patients with akinetic seizures.

The ketogenic diet is more expensive than ordinary meals, and its preparation requires intelligence and care. Rigid control must be enforced lest the effectiveness be diminished or lost. Therefore, it should be prescribed only for carefully selected children. The parents must have complete understanding and be willing to cooperate fully. The most suitable age of the child is between 2 to 5 years. Young infants may not tolerate the high fat content; older children may rebel and refuse to take the diet. Retarded or brain-damaged children may not cooperate in finishing their meals and may accept carbohydrate foods offered inadvertently.

Preferably the child should be hospitalized for the initiation of the dietary regime, which should be preceded by a period of total starvation (3 to 4 days) during which only water is given. If this is successful, the child is so hungry that he is ready and willing to eat what is served. The ketosis induced by the starvation is maintained as long as the dietary regime is not broken. Even minor infringement such as one cookie or a lump of sugar may diminish the effectiveness of the diet drastically. Like drug therapy, the diet should be continued for two to three years. In weaning from the diet, the proportion of fat should be decreased gradually over a period of weeks, lest sudden reversion of ketosis precipitate a convulsive attack.

The basic requirement of a ketogenic diet is to provide sufficient protein and calories for growth and maintenance with a fat to protein-carbohydrate ratio of 4:1 by weight. The procedure of calculation and a list of interchangeable dietary items have been described in detail by Livingston and Keith.

SURGICAL TREATMENT. With the advent of refined diagnostic techniques, the surgical treatment of certain types of focal epilepsy has become effective. This therapeutic approach requires a competent and experienced team which usually is available only in large medical centers. Indications for surgical therapy are clear in patients with progressive lesions of the brain (tumor, abscess, hematoma, and vascular malformation). For chronic epilepsy due to static or atrophic lesions, the primary treatment is medical, and surgery should be considered only when drug, dietary, and other therapeutic measures have failed after adequate trial.

The indication for surgery is limited further to cases in which clinical and laboratory studies clearly point to a well-localized lesion in a surgically accessible site in one cerebral hemisphere. Bilateral, diffuse, or subcortical lesions are contraindications for surgery, as are the genetic epilepsies.

The general status of the patient, his physical and mental deficits other than epilepsy, and the anticipated disability to surgical intervention should also be carefully evaluated before such treatment is recommended.

When surgery is indicated, exact cortical localization of the epileptogenic focus or foci must be accomplished through clinical and special radiographic and electrographic studies carried out preoperatively as well as during the operation.

A number of effective procedures have been developed: techniques for local excision, total lobectomy, and hemispherectomy have been perfected. The tendency has been toward wider excision of tissues surrounding the epileptogenic focus. In competent hands the surgical mortality is about 1 to 2 percent; complete control or marked improvement is obtained in more than 50 percent of properly selected cases.

Febrile Convulsions

Convulsive disorder can be divided into two major categories; the acute sporadic and the chronic paroxysmal. To the former belong the febrile convulsions of infancy and childhood. By definition, febrile convulsions are provoked by hyperthermia associated with an acute illness of extracranial origin. Acute convulsions associated with intracranial diseases of infectious, toxic, metabolic, vascular, and neoplastic origin are also classified in the first group but will not be considered here.

Although febrile convulsions are the most common seizure disorder in childhood its incidence is not accurately known but estimated to be around 5 percent. They commonly occur between 6 months to 3 years with the peak incidence at 18 months. The incidence in boys is slightly greater than in girls. There is a high familial incidence of febrile convulsions (around 30 percent) and of other epileptic disorders (around 15 percent) suggesting the importance of genetic predisposition.

DIAGNOSIS AND DIFFERENTIAL DIAGNOSIS. The most common cause of febrile convulsions is acute upper respiratory infection. A sudden sharp rise of temperature appears more important than the height of fever, as the threshold for convulsion differs in individual patients.

In an infant with fever and convulsions, the diagnosis of "benign febrile convulsion" must be differentiated from other acute convulsions. Of particular importance is the possibility of primary intracranial disease (e.g., meningitis) which demands immediate diagnosis and specific therapy.

When febrile convulsion is diagnosed with reasonable assurance, a second step must be taken to differentiate "benign" (or "typical") from "nonbenign" (or "atypical") febrile seizure. This is important in both management and prognosis.

Any child presenting a febrile convulsion deserves a careful work-up and planned follow-up. Laboratory studies should include examination of the cerebrospinal fluid; measurement of blood glucose, calcium, phosphorus, phosphatase, and urea nitrogen; radiographs of the skull; and an electroencephalogram.

Benign febrile convulsions most commonly occur in neurologically normal children within the age of 6 months to 3 years. In addition the following criteria are helpful in differentiating benign febrile convulsions from the nonbenign group:

1. Positive family history of febrile convulsions
2. An abrupt rise of temperature over 103° F inciting a generalized convulsion seldom longer than a few minutes in duration
3. No neurologic abnormality after the attack
4. Normal laboratory studies including electroencephalogram

In contrast children with *nonbenign* febrile convulsions often have a lowered seizure threshold which may be related to a preexisting but subclinical condition such as prematurity or birth trauma. In these cases fever acts as a trigger and the convulsive episodes are more prone to be repetitive with lowering degree of fever each time and finally with no fever at all. In this group we should also include those children who were neurologically normal but have sustained brain insult as a sequel to their first febrile convulsion. Helpful criteria in identifying the nonbenign group are:

1. Asymmetric or focal seizure with or without Todd's paralysis
2. Seizures longer than 30 minutes
3. Repeated seizures during one febrile illness
4. Presence of neurologic deficits before, during, or after the seizure
5. Persistent and significant EEG abnormalities
6. Onset of seizure before 6 months or after 3 years of age

Electroencephalogram. This test should not be used too soon following a seizure on in phase of fever. The optimum time for the test is a week following the initial attack; however, a single examination is of little assistance in prognosis. A serial study should be performed in children with recurrent febrile convulsions. Abnormal EEG's are found in about 25 percent of children with febrile convulsions and 10 percent have shown definite epileptiform activity.

PROGNOSIS. Febrile convulsions are not necessarily benign. The child may experience subsequent febrile seizures, develop afebrile seizures (epilepsy), or manifest signs of underlying brain dysfunction.

1. *Recurrent febrile seizures.* The risk of further febrile convulsions seems to increase with each additional attack: 35 percent recurrence after the first seizure; 47 percent after the second, and 60 percent after the third.
2. *Recurrent afebrile seizures or epilepsy.* From a 15- to 22-year longitudinal study, Livingston found the incidence of chronic epilepsy in the "benign" group was 2.9 percent and 97 percent in the "nonbenign" group. Psychomotor epilepsy has been found to occur more frequently

in children with a history of "benign" febrile convulsions.

3. *Brain dysfunction.* The nagging question regarding the possibility of brain damage and mental retardation as sequelae of febrile convulsions cannot be easily answered, as carefully planned, long-term follow-up studies are sadly lacking. Of the overall febrile convulsion group, the incidence of mental retardation has been reported as 6 to 8 percent and behavior disorder as 10 percent. It is unknown what proportion of these belong to the benign and nonbenign group of febrile convulsions.

In our experience, subtle changes of brain function are more common than straightforward mental retardation. These include behavior disturbance, speech disorder, learning deficits, and autonomic dysfunctions. The latter may manifest as sleep disturbance, and visceral, sensory, vasomotor, or other autonomic seizure equivalents. Fortunately, many of these symptoms are age-determined and tend to improve, even disappear with CNS maturation.

TREATMENT. The treatment of febrile convulsions should be directed at the control of the convulsions, the lowering of fever, the treatment of the underlying infection, and the use of maintenance anticonvulsants. There is a difference of opinion as to the value of long-term prophylactic anticonvulsant therapy. The difficulty in distinguishing the benign from the nonbenign febrile convulsion and identifying the complications that may result from a seizure has prompted us to recommend that all children be treated with daily anticonvulsant medication until at least 6 years of age after the initial febrile convulsion.

Migraine

Migraine is a paroxysmal disorder characterized by recurrent headaches, classically unilateral, often preceded by visual aura and followed by nausea and vomiting. A family history (sibling or parents) of headache described as migrainous is high. It is a common pediatric problem. From reliable longitudinal follow-up study it has been shown that in children with true migraine about 50 percent had hemicrania; 90 percent had nausea and vomiting; 60 to 70 percent had positive family history.

INCIDENCE. The diagnosis of migraine in infancy and early childhood is less certain because of incomplete clinical picture. Although classical hemicrania has been reported in a 2½-year-old, migraine is more competently diagnosed after the age of 5 years. The incidence in children is about 5 percent; it increases in older children to 10 percent. In the latter age group the symptomatology is closely similar to that of the adult patients.

It is interesting to note that the incidence in children is higher in boys than girls; but in adults it is higher in women than men.

ETIOLOGY AND PATHOGENESIS. The cause and mechanism of migraine are not completely understood. The consensus is that migraine is primarily a hereditary instability of the autonomic functions with secondary effects on cerebral and cranial circulation. The chain of events in the symptomatology is believed to arise under the influence of an active substance such as histamine or a neurohumor such as serotonin.

The paroxysmal attacks are often precipitated by emotional upsets, acute anxieties, traveling sickness, or physical exhaustion. Allergic disorders are common in migraine patients and their relatives. It has long been suspected that there might be a relationship between migraine and epilepsy. Although classic migraine and epilepsies are different clinically, the variants of these disorders are remarkably similar. A history of migraine is more common in the families of epileptic patients than normal population. According to Wolff, there are three phases in a migraine attack: (1) Vasoconstriction of intracranial arterioles resulting in cerebral ischemia. In the majority of cases, this occurs in the distribution of the common carotid system, thus evoking cortical and retinal phenomena as visual disturbances, paresthesias and visceral symptoms. In rare cases the basilar system is involved and the clinical picture in a child is that of "benign paroxysmal vertigo." (2) Vasodilatation of the extracranial vessels resulting in pressure upon sensitive nerve endings in the walls of the distended arterioles producing headaches of throbbing nature. (3) Exudation and tissue edema results in persisting head pain.

CLINICAL PICTURE. An aura or prodrome may or may not be present. The onset is usually sudden. Visual symptoms are seldom seen in young children. In older children, dimness or loss of vision and visual field defects are more common than circumscribed scotomas. Transient numbness and tingling of a limb or of the face, followed by clonic movements may precede the headache. Hemiplegia, ophthalmoplegia, and dysphasia lasting for varying periods are less common. Although hemicrania is characteristic of migraine, the headache in children may be bilateral or in the posterior aspect of the head and neck. Hemicrania, when present, is commonly preceded by pain behind the eye of the involved side. Closely following the onset of headache, nausea appears and vomiting is often distressing. After the vomiting, the headache may be instantly relieved; or if the patient falls asleep, he may awaken in an asymptomatic state. Attacks may be precipitated by mental tension, physical exertion, emotional stresses, and special sensory stimuli (bright lights, cinema and television, and loud noises). Attacks are often diminished in frequency and severity during vacation periods.

As a rule, between attacks, the physical and neurologic findings are normal and laboratory studies noncontributory.

ELECTROENCEPHALOGRAM. The EEG in children with migraine may be normal, but a significant number show various types of abnormalities, including focal and paroxysmal patterns. This fact often renders the EEG of little value in differentiating convulsive equivalent states from migraine headaches.

DIAGNOSIS. The diagnosis depends entirely upon the history. The most important features are the characteristic triad of symptoms, the chronic recurrent course, and the positive family history. At least two, preferably more, of these criteria should be satisfied before a diagnosis of migraine may be seriously considered.

DIFFERENTIAL DIAGNOSIS. While the diagnosis in cases of classical migraine offers no difficulty, atypical forms may be confused with convulsive equivalent syndrome or autonomic epilepsy. Headache and visceral symptoms are common features of both conditions. The incidence of convulsive equivalent epilepsy, however, is 10 or more times greater than migraine in the pediatric age group. A positive family history for migraine is helpful. Therapeutic response to antimigraine or anticonvulsant medication may clarify the diagnosis in difficult cases. In some instances it may be impossible to differentiate atypical migraine from atypical convulsive equivalent syndrome.

Headache is a common pediatric complaint, and its evaluation and diagnosis can be difficult. Consideration must be given to such conditions as intracranial mass lesions, vascular malformations, and functional disorders. Headache may also have its origin in multiple extracranial causes.

PROGNOSIS. The prognosis of childhood migraine is generally favorable but it is not uncommon for the headaches to persist into adult life.

PREVENTION AND TREATMENT OF ATTACK. The frequency and severity may be diminished if all factors known through experience to provoke attacks are avoided or minimized as much as possible. Premedication in anticipation of mental tension, physical or physiologic stress, or emotional excitement may be justified.

Ergotamine preparations have been widely used for the treatment of migraine. Cafergot, which is a mixture of 1 mg ergotamine tartrate and 100 mg caffeine in one tablet, may be given orally. One or two tablets are given as initial dose according to size of child. This can be repeated in 15 to 30 minutes for two or three times. Ergomar can be given sublingually and cafergot suppositories may be used rectally. These drugs must be given during the vasoconstriction phase. Once headache is established the attack runs its course and is little effected by ergot preparations.

For relief of well-developed migraine symptoms appropriate doses of salicylates and codeine, and induced sleep in a darkened quiet room are often followed by relief. In this writer's experience, the judicious use of Dilantin or Mebaral in adequate doses between migraine attacks has often led to long periods of remission.

Narcolepsy

Narcolepsy is a syndrome of paroxysmal episodes of irresistible sleep which may be associated with transient episodes of weakness or cataplexy.

ETIOLOGY. This condition is believed to result from disturbance of the sleep-wakefulness mechanism of the reticular activation system in the diencephalon. A primary and a secondary or symptomatic type are distinguished. In primary narcolepsy, a familial incidence has been estimated at around 10 percent. Inheritance is by autosomal transmission as a simple dominant factor. Secondary or symptomatic narcolepsy may be caused by diffuse or localized brain lesions, encephalitides being the most common. Head trauma, tumors in the region of the third ventricle, and the Pickwickian syndrome are among the less frequent causes.

INCIDENCE. This is a relatively rare condition, and no exact incidence is available. In Sours' series of 75 cases of primary narcolepsy, one-third were from 11 to 15 years of age at the time of onset. It predominates in males by a 3:2 ratio. Higher incidence in the Negro race has been observed by Ford.

CLINICAL MANIFESTATIONS. The onset is insidious and may coincide with major physiologic changes of life such as puberty. The somnolence has been described in an irresistible urge to sleep. The change from wakefulness to sleep is gradual. It usually occurs in hypnapagogic situations, although some patients may fall asleep while engaged in physical activities. Between episodes the patient may be alert but more often is drowsy.

Cataplexy may occur spontaneously, or more often is brought on by laughter, anger, or surprise. It is a sudden decrease or abrupt loss of muscle tone; the child sinks limply to the ground without loss of consciousness. The attack is usually brief and is followed by full recovery. Two other manifestations—namely, sleep paralysis and hypnapagogic hallucinations—are rare in children.

In the secondary type, the paroxysmal somnolence tends to last longer than in the primary type. Other symptoms of encephalopathy such as mental retardation, motor, speech, and behavior disorders may be present. The Pickwickians are characteristically obese and show cyanosis, hypercapnia, right heart hypertrophy, and congestive heart failure. The secondary narcoleptics do not exhibit cataplexy.

LABORATORY DATA. In primary narcolepsy, the EEG shows normal sleep activity during the narcoleptic attack, and the waking record is usually normal. When photic stimulation is used, two-thirds of the patients show poor following, considered indicative of lower reactivity of the nervous system. In the secondary narcolepsy, the EEG may be abnormal, depending upon the type of the underlying cerebral abnormality.

DIAGNOSIS. The diagnosis of narcolepsy suggests itself when the cardinal symptoms are present. The possibility of a hypothalamic neoplasm and other cerebral lesions should be excluded.

PROGNOSIS. In most cases the disorder does not interfere too much with the child's activities but is often responsible for poor schoolwork. Spontaneous remission occurs in many cases.

TREATMENT. The amphetamines, Dexedrine or Benzedrine sulfate, 10 mg, after breakfast and lunch, or Ritalin (methylphenidate hydrochloride) in the same dosage, are effective in alleviating the sleepiness and the cataplexy.

REFERENCES

EPILEPSY

General

Chao, D., Druckman, R., and Kellaway, P. Convulsive Disorders of Children. Philadelphia, W. B. Saunders Co., 1958.
Farmer, T. W., ed. Pediatric Neurology. New York, Paul B. Hoeber, Inc., 1964.
Ford, F. Diseases of the Nervous System in Childhood and Adolescence. Springfield, Ill., Charles C Thomas, Publ., 1966.
Gibbs, F. A., ed. Molecules and Mental Health. Philadelphia, J. B. Lippincott Co., 1959.
——— and Gibbs, E. L. Atlas of Electroencephalography, 2nd ed. Cambridge, Mass., Addison-Wesley Press, Inc., Vol. 2, 1952.
Jeavons, P. M., and Bower, B. D. Infantile Spasms: A review of the literature and a study of 112 cases. Clinics of Developmental Medicine, No. 15. Medical Education and Information Unit of the Spastic Society in Association with William Heinemann Medical Books, Ltd., London, 1964.
Lennox, W. G., and Lennox, M. A. Epilepsy and Related Disorders. Boston, Little, Brown and Co., 1960.
Livingston, S. The Diagnosis and Treatment of Convulsive Disorders in Children. Springfield, Ill., Charles C Thomas, Publ., 1954.
——— Living with Epileptic Seizures. Springfield, Ill., Charles C Thomas, Publ., 1963.
Millichap, J. G. Febrile Convulsions. New York, The Macmillan Co., 1968.
Penfield, W., and Jasper, H. H. Epilepsy and the Functional Anatomy of the Human Brain. Boston, Little, Brown and Co., 1954.
Robb, P. Epilepsy: A review of basic and clinical research. NINDB Monogr. No. 1, Public Health Service Pub. No. 1357, U.S. Dept. of Health, Education and Welfare, 1965.
Tower, D. B. Neurochemistry of Epilepsy. Springfield, Ill., Charles C Thomas, Publ., 1960.

Classification and Etiology

Burke, J. B. Significance of neonatal convulsions. Arch. Dis. Child., 29:342, 1954.
Caveness, W. F. Sequelae of cerebral concussion. New York J. Med., 61:1871, 1961.
Chao, D. Subacute inclusion body encephalitis. J. Pediat., 61:501, 1962.
Christensen, E., and Husby, J. Chronic subdural hematoma in infancy. Acta Neurol. Scand., 39:323, 1962.
Craig, W. S. Convulsive movements occurring in the first 10 days of life. Arch. Dis. Child., 35:336, 1960.
Edgar, G. W. F., and Post, P. J. J. Amaurotic idiocy and epilepsy. Epilepsia, 4:251, 1963.
Evans, J. H. Post-traumatic epilepsy. Neurology, 12:665, 1962.
Fowler, M. Brain damage after febrile convulsions. Arch. Dis. Child., 32:67, 1957.
Friedlander, W. J. Epilepsy. Amer. J. Psychiat., 120: 674, 1964.
Gastaut, H. et al. A proposed international classification of epileptic seizures. Epilepsia, 5:297, 1964.
——— and Tassinari, C. A. Triggering mechanism in epilepsy, the electroclinical point of view. Epilepsia, 7:85, 1966.
Gerken, H., Doose, H., Volzke, E., Volz, C., and Hien-Volpel, K. F. Genetics of childhood epilepsy with photic sensitivity. Lancet, 1:1377, 1968.
Gibbs, F. A., and Gibbs, E. L. Age factor in epilepsy. New Eng. J. Med., 269:1230, 1963.
Lennox, W. G., Gibbs, E. L., and Gibbs, F. A. Inheritance of cerebral dysrhythmia and epilepsy. Arch. Neurol. Psychiat., 44:1155, 1940.
Low, M. L., Bosma, J. F., and Armstrong, M. D. Studies on phenylketonuria. VI. EEG studies in PKU. Arch. Neurol. Psychiat., 77:359, 1957.
Marson, C. A. A newly proposed classification of epileptic seizures: neurophysiological basis. Epilepsia, 6:275, 1965.
Metrakos, K., and Metrakos, J. D. Genetics of convulsive disorders: II. Genetic and electroencephalographic studies in centrencephalic epilepsy. Neurology, 11:474, 1961.
Rodin, E. A. Familial occurrence of the 14 and 6 positive spike phenomenon. Paper presented at the Eastern Association of EEG Meeting, New York City, 1963.
Schwartz, J. F. Photosensitivity in a family. Amer. J. Dis. Child., 103:90, 1962.
Sorel, L. The descendants of epileptic parents. Epilepsia, 10:91, 1969.
Symonds, C. Classificaiton of the epilepsies. Brit. Med. J., 1:1235, 1955.

Clinical

Aigner, B. R., and Mulder, D. W. Myoclonus, Arch. Neurol., 2:600, 1960.
Barslund, I., and Danielsen, J. Temporal epilepsy in monozygotic twins. Epilepsia, 4:138, 1963.
Bray, P. F. Temporal lobe epilepsy syndrome. Pediatrics, 29:612, 1962.
Chao, D. Seizures in infancy and early childhood. Med. Clin. N. Amer., p. 399, 1958.
——— Sexton, J. A., and Pardo, L. S. Temporal lobe epilepsy in children. J. Pediat., 60:686, 1962.
——— Taylor, F. M., and Druckman, R. Massive spasms in infancy and childhood. J. Pediat., 50:670, 1958.
Charlton, M. H., and Yahr, M. D. Long-term follow-up of patients with petit mal. Arch. Neurol., 16:595, 1967.
Currier, R. D., Kovi, K. A., and Saidman, L. J. Prognosis of "pure" petit mal. Neurology, 13:959, 1963.
Debiolley, D. Petit mal variant or Lennox syndrome. Electroenceph. Clin. Neurophysiol., 23:282, 1967.
Epstein, M. H., and O'Connor, J. S. Destructive effects

of prolonged status epilepticus. J. Neurol. Neurosurg. Psychiat., 29:251, 1966.

Frantzen, E., Lennox-Buchthal, M., and Nygaard, A. The electroencephalogram in children with febrile convulsions. Electroenceph. Clin. Neurophysiol., 23:389, 1967.

——— Lennox-Buchthal, M., and Nygaard, A. Longitudinal EEG and clinical study of children with febrile convulsions. Electroenceph. Clin. Neurophysiol., 24: 197, 1968.

Friderichsen, C., and Melchior, J. Febrile convulsions in children, their frequency and prognosis. Acta Paediat., Suppl. 100, 1954.

Gastaut, H. et al. Childhood epileptic encephalopathy with diffuse slow spike-waves (otherwise known as "petit mal variant") or Lennox syndrome. Epilepsia, 7:139, 1966.

——— Startle disease (pathological surprise reaction). Electroenceph. Clin. Neurophysiol., 23:494, 1967.

Gibberd, F. B. The prognosis of petit mal. Brain, 89: 531, 1966.

Hammill, J. F., and Carter, S. Febrile convulsions. New Eng. J. Med., 274:563, 1966.

Jaffe, R. J. Ictal behavior disturbance as the only manifestation of seizure disorder: a case report. J. Nerv. Ment. Dis., 134:470, 1962.

Lennox, W. G. Significance of febrile convulsions. Pediatrics, 11:341, 1953.

Livingston, S. Infantile febrile convulsions. Develop. Med. Child Neurol., 10:374, 1968.

Lombroso, C. T., and Lerman, P. Breathholding spells (cyanotic and pallid infantile syncope). Pediatrics, 39: 563, 1967.

Meyer, A., Beck, E., and Shepherd, M. Unusually severe lesions in the brain following status epilepticus. J. Neurol. Neurosurg. Psychiat., 18:24, 1955.

Niedermeyer, E. The Lennox-Gastaut syndrome: a severe type of childhood epilepsy. Electroenceph. Clin. Neurophysiol., 24:283, 1968.

Peterman, M. G. Febrile convulsions in children. J.A.M.A., 143:728, 1950.

Rogina, V., and Serafetinides, E. A. Epilepsy and behavior disorder in patients with generalized spike and wave complexes. Electroenceph. Clin. Neurophysiol., 14:376, 1962.

Samson, J. H., Apthorp, J., and Finley, A. Febrile seizures and purulent meningitis. J.A.M.A., 210:1918, 1969.

Steinschneider, A., Ginsberg, T., George, E. D., and Lipton, E. L. Febrile convulsions. Neurology, 14:362, 1964.

Swanson, P. D., Luttrell, C. N., and Magladery, J. W. Myoclonus. Medicine, 41:339, 1962.

Yanai, N. Febrile convulsions in children. Develop. Med. Child Neurol., 10:255, 1967.

Treatment

Bell, D. S. Dangers of treatment of status epilepticus with diazepam. Brit. Med. J., 1:159, 1969.

Carson, M. J. Treatment of minor motor seizures with nitrazepam. Develop. Med. Child Neurol., 10:772, 1968.

Carter, S., and Gold, A. P. Seizures in childhood. New Eng. J. Med., 278:315, 1968.

——— and Gold, A. P. Care of the critically ill child: management of status epilepticus. Pediatrics, 44:732, 1969.

Chao, D. Overall management of the epileptic child. Med. Clin. N. Amer., p. 461, 1958.

——— Drug therapy in paroxysmal disorders. Pediat. Clin. N. Amer., p. 3, 1963.

——— and Plumb, R. Diamox in epilepsy—a critical review of 178 cases. J. Pediat., 58:211, 1961.

Connelly, J. P. et al. Control of refractory epilepsy. Clin. Pediat., 2:624, 1961.

Gold, A. P., and Carter, S. Pediatric neurology. *In* Shirkey, H. C., ed., Pediatric Therapy. St. Louis, C. V. Mosby Co., 1968.

Gordon, N. Folic acid deficiency from anticonvulsant therapy. Develop. Med. Child Neurol., 10:497, 1968.

Hammill, J. F., and Carter, S. Febrile convulsions. New Eng. J. Med., 274:563, 1965.

Keith, H. M. Convulsive disorders in children with special reference to treatment with ketogenic diet. Boston, Little, Brown and Co., 1963.

Livingston, S., Villamater, C., Sakata, Y., and Pauli, L. L. Use of carbamazepine (Tegretol) in epilepsy. J.A.M.A., 200:116, 1967.

Nicol, C. F., Tutton, J. C., and Smith, B. H. Parenteral diazepam in status epilepticus. Neurology, 19:332, 1969.

Nygaard Jensen, O., and Vendeline Olesen, O. The clinical importance of folic acid in patients treated with anticonvulsant drugs. Excerpta Medica, Amsterdam, Int. Congr. Ser., 193:260, 1969.

Merritt, H. H. Medical treatment in epilepsy. Brit. Med. J., 1:666, 1958.

Penfield, W., and Paine, K. Results of surgical therapy of focal epileptic seizures. Canad. Med. Ass. J., 73: 515, 1955.

Peterson, W. G. Clinical study of Mogadon, a new anticonvulsant. Neurology, 17:878, 1967.

Prensky, A. L., Raff, M. C., Moore, M. J., and Schwab, R. S. Intravenous diazepam in the treatment of prolonged seizure activity. New Eng. J. Med., 276:779, 1967.

Rasmussen, T. Surgical aspects of focal epilepsy. Electroenceph. Clin. Neurophysiol., 15:1050, 1963.

Reynolds, E. H., Miller, C. G., and Matthews, D. M. Anticonvulsant therapy, folic acid and vitamin B_{12} metabolism and mental symptoms. Epilepsia, 7:261, 1966.

Sansoy, O. M., and Whorton, D. Chlordiazepoxide hydrochloride in treatment of convulsive disorders. Rocky Mount. Med. J., 63:56, 1966.

Scholl, M. L. Treatment of seizure disorders. New Eng. J. Med., 269:1424, 1962.

Walker, A. E. Surgical treatment of epilepsy. *In* Livingston, S., ed., Convulsive Disorders in Children. Springfield, Ill., Charles C Thomas, Publ., 1954, Chap. 14.

Wilder, R. M. The effect of ketonemia on the course of epilepsy. Mayo Clin. Proc., 2:307, 1921.

Wilson, P. J. E. Cerebral hemispherectomy for infantile hemiplegia. Brain, 93:147, 1970.

MIGRAINE

Berman, B. A. Migraine in children. Ann. Allerg., 21:91, 1963.

Bille, B. Migraine in children. Acta Paediat. Scand., 51: 614, 1962.

Bruyn, G. W., and Weenink, H. R. Migraine accompagnée. A critical evaluation. Headache, 6:1, 1966.

Chao, D. et al. The migraine syndrome. IV. Headache in children. Headache, 3:1, 1963.

Fenichel, G. M. Migraine as a cause of benign paroxysmal vertigo of childhood. J. Pediat., 71:114, 1967.

Gold, A. P., Chutorian, A. M., and Carter, S. Migraine and allied head pains in children. *In* Friedman, A. P., and Haims, E., eds., Headaches in Children. Springfield, Ill., Charles C Thomas, Publ., 1967.

Hinrichs, W. L., and Keith, H. M. Migraine in childhood: a follow-up report. Mayo Clin. Proc., 40:593, 1965.

Holguin, J., and Fenichel, G. Migraine. J. Pediat., 70: 290, 1967.

Macoun, S. Migraine in school children. Develop. Med. Child Neurol., 5:62, 1963.

Mitchell, R. Migraine in childhood. Develop. Med. Child Neurol., 9:641, 1967.

Ohta, M., Araki, S., and Kuriowa, Y. Familial occurrence of migraine with a hemiplegic syndrome and cerebellar manifestations. Neurology, 17:813, 1967.

Vahlquist, B., and Hackzell, G. Migraine of early onset. A study of 31 cases in which disease first appeared between 1 and 4 years of age. Acta Paediat., 38:622, 1949.

Weil, A. A. EEG observation on "dysrhythmic" migraine. J. Nerv. Ment. Dis., 134:277, 1962.

Whitehouse, D., Pappas, J. A., Escala, P. H., and Livingston, S. Electroencephalographic changes in children with migraine. New Eng. J. Med., 276:23, 1967.

Wolff, H. G. Headache and Other Head Pains. New York, Oxford Univ. Press, 1948, p. 268.

NARCOLEPSY

Salfield, D. J. Narcolepsy in a child under 7 years old. Arch. Dis. Child., 35:538, 1959.

Sours, J. A. Narcolepsy and other disturbances in the sleep-waking rhythm: a study of 115 cases with review of the literature. J. Nerv. Ment. Dis., 137:525, 1963.

Spier, N., and Karelitz, S. The Pickwickian syndrome. Amer. J. Dis. Child., 99:822, 1960.

Yoss, R. E., and Daly, D. D. Criteria for the diagnosis of the narcoleptic syndrome. Mayo Clin. Proc., 32: 320, 1957.

——— and Daly, D. D. Narcolepsy in children. Pediatrics, 25:1025, 1960.

Chapter 10 THE PERIPHERAL NEUROPATHIES

NIELS L. LOW

Polyneuritis

The peripheral nervous system may be affected by toxic agents, inflammatory diseases, and metabolic disorders of known and unknown causes. Diseases of peripheral nerves are classified as acute, chronic, and recurrent neuropathies. Single nerve involvement is termed mononeuritis; disease of multiple peripheral nerves, cranial nerves, or both is called polyneuritis.

Acute Polyneuritis

Synonyms for acute polyneuritis are polyneuropathy, polyradiculoneuropathy, infectious neuronitis, schwannitis, and Guillain-Barré syndrome.

ETIOLOGY. In the vast majority of patients, the cause is unknown. Since polyneuropathy of unknown origin is frequently preceded by an infection, it is commonly called postinfectious polyneuritis. However, etiologic delineation can be established in some cases, and it is above all of importance because of the possible therapeutic implications. Specific bacterial and viral agents known to produce this condition include diphtheria with its particular affinity for the ninth and tenth cranial nerves leading to impairment of gag, swallow, and phonation. Infectious mononucleosis, rubeola, rubella, Coxsackie, and other viral infections have been known to produce the clinical picture of polyneuritis. Metabolic and toxic states may likewise produce a neuropathy. Diabetes and lead, common in adults, are rarely observed in children. Mercury and other heavy metal toxins are also possible etiologic factors. Thallium toxicity is considered when the paresis is associated with alopecia and optic atrophy.

Tick paralysis is an uncommon form of very acute and overwhelming polyneuropathy that is apparently due to an unknown toxin released by the wood tick during a feeding on the human host. Tick paralysis causes respiratory muscle paralysis which can be fatal. Removal of the tick results in prompt improvement and full recovery. The search for ticks, especially in the region of the head and neck in children, is imperative whenever tick exposure was possible.

PATHOLOGY. The earliest changes in the peripheral or cranial nerves are edema with early disintegration of myelin and axis cylinders. Phagocytosis and proliferation of Schwann cells occur later, while macrophages with myelin inclusion are seen only in those patients who die late in the disease. Marked involvement of the roots of cranial nerves and of the ventral roots along the spinal axis is common. Both the degree of elevation of CSF protein and the presence of meningeal signs are apparently related to the extent of root involvement, termed polyneuroradiculitis.

CLINICAL MANIFESTATIONS. The clinical picture of this syndrome is variable but is usually characterized by acute ascending motor paralysis, motor and sensory findings of peripheral nerve distribution, and cranial nerve involvement. A respiratory or gastrointestinal infection frequently precedes the disease by a few days to two weeks. Boys and girls are equally affected during the various age groups of childhood and adolescence.

Mode of Onset. Muscle weakness normally precedes sensory symptoms, but paresthesia in hands and feet may be the initial complaint. Weakness, usually first apparent in the lower extremities, may manifest itself from the onset as a quadriparesis.

Motor Manifestations. Paresis may remain mild or, more commonly, becomes profound. It is usually ascending, symmetric in distribution, and the distal parts of the extremities are more severely affected than the proximal muscle groups. With involvement of the intercostal nerves, respiratory paralysis will occur with varying degrees of reduction in vital capacity. Atrophy of the skeletal muscles in the affected areas tends to occur early, especially in the intrinsic muscles of the hands and in the calves. The muscle weakness is of the flaccid type.

Cranial Nerves. Any motor nerve from the third to the twelfth may be involved with resultant paresis in the corresponding muscles. Bilateral facial nerve paresis occurs in approximately one-third of the affected children; unilateral facial weakness is less common. Involvement of the ninth and tenth nerves has greater clinical significance because of the potential consequence of impaired gag, swallow, and cough. Other cranial nerves are rarely involved, but complete ophthalmoplegia may occur. Papilledema is occasionally observed; it is unrelated to cerebrospinal fluid pressure but is often associated with an elevated protein content of the fluid.

Autonomic System. Postural hypotension in some children is due to impairment of the preganglionic nerves in the ventral roots with subsequent reduction of vasoconstriction. Absent or reduced sweating in the involved areas is presumably due to a similar process. The mechanism leading to the arterial hypertension observed occasionally is unclear.

Sensation. A reliable sensory examination in young children may be difficult or impossible. Paresthesia, impaired sensation, or both are common findings but may be absent even in the older, more reliable child. Position sense is the most frequently impaired sensory modality, followed by vibration, pain, and touch in descending order of frequency.

Reflexes. The deep tendon reflexes are usually absent, but incomplete loss does occur. There is an approximate correlation between degree of weakness and loss of reflexes. Abdominal and cremasteric reflexes may also disappear during the early stages of the disease process.

Bladder and Bowel Dysfunction. Urinary incontinence or retention may occur transiently. Constipation is common; it is related to weakness of the abdominal muscles as well as the difficulty of defecating in the recumbent position. Fecal incontinence with absent anal reflex is uncommon.

Meningeal Signs. Slight nuchal pain and rigidity are commonly observed. Positive Kernig and Brudzinski signs are found in a moderate number of children.

LABORATORY FINDINGS. Most children with acute polyneuritis have a normal peripheral blood count, urinalysis, and sedimentation rate. The cerebrospinal fluid (CSF) should always be examined in a suspected case of polyneuropathy. The pressure of the fluid is usually normal, but a pleocytosis of 50 or even 200 to 300 white blood cells does not exclude the diagnosis of polyneuritis. Approximately three-fourths of these children show an elevated protein content in the CSF. This increase of protein may only be slight, but values occasionally exceed 400 mg per 100 ml. Most commonly, there is a slight rise of protein during the first one or two weeks of the disease, with a peak concentration at about four weeks, followed by a gradual decline over several more weeks. This frequent dissociation between a normal cell count and an elevated protein was described initially by Guillain, Barré, and Strohl, and polyneuritis is often called the Guillain-Barré syndrome. Because these laboratory findings are not present routinely and the dissociation does not signify a special or separate clinical entity, it is probably wise not to use that eponym. The CSF sugar should always be in the normal range. Electrical testing is a useful ancillary procedure. Electromyography may show fibrillation and positive potentials; and on contraction of the muscle abnormalities of the motor unit, the type characteristic of denervation may be evident. Conduction velocity of the motor nerve is usually decreased, and the chronaxie values are elevated.

DIAGNOSIS. When a child presents with muscle weakness associated with loss or reduction of tendon reflexes, acute polyneuritis should be suspected whether or not there are sensory changes. Electromyographic studies will reveal evidence of denervation, and conduction velocity of the nerve may be decreased. The flare reaction on the skin obtained by scratch or intradermal injection of histamine may be absent. Tests for diphtheria and infectious mononucleosis should be performed. Appropriate serologic tests for viral infections should be made. Diabetes should be excluded, and a detailed history should be taken for exposure to possible toxins such as mercury, lead, or thallium supported by laboratory tests as indicated. Primary disease of muscle and of the anterior horn cells of the spinal cord may give a clinical picture that simulates polyneuritis. Muscular dystrophy is differentiated by its slow development and tendency to involve proximal more than distal musculature. Polymyositis may be diffcult to distinguish, but the deep tendon reflexes are usually retained. Electromyography is frequently of value in distinguishing muscle from peripheral nerve disease. Infantile spinal muscular atrophy (Werdnig-Hoffmann disease), characterized by muscle weakness secondary to anterior horn cell disease, is distinguished from polyneuropathy by its early age of onset, progressive course, tongue involvement, and absence of sensory findings.

COURSE AND OUTCOME. The clinical course is variable. The appearance of paresis may be very insidious but is usually progressive and tends to reach a peak within 7 to 10 days. Approximately one-half of the children show clinically recognizable improvement by the end of the second week of the illness. The period necessary for complete recovery varies from 2 to 18 months. Muscle strength returns much more rapidly than the tendon reflexes. Complete recovery without residua is the most common end result. With proper management and detailed attention to respiratory problems and complications, the mortality should be less than 5 percent.

MANAGEMENT. A therapeutic program recognizes the multiple etiologies and, when present, corrects or removes such factors. General supportive or symptomatic care may be lifesaving and is essential to achieve maximum rehabilitation. A supportive program should include complete bed rest, adequate hydration and nutrition, skillful nursing care, prevention of contractures and deformities, and the use of an indwelling catheter in the presence of urinary retention. Analgesics may be required for pain resulting from root involvement. Tracheostomy and/or a respirator may be lifesaving in the presence of respiratory difficulties. Physiotherapy is essential in all phases of the disease. Early in the course, it is limited to proper positioning and passive full range of motion; later, an active program of exercises, gait training, and bracing is employed.

Chronic and Recurrent Polyneuropathies

Occasionally, children are seen who develop polyneuropathy with a long, protracted chronic course. This neuropathic weakness leads to progressive atrophy and severe disability over a number of years. The cause of this form of chronic disease of the peripheral nervous system is unknown, and the mechanism is poorly understood.

Another group of children suffer from repeated attacks of apparently acute polyneuritis with incomplete recovery between attacks. The residua of these recurrences tend to increase with each exacerbation. It is not known whether the chronic and the recurrent types are two different forms of one disease or represent separate entities.

Some patients with "idiopathic" chronic or relapsing polyneuritis benefit from treatment with adrenocortical steroids. If an initial attempt over a period of a month of therapy results in improvement, the steroids may be required for months to years. In a 6-year-old child, prednisone is initially given in the dosage of 40 to 60 mg daily and, after the first 4 to 6 weeks, is gradually reduced to 20 mg a day.

Special Clinical Entities

Chronic hypertrophic polyneuropathy of Dejerine-Sottas is a familial disease of dominant inheritance characterized clinically by onset in childhood of slowly progressing weakness and sensory phenomena in the distal parts of the extremities. The disease is usually fatal by the second or third decade of life. The typical pathologic findings are axonal destruction and proliferation of Schwann cells leading to thickened palpable peripheral nerves. These changes may be diffuse along the entire length of nerves or may be of nodular or intermittent distribution.

Charcot-Marie-Tooth disease or peroneal muscular atrophy is also a familial disease with an autosomal mode of inheritance. It involves predominantly the lower parts of the legs and the small muscles of the hands. The clinical spectrum is variable; only the peripheral nerves may be affected, or the cord and probably even the muscles may also be involved. Peroneal atrophy progresses much slower than the previously mentioned hypertrophic neuritis. The differential diagnosis between Charcot-Marie-Tooth disease and the various hereditary forms of spinal degenerative disease may be very difficult, and at times impossible. One form may gradually change into the other in a given patient, and both forms may be seen in different members of a family. No specific therapy is available for this condition.

Progressive involvement of peripheral nerves is not uncommonly seen in periarteritis nodosa and less frequently in lupus erythematosus. *Chediak-Higashi syndrome* is a rare entity characterized by progressive neuropathic weakness and peroxidase-positive inclusions in leucocytes. *Acanthocytosis* (Bassen-Kornzweig disease), a recessively inherited disorder in the metabolism of beta-lipoproteins, is manifested by a celiac syndrome in early childhood, followed by polyneuropathy and deformity of erythrocytes. *Refsum syndrome* is a recessively inherited progressive form of polyneuritis with ataxia, retinitis pigmentosa, pupillary abnormalities, deafness, electrocardiographic changes, epiphyseal dysplasia, and ichthyosis. It is associated with an inborn error of metabolism with an inability to oxidize phytanic acid to dicarboxylic acid.

Acute attacks of the acute intermittent form of porphyria, rarely observed in children, are usually associated with polyneuritis. Abdominal pain is a prominent symptom in addition to marked irritability, convulsions, and sometimes psychosis. Increased urinary porphobilinogen is found during the acute episodes.

Heredofamilial neuritis with brachial predilection is characterized by recurrent neuropathy involving the shoulder and arms. The facial appearance of involved persons is conspicuously similar. The disease has a dominant inheritance and does not tend to progress to chronic disability.

Cranial Nerve Palsies

Cranial nerve palsies may occur with polyneuritis or may be manifestations of other disease states. Cranial nerves are characteristically involved in brainstem tumors and are frequently affected by acute poliomyelitis and some progressive degenerative diseases. Facial weakness may be due to primary muscle disease. Myasthenia gravis typically manifests itself in weakness of the extraocular muscles. Isolated impairment of one or both abducens nerves is usually secondary to increased intracranial pressure but occasionally its involvement is benign and unrelated to increased pressure. The third, fourth, fifth, and sixth cranial nerves may be involved in disease such as thrombosis, injury, or tumors in and around the cavernous sinus.

Isolated peripheral facial weakness may be present from birth or acquired. If congenital, it may be part of or the only manifestation of Möbius' syndrome. Acquired facial palsy may be present from birth and result from forceps pressure on the facial neve. In such patients full recovery can be expected. Isolated, acquired neuritis of the seventh cranial nerve is called *Bell's palsy*. The clinical signs of Bell's palsy are obliteration of the nasolabial fold on the affected side, a pulling of the corner of the mouth to the opposite (stronger) side, incomplete closure of the eyelid, and the inability to wrinkle the forehead on the same side. Retroauricular pain may be present, and taste may be impaired over the anterior two-thirds of the ipsilateral side of the tongue. The cause is unknown in most instances, but the palsy frequently follows mild respiratory infections. The association with purulent otitis media, acute mastoiditis, or parotitis is uncommon. Herpes zoster, syphilis, and sarcoidosis are rare causes. If there is no specific cause, recovery within a few weeks to several months can be expected in the vast majority of cases. It has not been established whether treatment with ACTH, adrenocortical steroids, or surgical decompression is helpful.

References

POLYNEURITIS

Adler, K. Tick paralysis. Canad. Med. Ass. J., 94:550, 1966.

Appenzellar, O., and Marshall, J. Vasomotor disturbance in Landry-Guillain-Barré syndrome. Arch. Neurol., 9: 368, 1963.

Birchfield, R. I., and Shaw, C. M. Postural hypotension in the Guillain-Barré syndrome. Arch. Neurol., 10: 149, 1964.

Dunn, H. G., Buckler, W. St. J., Morrison, G. C. E., and Emory, A. W. Conduction velocity of motor nerves in infants and children. Pediatrics, 34:708, 1964.

Guillain, G., Barré, J. A., and Strohl, A. Sur un syndrome de radiculo-névrite avec hyperalbuminose du liquide céphalo-rachidien sans réaction cellulaire. Bull. Soc. Med. Hop. Paris, 40:1462, 1916.

Haymaker, W., and Kernohan, J. W. The Landry-Guillain-Barré syndrome. Medicine, 28:59, 1949.

Low, N. L., Schneider, J., and Carter, S. Polyneuritis in children. Pediatrics, 22:972, 1958.

Peterman, A. F., Daly, D. D., Dion, F. R., and Keith, H. M. Infectious neuronitis in children. Neurology, 9:533, 1959.

Seto, D. S. Y., and Freeman, J. M. Lead neuropathy in childhood. Amer. J. Dis. Child., 107:337, 1964.

CHRONIC AND RECURRENT POLYNEUROPATHIES

Austin, J. H. Observations on the syndrome of hypertrophic neuritis. Medicine, 35:187, 1956.

Dejerine, J., and Sottas, J. Sur la névrite interstitielle, hypertrophique et progressive de l'enfance. C. R. Soc. Biol., 5:63, 1893.

Donohue, W. L., and Bain, H. W. Chediak-Higashi syndrome: A lethal familial disease with anomalous inclusions in the leukocytes and constitutional stigmata: report of a case with necropsy. Pediatrics, 20: 416, 1957.

Haase, G. F., and Shy, M. Pathological changes in muscle biopsies from patients with peroneal muscular atrophy. Brain, 83:631, 1960.

Higashi, O. Congenital gigantism of peroxidase granules; the first case ever reported of qualitative abnormality of peroxidase. Tohoku J. Exp. Med., 59:315, 1954.

Jacob, J. C., Andermann, F., and Robb, J. P. Heredofamilial neuritis and brachial predilection. Neurology, 11:1025, 1961.

Refsum, S. Heredopathis atactica polyneuritiformis. Acta Psychiat. Neurol. Scand. (Suppl.), 38:308, 1946.

Richterich, R., van Mechelen, P., and Rosse, E. Refsum's disease (heredopathia atactica polyneuritiformis): An inborn error of lipid metabolism with storage of 3, 7, 11, 15-tertra-methyl hexadecanoic acid. Amer. J. Med., 39:230, 1965.

Schwartz, J. F., Rowland, L. P. et al. Bassen-Kornzweig syndrome: Deficiency of serum β-lipoprotein. Arch. Neurol., 8:438, 1963.

Taylor, R. A. Heredofamilial mononeuritis multiplex with brachial predilection. Brain, 83:113, 1960.

CRANIAL NERVE PALSIES

Boone, P. C. Bell's palsy. Acta Neurochir., 7:16, 1959.

Evans, P. R. Nuclear agenesis. Arch. Dis. Child., 30: 237, 1955.

Henderson, J. L. The congenital facial diplegia syndrome. Brain, 62:381, 1939.

Chapter 11
INFECTIONS OF THE NERVOUS SYSTEM

DAVID B. CLARK

Craniospinal Focal Sepsis

Any portion of the brain, spinal cord, or meninges may be the site of abscess formation. Epidural abscess, usually small and often granulomatous, lies between skull and dura; in the vertebral column it is also called pachymeningitis spinalis. Subdural abscess or subdural empyema lies between dura and arachnoid. Brain abscess and intramedullary abscess are within the brain and spinal cord, respectively. Ventriculitis, an inflammation of the walls of the cerebral ventricles, may go on to filling of the ventricular system with pus, a pyocephalus. Subarachnoid loculations are circumscribed poolings of pus within the subarachnoid space; like ventriculitis and pyocephalus, they usually result from an inadequately treated meningitis. Meningitis circumscripta is the patch of localized meningitis often found above a brain abscess.

All of these conditions are secondary complications rather than primary illnesses. Craniospinal abscess is not a primary disease. It results from infection of the nervous system and its membranes by: (1) direct, penetrating trauma; (2) direct extension, by involvement of contiguous layers or along infected and thromboid veins, from paracranial and spinal foci in sinuses, mastoid air cells, scalp infections, spondylitis, or pleural or perirenal infections; and (3) hematogenous or metastatic spread from distant sites, usually in lung, heart, or bone, or cutaneous infections. Much more rarely, a primary pyogenic meningitis or infection via a congenital dermal sinus is responsible. Less than 10 percent of all craniospinal abscesses are without demonstrable primary sources. They are, in most cases, avoidable illnesses. They are always serious, their outcome if untreated or poorly treated being death or severe handicap. The physician has therefore the dual responsibility of preventing them where possible by prompt eradication or primary foci and, where this has failed, of recognizing abscess early and treating it vigorously.

EPIDEMIOLOGY. Incidence is very difficult to determine. For the antibiotic era, a figure between 1.5 and 3.0 per 10,000 hospital admissions is a fair approximation, at least for large general hospitals with active pediatric, neurosurgical, and neurologic services. There is no certain evidence that antibiotics have altered incidence materially. Modern therapy has not significantly affected routes of infection; metastatic abscess continues to outnumber abscess developing by extension by about 2:1.

Males outnumber females, but this is apparently an expression of greater vulnerability of the male to infections rather than of greater frequency of trauma. Race and socioeconomic factors are of importance only in that the better medical care available to some racial, cultural, or economic groups tends to remove potential primary sources early.

No age is spared, but craniospinal abscess is rare below 1 year and is predominantly a disease of the early decades of life. A third of all cases fall in the pediatric age group. The type and location of abscesses are to some degree age-dependent, expressing the age preference of the primary infection. Subdural empyema and pyocephalus, which often complicate meningitis, are, like meningitis itself, common in very young children, while brain abscess secondary to otitis media, sinusitis, and mastoiditis is more frequent in older children or adolescents.

BACTERIOLOGY. Almost any pyogen may be responsible: anaerobic or microaerophilic streptococci, pneumococci, staphylococci, and gram-negative bacilli are the most common. Fungi (actinomycetes, aspergillus, leptothrix, and nocardia) and even protozoa, particularly *Entamoeba histolytica,* are reported.

In many cases, more than one organism is present. Most abscesses, particularly brain abscess, will sterilize themselves in time, the hardier organisms persisting longer. Since sterilization is hastened by antibiotics, culturally negative abscesses are more and more frequently encountered, and great care must be taken to culture and to examine stained smears of pus if organisms are to be identified.

PATHOLOGY AND PATHOGENESIS. A fully formed brain abscess consists of a center of broken down leucocytes, tissue debris, and microorganisms, surrounded by a zone of granulation tissue and fat-laden phagocytes, and then a capsule of collagenous and glial fibers. Most peripherally there is a zone of edema, with inflammatory exudate about blood vessels, and some breakdown of white matter. Daughter abscesses may form in the capsule or surrounding edematous zone. Brain abscesses range in size from miliary foci to large structures containing 40 to 60 ml, the average being 15 to 30 ml. Walls of chronic abscesses may calcify.

Subdural empyema is initially an unencapsulated mass of pus, or infected meningitic effusion, which can flow freely in the subdural space, usually above the cerebral hemispheres or in the interhemispheric cleft; in time, it becomes encapsulated, principally from the dural side. Epidural abscess is usually much smaller, frequently a granulomatous mass with small droplets of pus rather than a single large abscess.

Both dead brain tissue and bacteria are required for the development of a brain abscess. Infective emboli provide these in metastatic abscess, septic thrombi in abscess by extension; in traumatic abscess, brain tissue is killed and infected by the same wound. Cranial epidural abscess usually occurs by direct extension from skull foci; subdural abscesses may also develop from direct extension or evolve from an infected effusion. Spinal epidural abscess is often metastatic.

All forms damage the nervous tissue by direct destruction of tissue, edema, compression, and vascular damage leading to tissue necrosis, and to some degree at least by toxemia.

Clinical Types

Cranial Epidural Abscess

This usually develops by direct extension from sinusitis, mastoiditis, or dental infections. The abscess is usually small and granulomatous. Symptoms, if not confused by those of the primary infection, are rather slight, consisting of headache, with pain and tenderness often localized at the site, fever rarely above 100° F, and a mild leucocytosis and elevated ESR. Physical signs are those of the primary illness, and frank neurologic signs are rare or absent.

The commonest and most important site of cranial epidural abscess is along the lateral and sigmoid sinuses. It develops as a complication of otitis or mastoiditis, and is a leading childhood cause of benign increased intracranial pressure, so-called pseudotumor cerebri. The sinus may be thrombosed or only compressed by granulation tissue. Frank otitis or mastoiditis need not be present, but scarred or perforated tympanic membranes and x-ray changes in the mastoid cells are constant. The symptoms and signs are those of increased intracranial pressure, including headache, vomiting, diplopia due to abducens palsy, and papilledema, often of startling degree, in a child who does not usually appear seriously ill.

In most cases of cranial epidural abscess, the skull x-rays are abnormal, demonstrating either the primary focus—such as mastoiditis, sinusitis, or osteomyelitis—or sutural separation, or both. The EEG is mildly abnormal, but seldom diagnostic. The cerebrospinal fluid may be normal or under increased pressure; infrequently it may show a mild increase in protein or a slight pleocytosis.

The important diagnostic distinction is from other forms of focal intracranial sepsis such as cortical thrombophlebitis, subdural empyema, and brain abscess and from brain tumor. Focal neurologic signs, other than the false localizing sixth nerve palsies or increased pressure, are rarely if ever present, seizures are unusual, the cerebrospinal fluid except for pressure is normal or near normal, and the EEG is not sharply localizing; the reverse of all these is true for the other septic forms. The presence of a primary focus and signs of infection, the absence of localized neurologic deficit, and the speed of evolution distinguish it from brain tumor. In many cases a contrast study such as arteriography or ventriculography is necessary.

Some cases will respond to antibiotics alone, although curettage of the granuloma may be necessary. Mastoid granulomas, with benign increased intracranial pressure, may require repeated lumbar punctures or even ventricular or spinal shunting, to protect vision, and a mastoidectomy is necessary. The prognosis is good.

Cranial Subdural Empyema

Subdural empyema occurs in the infant usually as a sequelae of a missed or poorly treated meningitis, with an infected effusion. The symptoms are usually submerged in those of the meningitis; the patients presenting as chronically ill infants with enlarging heads, intermittent fever, vomiting, and seizures. Some degree of hemiparesis is usually present, and there is a marked pleocytosis of the cerebrospinal fluid with increased protein. The diagnosis is established by subdural taps, but brain abscess must often be excluded by ventriculography or angiography.

In older children, the source is more commonly sinusitis, mastoiditis, or scalp furuncles, and the interval between the original infection and the onset of symptoms may be many weeks. Patients are usually quite ill, fevers of 102° or 103° F being common. Lethargy, confusion, or stupor are present, cranial tenderness is marked, and hemiparesis and seizures are common. The CSF is regularly abnormal; pressure and protein are increased, and a considerable pleocytosis, including polymorphonuclear cells is present. EEG's may show voltage suppression, spikes, and slowing. The most important distinction is from brain abscess and septic cerebritis, both of which may also be present, and contrast x-ray studies, preferably arteriography are usually necessary.

Treatment is surgical drainage, which in both infant and adult is best done through multiple trephine holes or osteoplastic craniotomies, since the tendency of the pus to migrate between the hemispheres and into subarachnoid cisternae makes drainage at best difficult. Prolonged massive antibiotic therapy and supportive measures, including fluids, are generally necessary. Older children may make a good recovery, but infants are generally left with serious neurologic residuals.

Brain Abscess

Abscess within the brain, like the other forms of craniospinal focal sepsis, can develop (1) as a metastatic abscess, by hematogenous spread from a distant source; (2) by direction extension from paracranial foci in sinuses, mastoids, dental alveoli, and scalp infections; (3) by direct contamination of the brain from without, through wounds and congenital dermal sinuses; and (4) rarely, as a sequel of pyogenic meningitis. The great majority fall in the first two categories, and of these, metastic abscess is about twice as common as abscess due to direct extension.

The common sites of origin of metastatic abscess are in the heart and lungs; osteomyelitis, dental alveolar sepsis, skin infections, renal and perirenal abscess less frequently constitute such sites. Of the cardiac sources, acute bacterial endocarditis is less common than subacute bacterial endocarditis, and both are more prone to cause multiple miliary lesions than large solitary abscesses.

A more frequent cardiac source is any congenital cardiac malformation capable of producing a right-to-left shunt; congenital pulmonary AV fistulas, with an intact heart, may equally predispose to abscess. The mode of infection of the brain here is not completely explained. Despite the frequency of bacterial endocarditis in congenital heart disease, very few children who develop brain abscess have convincing evidence for endocarditis; the abscesses themselves are usually single and massive, and only rarely have autopsied patients had signs of endocarditis. The most plausible explanation is that, due to polycythemia, the very cyanotic child suffers recurrent miliary cerebral infarcts and, because of this shunt, recurrent bacteremias. If the two coincide, the necrotic segment of brain becomes infected and an abscess evolves. Three or four percent of all patients with cyanotic congenital heart disease or pulmonary AV fistulas will, if their condition is not relieved, develop brain abscess.

Pulmonary sources of brain abscess are most commonly bronchiectasis, lung abscess, and empyema. Since all are relatively uncommon in childhood, abscess complicating them is comparatively unusual. Pyelitis, perinephric abscess, osteomyelitis, dental alveolar sepsis, and furuncles are all occasional causes.

Mastoiditis and, in the older child or adolescent, frontal sinusitis lead as sources of abscesses forming by direct extension. Because of the nature and evolution of the lesion, all of these are liable to cause associated epidural granulations or subdural empyema as well. Traumatic abscesses may follow craniotomy or accidental head trauma. The latter are known for the chronicity of their course, many weeks or months intervening between injury and onset of symptoms. An interesting variety is the frontal abscess which follows penetrating wounds through the orbit, such as pencils perforating the orbital roof after falls. A rare cause is infection along a congenital dermal sinus, usually leading from the occipital to the midline cerebellar region.

Solitary brain abscess resulting from meningitis is less frequent than might be expected. Smith and Landing found only 2 in 34 autopsied cases of *H. influenzae* meningitis, and Swartz and Dodge only 1 dubious instance in 207 clinical cases of various causes. It is not, however, unusual to have the headache, slight fever, stiff neck, and mild pleocytosis of a rapidly developing abscess mistaken for meningitis, the signs and symptoms of the abscess being mistakenly interpreted as its source.

Traumatic abscess, or abscess developing by extension, is adjacent to the primary focus and usually solitary, though daughter abscesses may develop about it. Frontal sinusitis leads to frontal lobe abscess; mastoiditis to temporal lobe or cerebellar abscess. Metastatic abscess of any sort is solitary and supratentorial in about four-fifths of all cases. Only in the miliary abscesses of bacterial endocarditis and with certain fungi such as nocardia are multiple abscesses really common.

SYMPTOMS AND SIGNS. Occasionally an initial stage of brain infection, with headache, fever, and perhaps even a little stiff neck, may be identified. More often, the onset is insidious or so mixed with the symptoms of the primary illness as to be indistinguishable. Except for some traumatic abscesses, the duration from onset to severe symptoms is not long, two to six weeks at the most. The child is lethargic, eats poorly, and complains intermittently of headache. Fever due to the abscess itself is surprisingly slight, rarely over 100° or 101° F and often intermittent. A mild peripheral leucocytosis and anemia of infection may appear. Before long vomiting becomes evident, usually on arising and is seldom frequent or pernicious. Focal neurologic deficits and more obvious signs of increased intracranial pressure may develop progressively, or, more commonly, they are noted after the child has a seizure. These signs are, first, those appropriate to the region involved: hemiparesis, with sensory deficit in parietal lesions, visual field defects if temporal or occipital lobes become involved, and aphasias of varying degree, particularly with left-sided lesions. Posterior fossa or cerebellar abscesses produce ataxia and cranial nerve palsies and, especially if acute, skew deviations of the eyes. Second are the signs of increased intracranial pressure: papilledema, abducens palsies, and, in young children, sutural separation and Macewen's cracked-pot resonance. Third, and of great value, many patients describe or give evidence of localized percussion tenderness of the skull overlying the abscess.

DIAGNOSIS. The special diagnostic procedures of value, beyond physical examination and history, are: (1) blood count, ordinarily unrevealing except for moderate leucocytosis and perhaps anemia of infection; (2) elevated ESR; (3) x-rays, which may disclose a primary focus in sinuses, mastoids, and chest; x-rays of the skull usually are normal or show only separated sutures, although very old chronic abscesses sometimes are marked by curvilinear calcifications; and (4) EEG, which in 60 percent or more of the cases will demonstrate lateralized slowing, and finally a clear-cut focus of very slow (Fig. 73), usually high-voltage delta waves, due either to edema or probably to compression and disturbance of the reticular formation.

If abscess is seriously suspected, the CSF should ordinarily not be examined because of the danger of herniation. When done, the pressure is generally increased, and there is a mild to moderate increase in protein and cells, usually less than 50 and including a few polymorphonuclears. In the unruptured abscess the sugar content of the CSF is characteristically normal. Finding many cells is unusual, and cultures are regularly negative unless the abscess has begun to leak. This serious event causes sharp worsening of the clinical condition, high fever, marked stiff neck, and usually seizures and decerebration. Rupture is almost always into the ventricular system, rather than into the subarachnoid space.

If the story is clear-cut and the localization by symptoms, signs, EEG, and perhaps percussion tenderness is sharp, contrast studies may not be necessary but more commonly cerebral arteriography is the method of choice, except in very cyanotic cardiacs who may not tolerate it well and in abscesses placed far posteriorly in the occipital region where

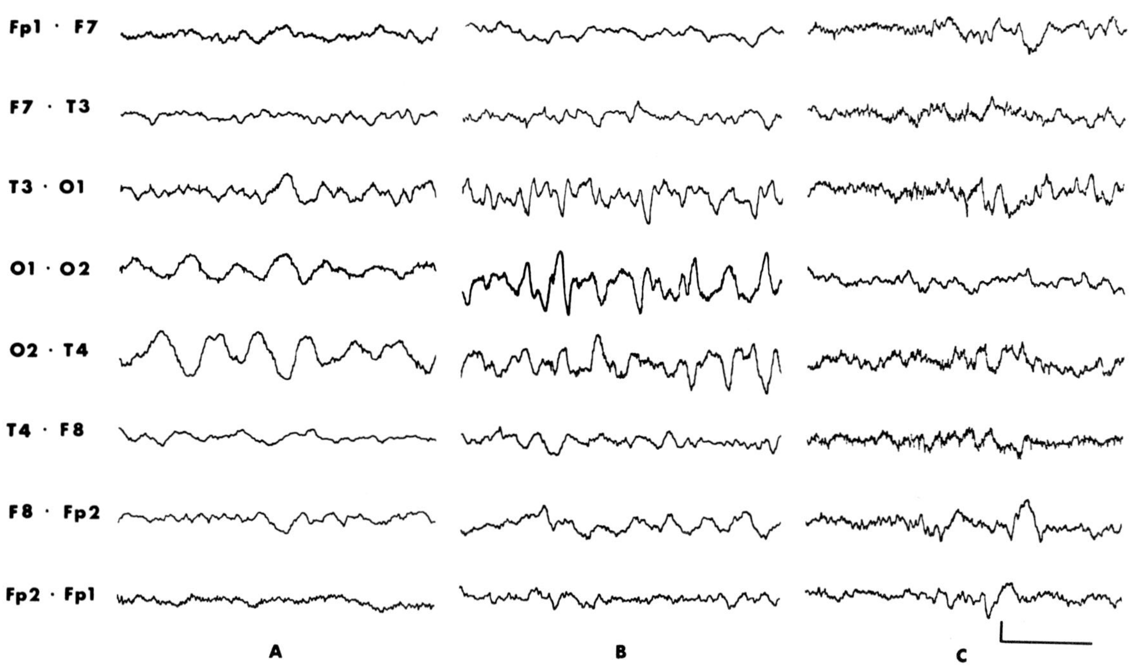

Fig. 73. EEG. Seven-year-old child with tetralogy of Fallot and right occipital lobe abscess. *A.* Before operation. *B.* One week after aspiration. C. Six months later. Note high-voltage slow focus, in leads 01-02 and 02-T4 disappearing on treatment.

localized deformity of the vessels may be difficult to define.

TREATMENT. The basis of treatment is surgical drainage. Some surgeons prefer trephination, tapping and drainage of the abscess, and instillation of a contrast material, usually Thorotrast, to label the abscess on successive skull films. The size of the abscess is then checked by x-rays at intervals (Fig. 74A and B), while the child is given antibiotics appropriate to the organisms cultured. If progressive shrinkage does not occur, the abscess is reaspirated until it does. Ordinarily two or three aspirations, over a period of a week to 10 days, are sufficient.

Total excision, preferred by other surgeons, requires that the abscess be well encapsulated, which is hastened by some days of antibiotic treatment before operation. In children with high intracranial pressure and advancing signs of intracranial decompensation, this time may not be available. Such preoperative antibiotic treatment also reduces edema and lessens the unavoidable destruction of brain tissue at the time of removal. It is also believed by some that total excision is attended by a lower incidence of seizures than is aspiration, though evidence for this is at best equivocal. Lastly, total excision avoids the possible delayed effects of retained thorium dioxide.

The author's preference is for aspiration, as a much shorter and simpler procedure with results which compare favorably with excision. In one instance, the very cyanotic cardiac patient, it is certainly superior, since these patients tolerate prolonged anesthesia poorly, and the tremendous congestion of their brain makes excision much more hazardous. Each case, however, must be considered on its own merits.

Massive antibiotic therapy is, with one exception, always necessary. It is determined when possible by knowledge or strong suspicion of the nature of the organism involved. When in doubt, or when organisms can be seen on smear but not cultured, combinations of antibiotics should be used. Treatment is maintained for at least three weeks after the abscess is removed or drained and the child appears clinically well. The one exception is in the child, usually a cardiac patient, whose diagnosis is in doubt, in whom abscess is suspected but not proved, and the signs are not yet clear enough to warrant operation. Under such circumstances antibiotics can indefinitely prolong but never cure the illness; they also obscure its symptoms beyond the point of possible diagnosis, even by angiography or ventriculography. When this situation occurs it is often necessary to stop all antibiotics, to watch the child closely with daily neurologic examinations and EEG's every three or four days, and thus permit definite, localizing findings to appear.

During treatment of abscess, the primary focus should be identified and treated. Curettage of mastoiditis or frontal osteomyelitis and treatment of pul-

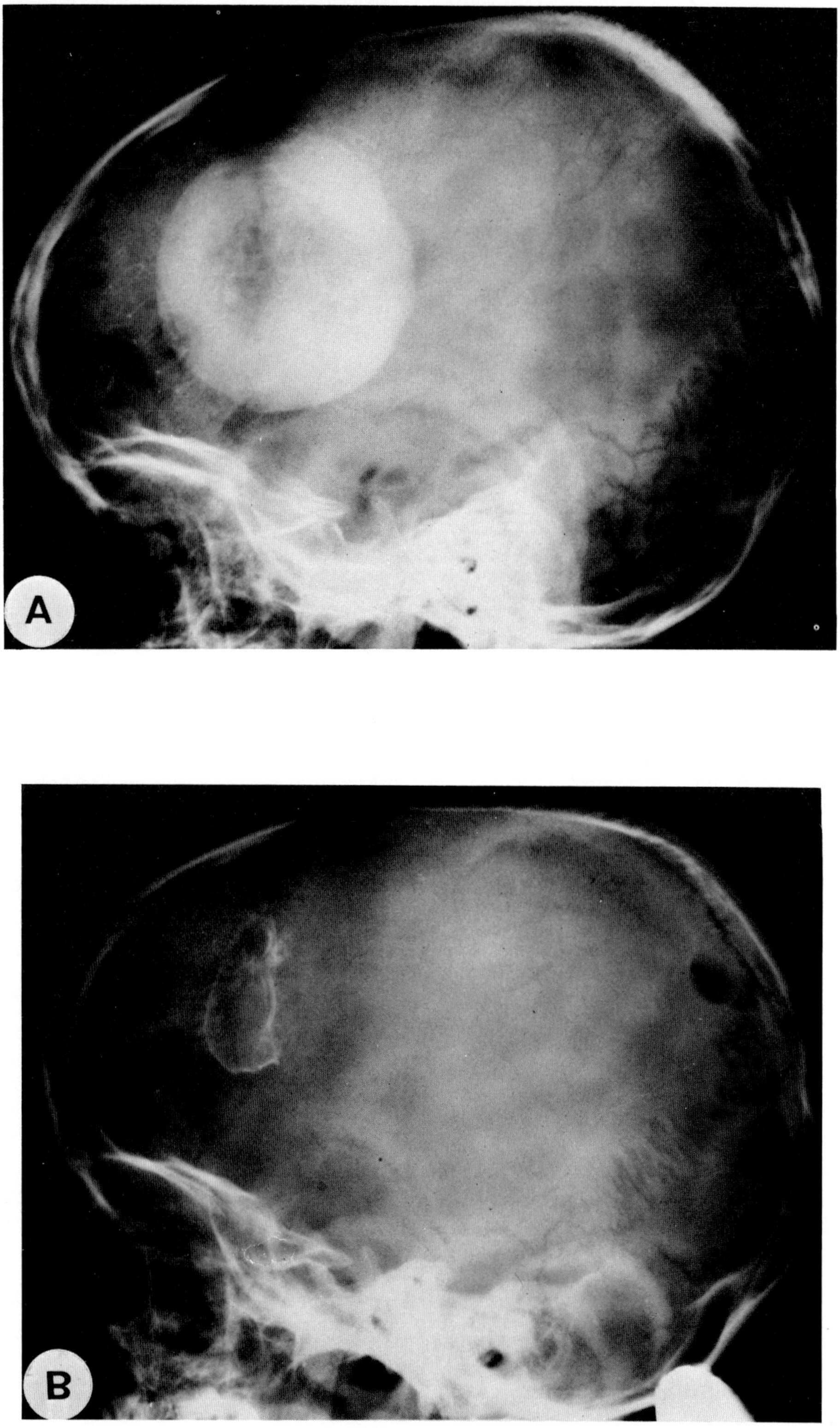

Fig. 74. *A.* Frontal abscess, aspirated and instilled with thorium dioxide. First day. *B.* After 10 days of antibiotic treatment and two additional aspirations.

monary infections should be pursued as rapidly as the patient's condition permits.

Lastly, it should not be forgotten that the incidence of seizures after brain abscess treated by any means is about 45 percent. Posterior fossa lesions and those restricted to the occipital and possibly the frontal poles are followed by seizures much less frequently than those in the central regions of the brain, but none is exempt. A good rule is to treat all patients with supratentorial lesions with anticonvulsants from time of operation for at least two years. Those who have seizures should be treated until seizure-free for three to five years.

PROGNOSIS. The mortality of brain abscess still exceeds 25 percent. With early recognition and prompt treatment, it can be brought well below this figure. It is always a serious life-threatening disease, and the neurologic residuals of hemiparesis, aphasic defects, seizures, learning impairment, and others are significant in one-half or more of the survivors.

Pyocephalus and Subarachnoid Loculations

Occasionally a young infant with severe or poorly treated meninigitis will develop a state in which the ventricles are filled with pus. A similar outcome may result from ascending infection in a meningomyelocele, the infection passing directly up the central canal and into the ventricles, without an intervening meningitis. There is always a severe ventriculitis and very extensive brain damage. The symptoms are persistent meningeal signs, enlarging head, "cerebral" cry, and signs of severe cerebral damage. Ventricular lavage and prolonged antibiotic therapy may in time clear the cerebrospinal fluid, but the end result is always bad and generally fatal.

Slowly resolving meningitis may also be accompanied by loculations of pus in subarachnoid cisterns, between the cerebral hemispheres, in the cavum septi pellucidi, or sometimes in the ventricles, usually in the temporal horns. These are usually small and generally respond in time to prolonged antibiotics. Their sudden rupture may account for brief exacerbation of meningeal signs, fever, and increase in cells in the CSF. Rarely, an intraventricular loculation may lead to localized enlargement of a part of the ventricular system, or a subarachnoid patch may be large enough to give local signs and permit surgical drainage.

Spinal Abscess

Abscesses involving the spinal cord are much rarer than intracranial abscess, the proportion being about 1 to 15. The causes, modes of development, and pathogenesis are, however, the same. Though any tissue or space may be involved, epidural abscess is the only one of practical importance. About half the cases are metastatic, the common sources being furuncles, bed sores, wound infections, or even infected acne. The other half develop by extension, from spondylitis or from pleural or perirental infections. Bacteriology is as variable as that of intracranial abscess, but staphylococci predominate because of the great frequency of primary cutaneous sources. The abscesses develop in the epidural space, posterior to the spinal cord and dura, and usually in mid or upper thoracic levels. Structurally, they may vary from frank, semifluid pus to thick granulations, with tiny droplets of enclosed pus. Acute forms begin with severe backache, local tenderness, fever of considerable degree, and leucocytosis. After two or three days to a week, sharp root or girdle pains appear. In another day or two, signs of spinal cord compression—stiffness and weakness of legs, heightened reflexes, and sphincter disorders—appear and are followed in hours to a day or two by complete paraplegia.

Epidural abscess developing from spondylitis may have a long phase of back pain and tenderness, but the time from root pains to complete paraplegia is often very short. In other instances, a slow, granulomatous infection may progress over weeks, months, or even years, simulating a spinal cord tumor.

The history of a previous infection, the back pain, worsened by flexion, local tenderness, and the evolution of signs of a spinal cord compression are generally present and highly suggestive. Plain x-rays will seldom do more than identify a primary focus, but lumbar puncture may either hit the abscess directly—and, unfortunately, be misinterpreted, since the pus is often so thick it will not flow through a needle—or demonstrate a low CSF pressure, with signs of spinal block, a very high protein, and increased cells, the Froin syndrome. Myelography is usually necessary to establish the lesion and its exact level.

Treatment is immediate surgical drainage and decompression, plus appropriate antibiotics. If decompression is done before paralysis or more than mild neurologic deficit has appeared, the results are excellent; if complete paraplegia has developed, complete recovery is less likely, and mortality may be high.

The important differential diagnostic possibilities include spinal cord tumor, metastatic tumor, and occasionally transverse myelitis due to viruses, spinal arteritis, or neuromyelitis optica. The importance of early decompression is so great that myelography should not be withheld if the least possibility of epidural abscess exists.

Intramedullary abscess is exceedingly rare, less than a dozen cases having been reported. It is diagnosed much as epidural abscess and, surprisingly, may respond well to midline myelotomy. Special note should also be taken of congenital dermal sinuses in the pilonidal area or thoracic region. The surface pore is often unimpressive, but the tract may lead to epidural space, to meninges, or into the cord itself. Recurrent meningitis or some form of spinal abscess almost always develops. The excision of such tracts, as soon as they are discovered, is very nearly an emergency procedure.

Encephalitis

HORACE L. HODES

Encephalitis may be caused by a variety of infectious agents including protozoa, fungi, bacteria, and viruses. The present discussion will be confined largely to this last group. Viral encephalitides are of two general types. In primary encephalitis there is direct invasion of the central nervous system by the virus, the pathologic changes being those of inflammation and neuronal injury. In secondary encephalitis the causative virus is not recoverable from the nervous system, some indirect mechanism apparently being responsible; the pathologic changes in this type are predominantly those of perivascular demyelination. A similar demyelinating process sometimes occurs in association with active immunization with viral antigens, notably after vaccination against smallpox and rabies.

Primary Viral Encephalitis

Viruses causing primary encephalitis in man include the following:

Von Economo's disease (virus not isolated)
Arthropod-borne encephalitides:
- *St. Louis encephalitis*
- *Western equine encephalitis*
- *Eastern equine encephalitis*
- *Japanese encephalitis**
- *Russian spring-summer encephalitis*
- *Murray Valley encephalitis (Australian X disease)*

Mumps
Herpes simplex
Infectious mononucleosis

Poliomyelitis, Coxsackie, and ECHO virus infections, rabies, and lymphocytic choriomeningitis belong in this group but are discussed elsewhere.

The pathologic picture in this group is in general similar for all the agents listed. Neuronal injury is apparent early in the disease, varying degrees of degeneration and necrosis of neurons and supporting cells being observed, followed by inflammatory changes. Neuronophagia, proliferation of glia, and perivascular infiltration with polymorphonuclear and mononuclear cells are seen. Areas of hemorrhage and necrosis in the ground substance of the gray and white matter are common, and cellular infiltration of the meninges is the rule.

* Originally designated Japanese B encephalitis.

Specific changes are seen in some of these infections such as the Negri bodies of rabies. Japanese encephalitis and Russian spring-summer viruses exhibit a particular tendency to attack the Purkinje cells of the cerebellum, whereas the related equine and St. Louis encephalitis viruses do not possess this property. For the most part it is, however, impossible to make an etiologic diagnosis from the pathologic changes.

The clinical picture is also nonspecific. The onset of symptoms may be gradual, following a prodromal illness resembling influenza. In other instances evidences of central nervous disorder appear with explosive suddenness. There may be fever, headache, and meningeal signs (stiff neck and Kernig and Brudzinski signs). Ataxia may be conspicuous. The sensorium is variably affected; there may be drowsiness and lethargy, followed by stupor and coma, or the patient may be excited, irritable, confused, or disoriented. Muscular twitchings, tremors, and convulsions may occur. Often there are bulbar symptoms —paralysis of the ocular or facial muscles or the muscles of deglutition. Respiration is commonly affected, becoming jerky or irregular. Profound variations in blood pressure and marked hyperthermia may occur. Involvement of the spinal cord may be revealed by paralytic and sensory disturbances or by loss of sphincter control. In infants, the onset is usually sudden and they are generally more severely affected than adults.

The blood commonly shows a moderate polymorphonuclear leucocytosis ranging between 10,000 and 15,000. The spinal fluid is under pressure and shows some elevation of protein and a pleocytosis (20 to 600 cells), mostly mononuclears; it may, however, be quite normal. The concentration of glucose is normal or slightly elevated and that of chloride is not affected. Electroencephalography shows widespread cerebral disturbance, irregular, slow, high-voltage complexes replacing the normal patterns.

Laboratory studies have shown that inapparent infections are common with all members of this group. The ratio of apparent to inapparent infections is highest with Eastern equine virus (1 in 18) and lowest with Japanese virus (1 in 500). In some inapparent cases it seems probable that infection gives rise to mild constitutional symptoms, but there is no evidence of invasion of the central nervous system.

The greater severity of the symptoms with Eastern equine encephalitis is notable; the fatality rate is higher, and permanent sequelae in the form of mental retardation, palsies, and convulsive disorders are more frequent. Such sequelae are also common in Japanese encephalitis in contrast to the Western equine and St. Louis virus infection. Clinical differentiation of the various types of encephalitis is, however, impossible; this must be made by recovery of virus or by antibody studies.

Primary encephalitis must be differentiated from a number of other conditions which affect the central nervous system. Helpful information may be revealed by a careful history. With a history of pica, lead poisoning is a strong possibility, and other evidences of this condition should be sought, particularly stippling of the red cells, lead lines in the bones, and the presence of an excess of lead in the plasma. The spinal fluid in lead encephalopathy is characterized by a relatively mild pleocytosis but a greatly increased concentration of protein. With a history of swimming in, or more particularly of falling into, stagnant water that may have been contaminated by animals, leptospirosis should be kept in mind. Tuberculous meningitis is readily confused with viral encephalitis. Evidence of tuberculosis elsewhere is important, particularly if the subject is an infant. A moderate decrease in glucose and in the chloride of the spinal fluid is characteristic of tuberculous meningitis as contrasted with viral encephalitis. Occasionally a low-grade bacterial meningitis will cause diagnostic difficulty, especially a mild meningococcal infection that may have been unrecognized. Such cases may present a predominantly lymphocytic reaction in the spinal fluid; the spinal fluid sugar is, however, likely to be reduced. Brain abscess may cause confusion at times; a history of preceding otitis media or of purulent meningitis may be helpful. Brain tumor may be a cause of difficulty, particularly when symptoms appear abruptly as may occur with pontine tumors. A pleocytosis of the spinal fluid may be observed with medulloblastoma; the mononuclear cells are not readily differentiated from lymphocytes unless a cell block is made.

The development of flaccid paralysis points to poliomyelitis as the cause of the disorder, though this has been observed in Coxsackie infections. Clinical evidence of mumps will also suggest the nature of the cerebral process, but by and large the identification of the agent rests with the virus laboratory. Recovery of virus from the blood is practical only in the case of Russian encephalitis, and from the spinal fluid in mumps and Coxsackie virus infections. A more practical procedure is the demonstration of a rising antibody titer in the blood or spinal fluid during convalescence; two specimens should be secured, one early in the disease and another two or three weeks later. Specific information can be obtained from neutralizing, hemagglutination-inhibiting, or complement-fixing antibodies, the last-named being the most useful.

Therapy for this group of infections is symptomatic. Sedation is often needed. When coma or bulbar symptoms are present, frequent aspiration may be needed to keep an open airway; tracheotomy may be necessary to remove secretions effectively. When tube feeding proves to be necessary, the danger of aspiration pneumonia must be borne in mind. Respiratory paralysis may require treatment in a tank respirator. Marked hyperthermia may be relieved by cold packs; it should be remembered that hyperthermia increases the need for water and electrolytes. Hypothermia has been employed in treating patients critically ill with viral encephalitis; its value is difficult to establish because of the variable course of these infections. Anticonvulsants should be given if there are seizures. In some types, such as mumps encephalitis, complete and relatively rapid recovery is the rule. In other types a variable percentage of the cases exhibit residual damage.

The specific types of primary encephalitis will now be considered.

VON ECONOMO'S DISEASE (ENCEPHALITIS LETHARGICA: EPIDEMIC ENCEPHALITIS, TYPE A). This form of encephalitis is almost certainly caused by a virus, but a causative agent has never been isolated. It is possible that the sleeping sickness epidemic of 1712 was this disease. The first modern cases were observed in 1915 in Rumania and subsequently in France. In 1917 it was well described by Von Economo in Vienna. The disease appeared in the United States in 1918, and up to 1926 it was observed in many parts of the world, but no new cases have been observed since that time. Nothing is known about the spread of the infection. Most cases were observed in the winter and spring months. All ages were affected, most of the cases being in young adults.

The disease affects the central nervous system only. Lesions are most conspicuous in nuclear masses such as the cranial nerve nuclei, the substantia nigra, globus pallidus and subthalamic nuclei, the medulla and pons. The white matter is rarely affected.

Clinically the disease is usually characterized by fever, headache, oculomotor palsies, and frequently somnolence. A small percentage of the cases exhibit pleocytosis of the spinal fluid early in the disease. Sequelae are frequent and include parkinsonism, sleep reversal, and serious personality changes and mental abnormalities which may be so severe as to reduce the child to a state of idiocy. Lesions in the region of the pituitary and hypothalamus have been known to cause obesity, diabetes insipidus, or sexual precocity.

The immediate mortality is between 20 and 40 percent, the ultimate mortality being considerably greater because of the progressive nature of the disease. Not more than 25 percent are well after three years, and it appears that even fewer make a complete recovery.

The diagnosis is easy if typical symptoms are present and an epidemic is in progress, difficult if this is not the case. The progressive nature of the disease and the characteristic late symptoms are important features. Late cases may strongly resemble the posttraumatic syndrome. Unless a clear history of a previous acute episode is obtained the diagnosis cannot be made with confidence.

Treatment is purely symptomatic. If there is excitement or choreiform movements, sedatives are indicated. Residual behavioral disorders require special treatment.

ARTHROPOD-BORNE VIRAL ENCEPHALITIDES (ARBOVIRUS ENCEPHALITIDES). These include St. Louis encephalitis, Western equine encephalitis, Eastern equine encephalitis, Japanese encephalitis, Russian spring-summer encephalitis, Murray Valley encephalitis. There are many common features. They all occur in epidemic as well as sporadic form, epidemics reaching their peak during the summer. In each instance, reservoirs of the virus exist among wild and domestic mammals and birds. Transmission of infection is accomplished by arthropod vectors, which usually become infected by feeding on the blood of birds, in which viremia is more prolonged than it is in mammals. The viruses in this group have a similar host range among laboratory animals; all produce fatal encephalomyelitis in mice. They are similar in size, and they produce similar pathologic changes in the central nervous system, primarily by direct invasion of neurons. Serologic tests indicate some degree of relationship between them. Outbreaks of St. Louis, and Western and Eastern equine encephalitis have occurred in many parts of the United States.

Epidemiology. St. Louis encephalitis was first observed in Illinois in 1932; larger epidemics occurred the following year in St. Louis and Kansas City. Since then the disease has been observed sporadically and in local outbreaks in western Canada and many parts of the United States, although not as yet in the northeastern area. Reservoirs of infection exist in animals and in domestic and wild birds. Cox demonstrated its presence in horses, but it appears that birds form the main reservoir. Two vectors are concerned in its transmission. It has been found that in chickens and in wild birds various mites transmit the infection from bird to bird, inducing a long-standing viremia without encephalitis. Mites can also transmit the infection to their own offspring; thus a large reservoir in birds is readily maintained. Bird mites do not, however, bite mammals, and transmission to the latter occurs by mosquitoes (particularly *Culex tarsalis* and *C. pipiens*). Prophylaxis consists in measures for mosquito control and protection from mosquitoes.

Western equine encephalitis is in most respects similar to the St. Louis type. The infection was first recognized in horses by Meyer in California in 1930, the first human cases being described in 1938. Outbreaks have been observed in California, Washington, Montana, Saskatchewan, Manitoba, the Dakotas, Nebraska, and Texas. The disease is observed among horses, but there appears to be a bird reservoir. The infection has been found in mites from chickens, blackbirds, and tropical birds; they appear to cause transmission from bird to bird, transmission from bird to mammal being caused by mosquitoes (chiefly *C. tarsalis*).

Eastern equine encephalitis was first discovered in horses by Ten Broeck in 1933, the first human cases being recognized in 1938 in Massachusetts. Both in horses and in man the disease is exceptionally severe, with a high mortality and a strong probability of residual damage among survivors. In the 1947 Louisiana epidemic, 3,700 horses and mules died of this infection. Ten human cases were observed, nine of them in children, of whom seven died. Outbreaks of the disease among horses have occurred in the East, South, and Middle West, in the Caribbean, Panama, and Brazil. In some of these epidemics the disease has developed in humans; in others antibodies to the virus have been found in man. The most recent epidemic occurred in New Jersey in 1959; 31 human cases were observed, of whom 21 died and only one of the survivors escaped permanent central nervous system damage. Recovery of virus from the mites and lice of chickens as well as from those of wild birds suggests that birds are the main reservoir for this virus; pheasants bred for the market seem to be particularly susceptible. Mosquitoes are apparently responsible for transmission from bird to mammal as well as from bird to bird. *Culex melanura* is regarded as the most important vector, although evidence from the New Jersey epidemic pointed toward *Aedes sollicitans*.

Prophylactic vaccines have been developed for Western and Eastern equine encephalitides which are recommended for horses and mules in infected areas and have been used in persons closely exposed to these viruses in the laboratory. They are not recommended for general use. Greater reliance may be placed on mosquito control.

Japanese encephalitis, though not as yet reported in this country, has been recognized in eastern Asia since the end of the nineteenth century. It is found in Japan, Taiwan, Korea, eastern China, and Indonesia, and outbreaks have been observed as far west as India and as far east as Guam. In the Okinawa epidemic of 1945 infection was demonstrated in horses; pigs and other domestic animals were also incriminated as reservoirs of virus. However, it is probable that nestling wild birds, especially of the heron family, are the most important source of infection for the mosquito vectors and the subsequent spread of the disease to man. Many species of mosquitoes have been shown capable of transmitting the infection.

Australian X disease, an epidemic form of encephalitis, was first recognized in Australia in 1917. More recently, this disease has been renamed Murray Valley encephalitis. The virus which causes this form of encephalitis, Murray Valley virus, is closely related to but distinct from that of Japanese encephalitis.

Russian spring-summer encephalitis is another arthropod-borne disease which is caused by a virus possessing properties similar to those of the viruses under discussion. This disease, which is transmitted by a wood tick, occurs in eastern Russia and Siberia. Domestic animals and rodents serve as reservoirs for the virus. Human cases occur chiefly among forest workers, and the great majority of patients give a history of having been bitten by ticks 8 to 15 days before onset of symptoms.

MUMPS MENINGOENCEPHALITIS. Mumps virus is probably the most common cause of encephalitis in the United States and Canada. Between 30 and 50 percent of mumps patients show pleocytosis of the spinal fluid, but only 5 to 10 percent show clinical evidence of meningoencephalitis. Of importance is the fact that meningoencephalitis may be the only clinical manifestation of mumps; a large proportion of patients with so-called aseptic meningitis—acute nervous symptoms and a low-grade mononuclear pleocytosis in the spinal fluid—are infected by mumps virus.

In the great majority of cases the picture is that of a primary encephalitis; virus is present in the nervous system and can be recovered from the spinal fluid. The symptoms, though often marked, nearly always clear completely; they are largely meningeal, there being little evidence of brain involvement. The nervous manifestations tend to occur at the height of the parotitis. On rare occasions a secondary type of encephalitis develops after mumps. The pathologic changes resemble those of measles and other postinfectious encephalitides, the outstanding change being perivascular demyelination. In such cases the symptoms are encephalitic rather than meningeal. Paralysis, particularly of the cranial nerves, may develop and is sometimes permanent. Most of the rare fatalities occur in this type.

Symptoms of drowsiness, coma, or excitement, or the presence of paralytic manifestations do not in themselves indicate that the more serious type of encephalitis is present. Such cases often recover completely. Lennette has reported cases in which the muscles of the trunk and extremities were affected with flaccid weakness similar to mild paralytic poliomyelitis, most of which cleared up completely or almost completely in the course of months. By and large this is true of involvement of the cranial nerves. Deafness, however, when it develops is likely to be permanent, though in most instances it is unilateral.

The spinal fluid is generally under increased pressure and contains 50 to 500 cells, mostly lymphocytes. The protein is only moderately increased, and the sugar is normal or slightly elevated.

Diagnosis offers little difficulty when parotitis or orchitis is present. When these are absent it is often in doubt. A history of exposure to mumps is helpful. An important differential point between mumps and poliomyelitis is the character of the spinal fluid; early in poliomyelitis the cells in the spinal fluid may be predominantly polymorphonuclear, lymphocytes predominating at a later stage, whereas in mumps the cells are predominantly mononuclear from the start.

Convalescent gamma globulin from mumps patients has been employed in therapy, as have steroids. Evidence that they are of value is, however, unconvincing. General measures are adequate in the great majority of cases.

Herpes Simplex Encephalitis

The virus of herpes simplex is capable of producing encephalitis, which may occur at any age, sometimes in the newborn. In most instances there have been perpetic vesicles in the skin and mucous membranes, but in some this has not been the case, evidence of central nervous system disease being the only clinical manifestation.

Lesions are found chiefly in the cortex but also in the hypothalamus, medulla, pons, and caudate nucleus. There is widespread evidence of neuronal injury, with necrotic changes particularly in the cortical gray matter. Perivascular accumulations of lymphocytes and mononuclear cells are found; proliferation of oligodendroglia may be present, and there may be petechial hemorrhages. Spherical or elongated acidophilic inclusion bodies similar to those seen in other tissues may be found in the nuclei of ganglion cells of the cortex. The meninges may be intensely infiltrated with lymphocytes and mononuclear cells.

The symptoms are both meningeal and encephalitic. Headache and fever are commonly present. There may be convulsions and delirium leading to stupor and coma and perhaps to fatal termination. Palsies of the cranial nerves may occur. A focal variant with unilateral temporal lobe predilection is also seen. In such patients, the clinical manifestations may mimic a neoplasm and ancillary laboratory studies confirm the presence of a "mass" lesion. The spinal fluid may be normal or show a mononuclear pleocytosis with counts ranging from 50 to 600 cells, an increase in protein, and no reduction of glucose.

In the absence of other manifestations of herpes the diagnosis can be made only by biopsy or laboratory criteria—the recovery of herpes virus from the spinal fluid or demonstration of a rise of complement-fixing antibody in convalescence. The mortality is high and the sequelae serious. Florman's patient, who became ill at 11 days, survived but was later observed to be spastic and severely retarded.

Dr. B. E. Juel-Jensen has reported very recently that the antimetabolitic cytosine arabinoside (cytarabine) had brought about a "dramatic recovery" in five patients with severe forms of generalized *herpesvirus hominis* infection, and that the same result had been obtained in the case of a man suffering from early simian herpesvirus encephalitis. The patients were given cytarabine intravenously once daily for 5 days in doses ranging from 0.3 to 2.0 mg/kg/per day. No toxic effects were noted in the patients treated. More experience with this drug in the treatment of herpesvirus infections of the central nervous system will certainly be reported soon.

Infectious Mononucleosis

Neurologic complications of this disease have been reported since 1931 in the English and American literature. The clinical picture may be that of the Guillain-Barré syndrome, or there may be a meningoencephalitis with mononuclear pleocytosis in the spinal fluid. Bulbar symptoms are often present. Recovery is the rule, but permanent damage may occur; a few fatalities have been reported. Diagnosis depends on the presence of nervous symptoms in association with other symptoms of infectious mononucleosis, a typical blood picture and a positive Paul-Bunnell test. Specific laboratory procedures may serve to rule out other possibilities. Complement-fixation tests make possible the exclusion of mumps, herpes, and the anthropod-borne encephalitides. Coxsackie and ECHO viruses can be excluded by failure to recover them from spinal fluid or feces which have been inoculated into suckling mice or tissue cultures.

Postinfectious Encephalitis

Many acute infectious diseases, particularly those of viral origin, are followed by an acute encephalitis characterized by diffuse demyelination of the brain and spinal cord. Postinfectious encephalitis is also called secondary encephalitis, allergic encephalitis, and acute demyelinating encephalitis. It is seen most commonly following measles but may occur after chickenpox, rubella, smallpox, and vaccinia; some cases associated with mumps fall in this category. Similar involvement of the nervous system may occur after vaccination with antigens of various types. The incidence of such postvaccination encephalitis is higher after antirabies vaccination than with other commonly employed antigens.

The injury to the nervous system in these cases is not attributable to the presence of the infectious agent. Virus cannot be demonstrated in the nervous tissue when the disease is at its height; furthermore, the symptoms usually develop gradually during convalescence. Many theories have been advanced to explain this type of encephalitis. The most satisfactory one postulates a primary asymptomatic injury to the nervous system with the production of altered chemical substances which then act as antigens. Antibodies are then formed against these substances which react not only against this material but also with unaltered nerve cell constituents. The available evidence indicates that myelin may be involved in this reaction. Details of the experimental work supporting this view cannot be given here except to state that a disease very similar to postinfectious and postimmunization encephalitis has been produced in monkeys. Rivers and his co-workers accomplished this by repeated injections of homologous and heterologous nerve tissue. By the use of adjuvants with homologous nerve tissues the same result was achieved rapidly by Kabat et al. and by Morgan.

It should be noted that occasionally symptoms of central nervous system disease begin early in the course of a primary infection. In these cases the possibility cannot be excluded that encephalitis results from direct action of the virus on the central nervous system.

MEASLES ENCEPHALITIS. The incidence of measles encephalitis varies considerably from outbreak to outbreak. Published reports indicate an incidence as high as one case of encephalitis for each 600 cases of measles and as rare as one in 3,000. In our own experience the incidence has been approximately one case of encephalitis for every 1,200 of measles. Measles encephalitis is more likely to occur among children suffering from severe attacks of measles than among those with mild measles. Although no accurate statistical data are available, it appears that the incidence of encephalitis following modified measles is much lower than that following the natural disease.

Pathology. The brain is usually congested at postmortem, and a few petechial hemorrhages may be present over the cortex. On histologic examination the characteristic lesion is seen to be perivascular demyelination with phagocytosis of lipid material by the microglia. The myelin sheaths of the nerve fibers in the affected areas are destroyed. In the center of each demyelinated area there is generally a small, distended vein which shows endothelial and adventitial thickening. In early cases the axis cylinders are usually not severely affected, but in cases of long standing, secondary degeneration of these structures may be present. Demyelinated areas are infiltrated with microglial cells which contain lipid material. Similar cells are found in the perivascular spaces, and lymphocytic infiltration of these spaces may be seen. About the margins of the demyelinated areas there is usually proliferation of the astrocytes and glial fibers. The gray matter is in general much less severely involved than the white matter, but evidences of neuronal degeneration may be found. The meninges show little change. The distribution of the lesions described is not uniform; they may be most common in the brain, the spinal cord, or the cerebellum.

Symptoms. In rare instances symptoms of encephalitis begin at the height of the measles eruption or even during the prodromal period. The onset may be delayed as long as two weeks after the appearance of the eruption. However, it usually develops on the fourth to sixth day after the appearance of the exanthem, when the fever has fallen and the rash has begun to fade. The temperature rises again and may rapidly reach a peak of 104° to 105° F. Headache, vomiting, and stiffness of the neck are common. In some severe cases convulsions are the initial symptoms; in others there is gradually deepening drowsiness, followed by stupor and coma. Evidences of bulbar involvement may be present, such as irregularities in the rhythm and rate of respiration and difficulty in swallowing. Death may occur within a few days after onset. In some instances consciousness returns gradually, in others quite suddenly. The period of coma may vary from 12 or 24 hours to more than three weeks. In neurologic examination after consciousness is regained the child is sometimes found to be entirely normal; in other cases monoplegia, paraplegia, or hemiplegia of the upper motor neuron type is noted. Mental confusion, disorientation, loss of memory, and speech disturbances may be present. Changes in personality are quite common. Nystagmus, ataxia, and loss of muscle tone pointing to involvement of the cerebellum are sometimes seen. In a relatively small proportion of cases the nervous symptoms are due entirely to changes in the spinal cord. These patients may show the picture of transverse myelitis or of ascending myelitis without involvement of the pons, medulla, or cerebrum. Paraplegia, loss of sphincter control, and changes in the reflexes are common findings.

Diagnosis. The symptoms of central nervous system disease appearing during convalescence from a typical case of measles usually makes the diagnosis of measles encephalitis apparent. Confusion arises chiefly in those cases, actually uncomplicated, in which nervous symptoms accompany the febrile rise which immediately precedes or coincides with the appearance of the measles eruption. These symptoms usually disappear promptly, in contrast to measles encephalitis in which they commonly persist for more than 24 hours. In case of doubt, lumbar puncture should be performed. In about 80 percent of cases of measles encephalitis, an increase in protein concentration in the spinal fluid and a mononuclear pleocytosis are found.

Treatment. There is no specific treatment for measles encephalitis. Convalescent serum and gamma globulin have been employed but without demonstrable benefit. Some authors have employed steroids with what they have considered favorable results. On the other hand, Karelitz and Eisenberg in a retrospective study of 42 patients with measles encephalitis published in 1961 concluded that cortisone had failed to afford any advantage. Hypothermia has been used by a number of pediatricians, including the author, with variable results, probably in keeping with the natural variability of measles encephalitis.

Good general care is essential. Particular attention should be paid to providing adequate calories, fluids, minerals, and vitamins when the patient is unable to swallow because of paralysis of the pharyngeal muscles or because he is comatose. In these instances intravenous administration of fluids and tube feeding are required. The danger of aspiration has been referred to in the treatment of primary encephalitis (p. 168). The tank respirator should be employed to furnish artificial respiration when this is necessary. It should be emphasized that the course of measles encephalitis is strikingly unpredictable, and no child's condition should be regarded as hopeless so long as life exists.

Prognosis. Approximately 10 percent of the patients with measles encephalitis die in the acute phase of the disease. However, the general tendency is toward recovery. Many patients whose condition appears hopeless in the beginning recover completely. We have seen complete recovery in patients comatose for more than one month. Unfortunately, approximately 20 percent of the patients who survive the acute stage suffer permanent damage. The sequelae range from minor changes in personality to complete dementia and generalized paralysis. Weakness of one or more extremities, hemiplegia, and paraplegia may occur. Epilepsy may develop. Other sequelae include cerebellar ataxia, nerve deafness, and permanent injury to the optic nerves. Lesions in the region of the pituitary may lead to precocious puberty and other endocrine disturbances.

ENCEPHALITIS ASSOCIATED WITH VARICELLA, RUBELLA, AND SMALLPOX. Encephalomyelitis which in general resembles that following measles may occur in association with varicella. The symptoms generally begin between two days and two weeks after the appearance of the rash, but in very rare instances the neurologic symptoms precede the eruption. The incidence of encephalitis is much lower than among patients with measles. We encountered only 14 cases of varicella encephalitis during a period of 12 years at the Sydenham Hospital in Baltimore, although this hospital treated practically all complicated cases of varicella in a population of over one million. In general, chickenpox encephalitis resembles that of measles, but cerebellar symptoms are relatively more common. The course tends to be milder, and the prognosis is better. The mortality rate is low as compared with measles, and recovery is more likely to be complete. In some instances, however, mental defects, spastic paraplegia, and monoplegia have been noted.

Encephalitis is extremely rare in German measles. The symptoms begin some days after the acute phase. Complete recovery is the rule, but a few fatal cases have been reported.

Encephalitis associated with smallpox is similar to measles encephalitis. The incidence appears to vary from year to year. Marsden and Hurst reported 11 cases among 2,400 patients, but encephalitis did not occur among a series of 8,000 subsequent patients with smallpox. It is believed that the incidence of neurologic symptoms is not related to the severity of the smallpox. Four deaths occurred among Marsden and Hurst's 11 cases. The survivors usually recover completely or very nearly so. There is no specific treatment.

POSTVACCINAL ENCEPHALITIS. Encephalitis following vaccination against smallpox was first reported in 1907. This complication has been encountered most frequently in England, Germany, Austria, and The Netherlands, less frequently in the United States. During the spring of 1947 roughly four million people in New York City were vaccinated against smallpox. It was believed that approximately 45 cases of encephalitis could be attributed to vaccination, an incidence of about 1 per 100,000.

The pathologic features of postvaccinal encephalitis are similar to those which occur with measles and require no separate description. The incubation period is generally between 10 and 11 days after vaccination. Occasionally, the period has been as short as two days and as long as 25 days. The disease is very rare in children under 1 year of age and appears to be less common in persons who have been vaccinated previously. The onset is generally abrupt. Its clinical course and neurologic findings are similar to those of measles encephalitis, with the possible exception that involvement of the spinal cord occurs more frequently in postvaccinal encephalitis. Laboratory findings are like those of measles encephalitis.

ENCEPHALITIS FOLLOWING VACCINATION AGAINST RABIES. The condition has been observed only with vaccines which contain mammalian brain or spinal cord. The newer killed virus grown in embryonated duck eggs is virtually free of nerve tissue, and experience with it to date encourages the belief that this complication has been avoided. Encephalitis, always rare, is somewhat more frequently seen with attenuated living Pasteur vaccine than with the killed Semple vaccine. The clinical symptoms are similar to those of measles encephalitis except that cord symptoms are more frequent; sometimes only a transverse myelitis is seen. The onset usually occurs 10 to 20 days after vaccination is commenced; it may be abrupt or gradual. Paresthesia and pain in the extremities may be noted, followed by motor weakness, usually in the limbs; bladder function may be impaired. Bulbar symptoms may occur early; in other instances an ascending Landry type of paralysis has been observed. The spinal fluid is sometimes normal but may show a mild pleocytosis with excess of protein. Approximately 15 percent of the cases have been fatal, but recovered cases rarely show residual damage; only occasionally do paralytic phenomena persist.

PERTUSSIS ENCEPHALOPATHY. The effects of pertussis upon the central nervous system warrant separate consideration here. The brain may be affected in several different ways. In a few instances there are massive hemorrhages in the brain substance or in the meninges. Their cause is not clear, and they are variously explained as the result of damage to the vessels or of congestion due to paroxysms of coughing. Several writers have found inflammatory lesions in the cortex, but in the only case in which we found such lesions there was also bacterial endocarditis. A number of cases have been described in which there was extensive atrophy of the cerebral cortex due chiefly to loss of neurons. Whether this is to be regarded as a result of toxic encephalopathy or of disturbances of cerebral circulation, as some authors claim, is still uncertain. In our experience this process is rare.

The clinical manifestations of these lesions are not uniform. Convulsions are the commonest and usually the first symptoms of involvement of the brain. Exceptionally tetany has been observed. The convulsions may cease promptly and leave no sequelae, or the child may remain in a state of stupor and exhibit general muscular rigidity or hemiplegia. A great variety of neurologic syndromes are described, including tremors, loss of vision, mental defects, and paralysis. Meningeal symptoms may be encountered, usually with a lymphocytosis in the cerebrospinal fluid. The cases followed by generalized cerebral atrophy present a fairly typical picture. After a series of convulsions the child becomes comatose and remains unconscious for periods of weeks or months. There is progressive rigidity of all the muscles, which may reach extraordinary intensity. All cortical functions seem to be abolished. Death may be long deferred.

ENCEPHALOPATHY FOLLOWING PERTUSSIS PROPHYLAXIS. We have described above the manner in which injections of vaccines containing viruses may bring about injury to the central nervous system. It should be noted that similar damage has been reported following the use of bacterial vaccines and antitoxins. The administration of typhoid vaccine or of tetanus antitoxin has on rare occasions been followed by lesions of the brain, cord, and peripheral nerves. A number of authors have observed similar results following vaccination against pertussis. In 1948 Byers and Moll described 15 infants who had suffered convulsions and severe brain injury following such vaccination. The symptoms of involvement of the central nervous system began from 20 minutes to 72 hours after injection of the vaccine. Convulsions, irritability, drowsiness, and coma were observed. These explosive reactions occurred after the first as well as the second and third of the immunizing injections. Spinal fluid contained an increase concentration of protein in most of the cases in which it was examined, and a mononuclear pleocytosis was found in some. The eventual outcome was grave. Of 12 cases observed for a long period only one recovered completely. The remaining children suffered from various combinations of cerebral palsy, continuing convulsive seizures, cortical atrophy, and mental retardation.

The pathogenesis of the encephalopathy associated with pertussis vaccination is not clear. It is impossible to conceive of an allergic or hyperimmune antigen-antibody type of reaction occurring so abruptly after the first injection of vaccine. A number of observers have obtained toxic filtrates and endotoxins from *Haemophilus pertussis* which have produced fatal encephalopathy in animals. The reactions described here may have some such pathogenesis.

It should be stated that the incidence of pertussis vaccination encephalopathy is extremely low when the total number of vaccinations is considered. Certainly it is so low as to leave no doubt regarding the wisdom of continuing mass pertussis immunization programs. We should, however, interpret the data as indicating that pertussis immunization should not be continued if an injection of the vaccine is followed by very high fever, drowsiness, convulsions, or any other symptoms referable to the central nervous system.

Slow Viruses in Chronic and Subacute Encephalitides

ALEX J. STEIGMAN

It has recently been firmly established that the measles virus is an essential ingredient in the subacute progressive encephalitis which is variously called subacute sclerosing panencephalitis (SSPE), Dawson's inclusion encephalitis, and Van Bogaert's subacute sclerosing leukoencephalitis.

SSPE does not present as a concomitant or early sequel to measles. Many months or years may elapse between the occurrence of measles and the onset of SSPE. (For acute encephalitis in measles see p. 172.) In 1933 Dawson hypothesized that SSPE might be due to a virus because intranuclear inclusion bodies were observed in the neurons in this disease. The recent sequential findings which lead to the conclusion that measles virus is associated with SSPE are: (1) electron microscopic demonstration of structures consistent with the nucleocapsids of a paramyxovirus such as measles; (2) the detection of measles-like antigen by immunofluoresence in SSPE brains; (3) the presence of unusually high levels of antibody to measles virus in the blood and spinal fluid of patients; and (4) the isolation of wholly infectious measles virus from brain tissue of patients with SSPE. This was accomplished by cocultivating the diseased brain cells in vitro with laboratory-established tissue culture cell lines. Such a strain of SSPE measles virus has been adapted to baby hamsters; the virus produces CNS disease in these animals.

SSPE generally evolves in three clinical stages. Initially one notes changes in personality, behavior, and intellectual ability sometimes accompanied by mild transient seizures. Then more ominous signs appear of loss of memory, apathy, myoclonic jerks, chorioathetoid and dystonic movements. Finally stupor, perceptual blindness, and decorticate spasticity occur.

The first human subacute "degenerative" CNS disease to be associated with a previously unrecognized virus was Kuru. This exotic condition is confined to a specific group of cannibalistic natives of the New Guinea highlands. The patients have a protracted afebrile grotesque neurologic course ending in death, the spinal fluid showing no increase in cells or protein. When Kuru was successfully transmitted in series to nonhuman primates following a long incubation period, great impetus was given to restudy the role of viruses in other subacute and chronic "degenerative" diseases of the central nervous system in man.

There is now some evidence and much speculation regarding other subacute and chronic disorders of the CNS of man in which a viruslike transmissible agent is involved. Most recently, brain suspensions from patients with Creutzfeldt-Jakob disease (spongiform encephalopathy) has produced a similar disease following a long incubation period in chimpanzees; and experimental transmission from chimpanzee to chimpanzees has been accomplished.

Viral investigation requiring long-term observation of experimental animals is now in progress for a number of obscure human neurologic disorders such as amyotrophic lateral sclerosis, multiple sclerosis, neuromyelitis optica, and Schilder's disease. It is recognized that factors other than those which occur in an acute episodic viral disease may well be involved in slow viruses affecting the human central nervous system. The suspicion that long-acting slow viruses might be associated in some fashion with chronic neurologic disease was first substantiated in *scrapie*. Briefly this is a slowly progressive neurologic degenerative disorder of certain genetic strains of sheep and goats. The disease can be reproduced by injecting suspensions of central nervous tissue of affected animals into healthy sheep and goats. The incubation period is one to five years; the protracted clinical course is afebrile and lasts for months. When infectious brain tissue is inoculated into mice the incubation period may be half a year or longer. The mysterious viral and immunologic characteristics of scrapie do not here concern us, nor do the growing number of naturally occurring chronic neurologic diseases of other animals now ascribed to slow viruses.

References

CRANIOSPINAL FOCAL SEPSIS

Altrocchi, P. H. Acute spinal epidural abscess vs. acute transverse myeopathy: Plea for neurosurgical caution. Arch. Neurol., 9:17, 1963.

Dutton, J. E. M., and Alexander, G. L. Intramedullary spinal abscess. J. Neurol. Neurosurg. Psychiat., 17: 303, 1954.

Evans, W. The pathology and etiology of brain abscess. Lancet, 1:1231, 1931.

Garfield, J. Management of supratentorial intracranial abscess: review of 200 cases. Brit. Med. J., 2:7, 1969.

Greer, M. Benign intracranial hypertension. I. Mastoiditis and lateral sinus obstruction. Neurology, 12:472, 1962.

Haymaker, W. Fatal infections of the CNS and meninges after tooth extractions. Amer. J. Orthodont. Oral Surg., 31:117, 1945.

Heusner, A. P. Non-tuberculous spinal epidural infections. New Eng. J. Med., 239:845, 1948.

Jenkins, R. B., Augustin, G. J., Putnam, L. E., and Horiwitz, N. H. Intracranial extradural and subdural empyemas. Report of a case and review of the literature. Med. Ann. D.C., 37:472, 1968.

Liske, E., and Weikers, N. J. Changing aspects of brain abscess. Neurology, 14:294, 1964.

Pine, I., Atoynaton, I. H., and Margolis, G. The EEG

findings in 18 patients with brain abscess. Case reports and a review of the literature. Electroenceph. Clin. Neurophysiol., 4:165, 1952.

Sanford, H. N. Abscess of the brain in infants under 12 months of age. Amer. J. Dis. Child., 35:256, 1928.

Smith, J. F., and Landing, B. H. Mechanism of brain damage in H. influenzae meningitis. J. Neuropath. Exp. Neurol., 18:248, 1960.

Swartz, M. N., and Dodge, P. R. Bacterial meningitis: A review of selected aspects. New Eng. J. Med., 272: 725, 1965.

Tyler, H. R., and Clark, D. B. Incidence of neurological complications in patients with congenital heart disease. Arch. Neurol., 77:17, 1957.

ENCEPHALITIS

Cramblett, H. G., Stegmiller, H., and Spencer, C. California encephalitis virus infections in children. Clinical and laboratory studies. J.A.M.A., 198:108, 1966.

Field, E. J., and Raine, C. S. Experimental allergic encephalomyelitis. An electron microscopic study. Amer. J. Path., 49:537, 1966.

Ford, F. R. Diseases of the Nervous System in Infancy, Childhood, and Adolescence, 4th ed. Springfield, Ill., Charles C Thomas, Publ., 1959.

Hodes, H. L. Common types of encephalitis in children. New York J. Med., 50:2277, 1950.

LaMotte, L. C., Jr., Crane, G. T., Shriner, R. B., and Kirk, L. J. Use of adult chickens as arbovirus sentinels. 1. Viremia and persistence of antibody in experimentally inoculated adult chickens. Amer. J. Trop. Med., 16:348, 1967.

Neal, J. B. et al. Epidemic Encephalitis: Etiology, Epidemiology and Treatment. Reports of the Matheson Commission. New York, Columbia University Press, 1929, 1932, 1939.

——— Encephalitis: A Clinical Study. New York, Grune and Stratton, Inc., 1942.

Pierce, N. F., Portnoy, B., Leeds, N. E., Morrison, R. L., and Wehrle, P. F. Encephalitis associated with herpes simplex infection presenting as a temporal lobe mass. Neurology, 14:708, 1964.

ARTHROPOD-BORNE VIRAL ENCEPHALITIS (ARBOVIRUS ENCEPHALITIDES)

Casals, J. Viruses: The versatile parasites; the arthropod-borne group of animal viruses. Trans. N.Y. Acad. Sci., Ser. 2, 19:219, 1957.

Clarke, D. H. Two nonfatal human infections with the virus of Eastern encephalitis. Amer. J. Trop. Med., 10:67, 1961.

Cox, H. R., and Fite, G. L. Serological distinctions between viruses of encephalitis in St. Louis, 1933, equine encephalomyelitis and vesicular stomatitis. Proc. Soc. Exp. Biol. Med., 31:499, 1934.

Goldfield, M., and Rowan, F. The 1959 Outbreak of Eastern Encephalitis in New Jersey. Paper presented at Conference of State Health Laboratory Directors. Washington, D.C., Nov. 2, 1960.

Hodes, H. L. Common types of encephalitis in children. New York J. Med., 50:2277, 1950.

Olitsky, P. K., and Casals, J. *In* Rivers, T. M., and Horsfall, F. L., eds., Viral and Rickettsial Infections of Man, 3rd ed. Philadelphia, J. B. Lippincott Co., 1959, p. 269.

Smorodintseff, A. A. The spring-summer tick-borne encephalitis. Arch. Ges. Virusforsch., 1:468, 1940.

Ten Broeck, C., and Merrill, M. H. Serological difference between Eastern and Western equine encephalomyelitis virus. Proc. Soc. Exp. Biol. Med., 31:217, 1933.

MUMPS MENINGOENCEPHALITIS

Donohue, W. L. The pathology of mumps encephalitis with report of a fatal case. J. Pediat., 19:42, 1941.

Lennette, E. H., Caplan, G. E., and Magoffin, R. L. Mumps virus infection simulating paralytic poliomyelitis; a report of 11 cases. Pediatrics, 25:788, 1960.

HERPES SIMPLEX ENCEPHALITIS

Florman, A. L., and Mindlin, R. L. Generalized herpes simplex in an eleven-day-old premature infant. Amer. J. Dis. Child., 83:481, 1952.

Gajdusek, D. C., Robbins, M. L., and Robbins, F. C. Diagnosis of herpes simplex infections by the complement fixation test. J.A.M.A., 149:235, 1952.

Haymaker, W. Herpes simplex encephalitis in man, with a report of 3 cases. J. Neuropath. Exp. Neurol., 8:132, 1949.

INFECTIOUS MONONUCLEOSIS

Epstein, S. H., and Dameshek, W. Involvement of the central nervous system in a case of glandular fever. New Eng. J. Med., 205:1238, 1931.

Thelander, H. E., and Shaw, E. B. Infectious mononucleosis with special reference to cerebral complications. Amer. J. Dis. Child., 61:1131, 1941.

POSTINFECTIOUS ENCEPHALITIS

Ferraro, A. Pathology of demyelinating diseases as an allergic reaction of the brain. Arch. Neurol. Psychiat., 52:443, 1944.

Hurst, E. W. A review of some recent observations on demyelination. Brain, 67:103, 1944.

Kabat, E. A., Wolf, A., and Bezer, A. E. Rapid production of acute disseminated encephalomyelitis in rhesus monkeys by injection of heterologous and homologous brain tissue with adjuvants. J. Exp. Med., 85:117, 1947.

Morgan, I. M. Allergic encephalomyelitis in monkeys in response to injection of normal monkey nervous tissue. J. Exp. Med., 85:131, 1947.

Rivers, T. M., and Schwentker, F. F. Encephalomyelitis accompanied by myelin destruction experimentally produced in monkeys. J. Exp. Med., 61:689, 1935.

MEASLES ENCEPHALITIS

Appelbaum, E., Dolgopol, V. B., and Dolgin, J. Measles encephalitis. Amer. J. Dis. Child., 77:25, 1949.

Ford, F. R. Diseases of the Nervous System in Infancy, Childhood, and Adolescence, 4th ed. Springfield, Ill., Charles C Thomas, Publ., 1959.

——— and Guild, H. Precocious puberty following measles encephalomyelitis and epidemic encephalitis. Bull. Hopkins Hosp., 60:192, 1937.

Hamilton, P. M., and Hanna, R. J. Encephalitis complicating measles; a report on 241 cases collected from

the literature and on 44 additional cases. Amer. J. Dis. Child., 61:483, 1941.
Haymaker, W., and Smadel, J. The Pathology of the Viral Encephalitides. Washington, U.S. Army Med. Museum, 1943.
Hodes, H. L. Encephalitides and Postinfectious Encephalopathies. *In* McIntosh, R., and Hare, C. C., eds., Neurology and Psychiatry in Childhood. Res. Publ. Ass. Res. Nerv. Ment. Dis., Baltimore, Williams and Wilkins Co., 1954, Vol. 34.
——— Common types of encephalitis in children. New York J. Med., 50:2277, 1950.
Karelitz, S., and Eisenberg, M. Measles encephalitis; evaluation of treatment with ACTH and adrenal corticosteroids. Pediatrics, 27:811, 1961.
Litvak, A. M., Sands, I. J., and Gibel, H. Encephalitis complicating measles; report of 56 cases with follow-up studies in 32. Amer. J. Dis. Child., 65:265, 1943.
Shaffer, M. F., Rake, G., and Hodes, H. L. Isolation of virus from a patient with fatal encephalitis complicating measles. Amer. J. Dis. Child., 64:815, 1942.
Spragins, M., Shinners, B. M., and Rochester, B. Measles encephalitis; clinical and electroencephalographic study. Pediatrics, 5:599, 1950.

ENCEPHALITIS ASSOCIATED WITH VARICELLA, RUBELLA, AND SMALLPOX

Boughton, C. R. Varicella zoster in Sydney. II. Neurological complications of varicella. Med. J. Aust., 2:444, 1966.
Davison, C., and Friedfeld, L. Acute encephalomyelitis following German measles. Amer. J. Dis. Child., 55: 496, 1938.
Margolis, F. J., Wilson, J. L., and Top, F. H. Postrubella encephalomyelitis; report of cases in Detroit and review of literature. J. Pediat., 23:158, 1943.
Marsden, J. P., and Hurst, E. W. Acute perivascular myelinoclasis ("acute disseminated encephalomyelitis") in smallpox. Brain, 55:181, 1932.
Wilson, R. E., and Ford, F. R. The nervous complications of variola, vaccinia and varicella, with a report of cases. Bull. Hopkins Hosp., 40:337, 1927.
Zimmerman, H. M., and Yannet, H. Nonsuppurative encephalomyelitis accompanying chickenpox. Arch. Neurol. Psychiat., 26:322, 1931.

POSTVACCINAL ENCEPHALITIS

Fatal viral encephalitis following 17D yellow fever vaccine inoculation. Report of a case in a 3-year-old child. J.A.M.A., 198:671, 1966. (A joint statement.)
Greenberg, M., and Appelbaum, E. Postvaccinal encephalitis: a report of 45 cases in New York City. Amer. J. Med. Sci., 216:565, 1948.
Ministry of Health (Great Britain). Vaccination, report of the committee on vaccination. London, H. M. Stationery Office, 1928.

PERTUSSIS ENCEPHALOPATHY

Byers, R. K., and Moll, F. C. Encephalopathies following prophylactic pertussis vaccine. Pediatrics, 1:437, 1948.

SLOW VIRUSES IN CHRONIC AND SUBACUTE ENCEPHALITIDES

Byington, D. P., Castro, A. E., and Burnstein, T. Adaptation to hamsters of neurotropic measles virus from subacute sclerosing panencephalitis. Nature, 225:554, Feb. 1970.
Chen, T. T., Watanabe, I. et al. Subacute sclerosing panencephalitis: propagation of measles virus from brain biopsy in tissue culture. Science, 163:1193, 1969.
Conference on measles virus and subacute sclerosing panencephalitis. Neurology, 18:1 (Part 2), 1968.
Gadjusek, D. E., Gibbs, C. J., Jr., and Alpers, M. Transmission and passage of experimental "Kuru" to chimpanzees. Science, 155:212, 1967.
Gibbs, C. J., and Gadjusek, D. C. Infection as the etiology of spongiform encephalopathy (Creutzfeldt-Jakob disease). Science, 165:1023, 1969.
Payne, E. E., Baublis, J. V., and Itabashi, H. H. Isolation of measles virus from cell cultures of brain from a patient with subacute sclerosing panencephalitis. New Eng. J. Med., 281:585, 1969.

Chapter 12
DISEASES OF THE MUSCLES

J. GORDON MILLICHAP

Clinical disorders of muscle may involve primarily the muscle fiber or may be secondary to disease which occurs predominantly in organs other than muscle. In myopathies such as progressive muscular dystrophy and polymyositis the pathology is centered largely in the muscle, whereas in polyneuritis and progressive spinal muscular atrophy (Werdnig-Hoffmann disease), muscle dysfunction is secondary to lesions in the nerve and spinal cord. In both, hypotonia, weakness, atrophy, and contracture of muscles are the chief clinical manifestations.

The diagnosis of myopathy depends principally on the clinical features, but valuable additional information may be obtained from muscle biopsy, electromyography, nerve conduction velocities, radiographs of the soft tissues, and biochemical tests. Examples of the histologic and electrical changes characteristic of certain myopathies are shown in Figures 75 and 76. Muscle biopsy is most reliable when the specimen is taken in the early stages of disease and from muscle which is not completely atrophied. It may be helpful in the differentiation of polymyositis from muscular dystrophy, and in addition it reflects also the characteristic muscle changes due to lower motor neuron diseases. Electromyography is of particular value in the distinction of neuropathic from myopathic disorders. Decrease in nerve conduction velocity indicates peripheral nerve rather than anterior horn cell disease as a cause of neuropathic atrophy.

The interpretation of muscle histology and elec-

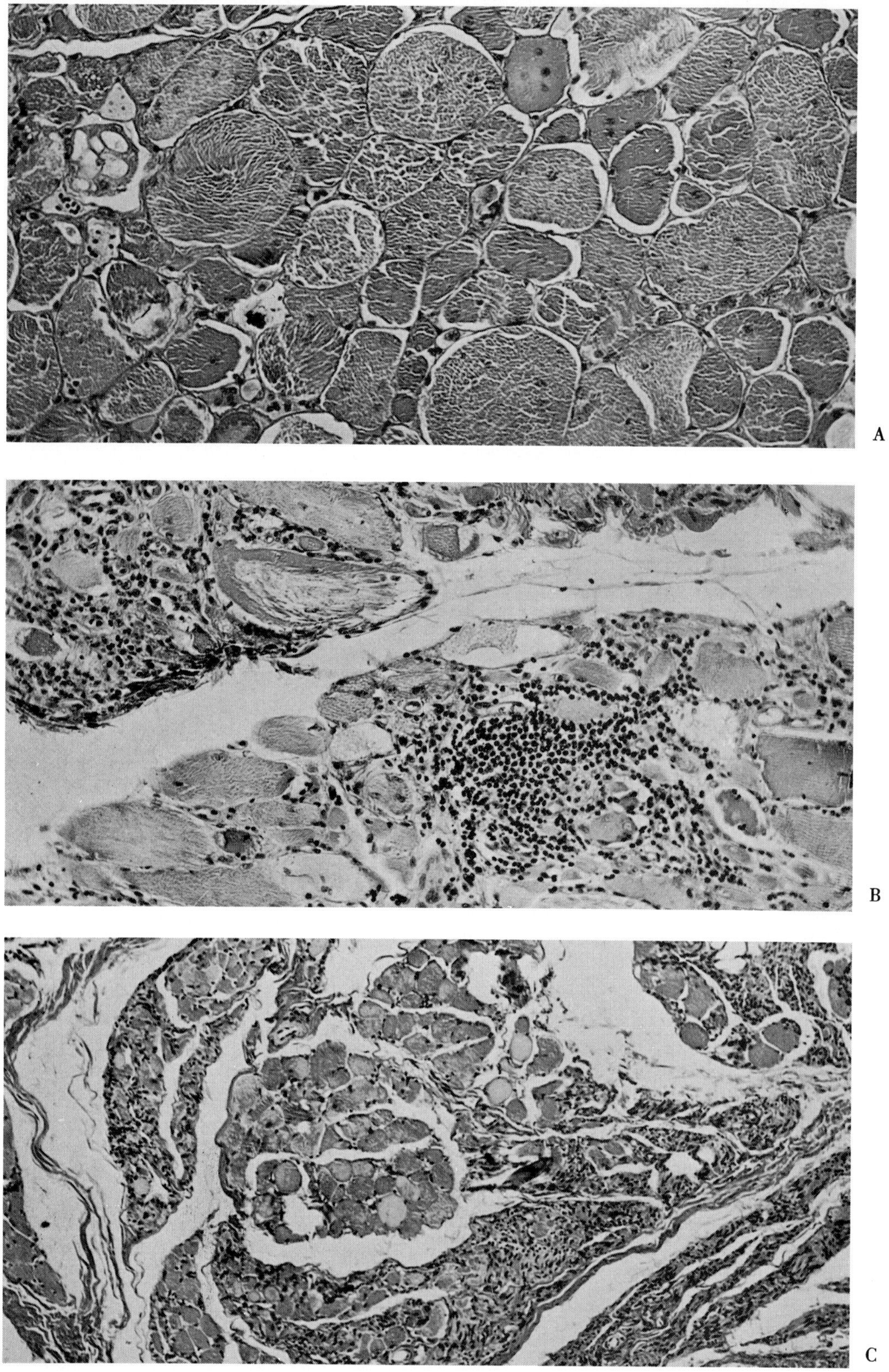

Fig. 75. *A.* Progressive muscular dystrophy. Section of muscle showing degeneration and variability of size of muscle fibers. *B.* Polymyositis. Section of muscle showing atrophy of fibers and infiltration with inflammatory cells. C. Infantile spinal muscular atrophy (Werdnig-Hoffman disease). Section of muscle showing groups of small atrophic fibers mixed with groups of normal fibers. (Courtesy of Raymond D. Adams, Boston.)

tromyography without reference to the clinical findings is sometimes difficult, and the occasional limitations of these methods of investigation must be recognized when diagnosis and prognosis are assessed.

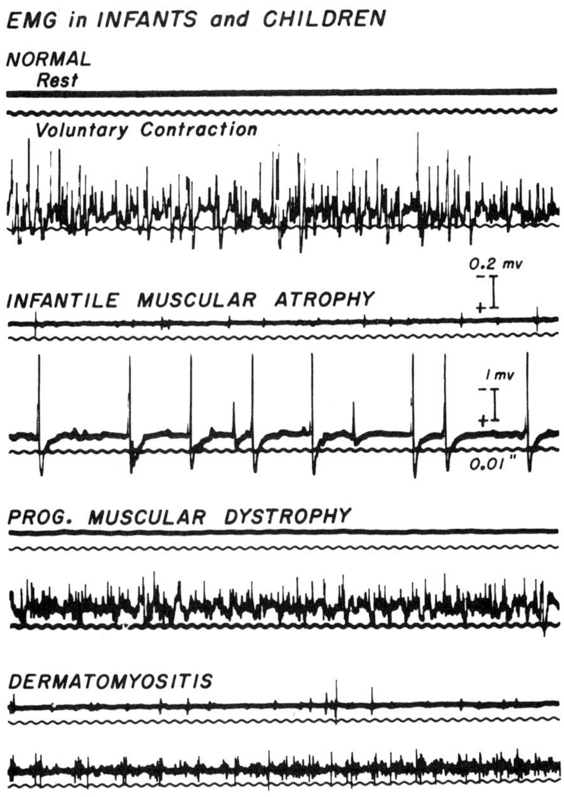

Fig. 76. Electromyograms in neuromuscular disease. Electric activity of quadriceps femoris muscle detected with a needle electrode inserted into the muscle and recorded by photographing the trace of a doublebeam cathode-ray oscilloscope on moving film. The lower beam of the oscilloscope traced a timing signal of 100 cycles per second. On the upper beam, an upward deflection indicates a change of voltage in the negative direction at the tip of the needle electrode.

A pair of records is shown for each patient. The upper record of each pair was obtained from the resting muscle; the lower record of each pair was obtained during voluntary contraction of the muscle. Amplification of the signal in the upper record of each pair is 5 times the amplification of the signal in the lower record. Calibrations are in millivolts and are the same for each pair of records.

Normal Infant. Upper record, no electric activity in the resting muscle. Lower record, numerous motor-unit action potentials during voluntary contraction.

Infantile Spinal Muscular Atrophy. Upper record, fibrillation potentials in the resting muscle. Lower record, greatly reduced number of motor-unit action potentials. A large, single, motor-unit action potential recurs in the range of the needle electrode.

Progressive Muscular Dystrophy. Upper record, no electric activity in the resting muscle. Minimal electric activity may occasionally be observed. Lower record, numerous motor-unit action potentials during voluntary contraction. These are shorter in duration and lower in amplitude than normal.

Dermatomyositis. Upper record, fibrillation potentials in the resting muscle. This is a much more common occurrence in polymyositis than in progressive muscular dystrophy. Lower record, numerous motor-unit action potentials during voluntary contraction. These are shorter in duration and lower in amplitude than normal. (Courtesy of Dr. E. H. Lambert, Mayo Clinic, Rochester, Minnesota.)

Limp Infant Syndrome

The limp infant (floppy child) syndrome is a term now used to describe all infants who have weak and hypotonic muscles, an increased range of joint movement or contracture, and various degrees of flaccid paralysis. In some infants hypotonia is marked and paresis slight, whereas in others muscular paralysis is profound. The symptoms may be obvious at birth or may present in late infancy. The prognosis is variable and dependent upon the underlying disease process. The disease may progress rapidly and death ensue early, but in some cases progression is slow, and in others the disease becomes arrested and recovery may be partial or even complete. This clinical picture may be produced by various diseases with primary lesions in the cerebrum, cerebellum, spinal cord, peripheral nerve, neuromuscular junction, or the muscle itself. Most commonly it is due to a degeneration or malformation of the anterior horn cells of the spinal cord (Werdnig-Hoffmann disease).

The differential diagnosis of the limp infant syndrome (Table 27) includes the following: infantile progressive spinal muscular atrophy of Werdnig and Hoffmann, congenital poliomyelitis, benign congenital hypotonia of Walton, congenital or early infantile muscular dystrophy of Batten and Turner, polymyositis, "central core" myopathy of Shy and Magee, glycogen storage myopathy, congenital universal muscular hypoplasia of Krabbe, congenital laxity of the ligaments, neonatal myasthenia gravis, infantile polyneuritis, hypotonic cerebral diplegia, cerebellar malformations, mongolism and others forms of mental deficiency, Lowe's syndrome, and various metabolic disorders, such as hypophosphatasia, rickets, and idiopathic hypercalcemia. In those cases described by Oppenheim which were characterized by improvement, the pathology was not recorded; the clinical picture and course correspond most closely to that of benign congenital hypotonia and universal musclar hypoplasia.

Benign congenital hypotonia is the term coined by Walton for a form of early amyotonia which characteristically improves with time and in which the muscle fibers occasionally may appear universally small for the age but usually show no structural abnormality. The infant is limp and hypotonic at birth, the deep tendon reflexes may be absent or depressed, but respiration is rarely affected. Sitting and walking are delayed, yet muscular wasting is not profound and the eventual development proves to be essentially normal.

Congenital universal muscular hypoplasia is a rare disorder described by Krabbe in which all skele-

TABLE 27. *Differential Diagnosis of the Limp Child Syndrome**

Cerebral Diseases (Atonic Diplegia)
- Cerebral malformations
- Cerebral damage from hypoxia
- Cerebral birth injury
- Mongolism
- Metabolic (Lowe's syndrome, hypophosphatasia, rickets, hypercalcemia)
- Familial dysautonomia

Spinal Cord Diseases
- Infantile spinal muscular atrophy (Werdnig-Hoffmann)
- Poliomyelitis
- Spinal and birth injury

Peripheral Nerve Disease
- Polyneuritis

Neuromuscular Junction Disorders
- Developmental
  - Congenital hypotonia?
- Metabolic
  - Myasthenia gravis

Muscle Disorders
- Myopathies
  - Infantile muscular dystrophy
  - Arthrogryposis multiplex congenita
  - "Central core" disease
  - "Nemaline" myopathy
- Other conditions
  - Glycogen storage disease of muscle
  - Polymyositis

*Modified from Grinker, Bucy, and Sahs.

tal muscles are small and weak but otherwise normal. Deep tendon reflexes are normal or depressed. Changes of dystrophy or neurogenic atrophy of muscle are absent on histologic examination. The condition is nonprogressive.

Congenital or infantile muscular dystrophy is sometimes familial and is characterized by weakness which involves principally the proximal muscle groups, present at or soon after birth, and progresses at varying rates but in most cases slowly. The muscles are atrophied and hypotonic, but all movements may be performed, though feebly. The deep tendon reflexes are depressed or absent. Contractures of limb muscles tend to appear late, with equal involvement of the intercostals and diaphragm. The pharyngeal muscles are not involved and dysphagia is not a symptom of the disease. The diagnosis rests on the histologic appearance of the muscle (Fig. 75) and on the clinical course. Soft tissue radiographs may demonstrate severe wasting of muscles and thus aid in the differentiation of this disorder from benign congenital hypotonia.

"Central core" disease is a nonprogressive myopathy which is present at or shortly after birth, involves proximal muscle groups, and is said to have a distinctive histologic appearance of the muscle. Shy and Magee described five patients with this disorder in three generations of a family. Sitting and walking were delayed, and although all patients were ambulatory, running and climbing stairs were never performed without difficulty. Deep tendon reflexes were active, and the muscles supplied by cranial nerves were spared. On biopsy examination of muscles, a central core of closely set myofibrils with an amorphous appearance and altered staining qualities was interpreted as a characteristic feature of the disease.

"Nemaline" myopathy is another rare, nonprogressive, congenital myopathy which may be distinguished only by muscle biopsy. Engel et al. have reported female patients, age 4 years and 16 years, with mild weakness and wasting of proximal muscles which, on histologic examination, show rod-shaped structures in the fibers.

Myotubular and mitochondrial myopathies are two of the more recently described congenital myopathies. They may present the classical features of the limp infant syndrome. Diagnosis is only possible by muscle biopsy.

Congenital Defects of Skeletal Muscles

Single muscles or groups of muscles occasionally fail to develop. Most frequently it is the pectoralis major, particularly the lower sternocostal portion, which is deficient. Congenital absence of muscles is clearly evident when the hands are pressed together while the elbows are abducted. Other muscles which may fail to develop include the trapezius, serratus anticus, and quadratus femoris.

Defects of skeletal muscles may occur together with other congenital abnormalities. Agenesis of the pectoral muscle is sometimes associated with malformation of a rib, a defect of the mammary gland, and scoliosis. Congenital absence of the abdominal muscles is most frequently seen in boys. There are concomitant genitourinary anomalies including enlargement of the bladder, dilation of the ureters, hydronephrosis, and cryptorchidism. The weakened abdominal wall is deeply furrowed, defecation and coughing are hampered, and death from pulmonary complications often results in early infancy.

Congenital Defects of Cranial Muscles

Congenital ptosis due to weakness of the levator palpebrae may occur as an isolated anomaly and without involvement of other muscles supplied by the oculomotor nerve. In some cases muscular dystrophy or myasthenia gravis has developed in later life, and a primary myopathy affecting the levator muscle has seemed a more likely explanation than a lesion involving the third cranial nerve of its nucleus. In the rare "jaw-winking phenomenon" of Marcus Gunn, the ptosed eyelid is elevated when the mouth is opened or the jaw moved from side to side.

Congenital facial diplegia, or Möbius' syndrome, is characterized by bilateral weakness of the facial muscles and of the external rectus muscles of the eyes. It may occur alone or be associated with congenital malformations of the extremities. The condition is recognized soon after birth and has been explained by either a primary hypoplasia of cranial nerve nuclei or a primary deficiency of the muscles derived from the first two branchial arches. A dysgenesis of both neural and muscle tissue may occur concomitantly in some cases.

Congenital Clubfoot (Talipes)

The abnormal posture of the foot and ankle in this relatively common deformity is usually plantar flexion (talipes equinus) and less frequently dorsiflexion (talipes calcaneus), inversion and adduction (talipes varus), or eversion and abduction (talipes valgus). Two-thirds of the children are males, and in a small percentage the condition is familial. The anterior tibial and peroneal muscles are atrophic and may be replaced by adipose tissue. The mechanism of the muscular atrophy and antenatal contracture is not definitely determined, but occasionally the amyoplasia is secondary to a developmental defect of the anterior horn cells of the spinal cord or peripheral nerves.

Arthrogryposis Multiplex

Arthrogryposis multiplex congenita, also known as amyoplasia congenita or myodystrophia fetalis deformans, is characterized by deformity and rigidity of the extremities, the infant having the appearance of a wooden doll (Fig. 77). The limbs are fixed in almost any position, but most often the arms are rotated inward and extended at the elbows, with forearms pronated and hands flexed. Usually the lower extremities are flexed at the hips and externally rotated, the knees are either partly flexed or extended, and the feet are in equinovarus. The smallness of the limbs is contrasted with the unusually large and fusiform joints. The muscles are weak and hypotonic and the tendon reflexes are absent. The skin and subcutaneous tissues are thickened, wrin-

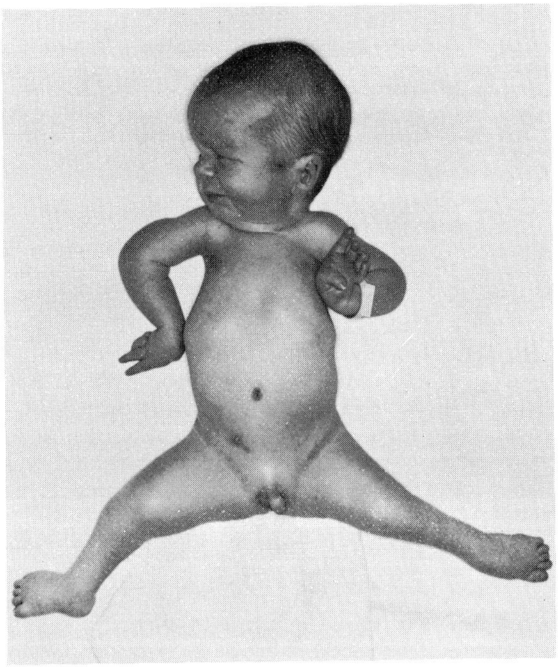

Fig. 77. Arthrogryposis multiplex congenita of the neuropathic type in an infant with unusual fixed postures.

kled, and flabby. Other congenital abnormalities are sometimes associated.

Fixation of joints is the most distinctive and constant clinical feature of the syndrome, but the underlying pathology is varied and may involve the spinal cord, muscles, or joints. When the disorder is associated with congenital muscular dystrophy, a characteristic posture of flexion at the hips and knees and adduction of the legs has been observed. When contractures are due to a primary defect in the anterior horn cells of the spinal cord or nerve roots, an attitude of extension and abduction of the legs is more frequent. Orthopedic treatment may effect some improvement in posture, but little or no change in muscle power is to be expected.

Congenital Muscular Hypertrophy

This may result from varied causes. In the syndrome described by DeLange, there is generalized, symmetric muscular hypertrophy, hypertonia, and an increase in muscle power. The head is small or deformed and the neck is usually retracted. Infants affected are mentally deficient and survive for only a few months. A congenital lesion of the brain consisting of polygyria, microgyria, and multiple cystic cavities has been described in some cases. In the Debré-Semelaigne syndrome there is an associated thyroid deficiency (cretinism). In a third variety of congenital muscular hypertrophy there are macroglossia and cardiomegaly in addition to the hypertrophied skeletal musculature.

Some infants with omphaloceles may have an associated muscular hypertrophy as well as macroglossia and hypoglycemia (Beckwith's syndrome).

Muscular Dystrophies

Progressive muscular dystrophy is a primary degenerative disease of skeletal muscles of unknown causation, characterized by muscular weakness and wasting. The great majority of cases of muscular dystrophy can be classified into three major groups, which are clinically and genetically distinct. These are the pseudohypertrophic, facioscapulohumeral, and limb-girdle types. A number of less common types may be distinguished on clinical criteria.

The pseudohypertrophic dystrophy of Duchenne is a rapidly progressive myopathy which usually begins in early childhood, has a strong familial incidence, and occurs predominantly in males (Fig. 78). It is transmitted as a sex-linked recessive character. The commonest presenting symptoms are an abnormal gait, slowness and clumsiness in walking and running, and a tendency to fall frequently. Sitting, standing, and walking are delayed, and often there is difficulty in climbing stairs. Muscular weakness always begins in the muscles of the pelvic girdle and is responsible for the waddling gait. The method of rising from the floor by "climbing up the legs" (Gower's sign), although not a pathognomonic sign, is characteristic and results from weakness of the lumbar muscles and glutei (Fig. 79). The foot assumes a talipes equinovarus position, and the patient tends to walk on his toes, owing to weakness of the anterior tibial and peroneal muscles. Muscles of the shoulder girdle become involved after three to five years. The deep tendon reflexes usually are depressed or absent but, rarely, are hyperactive in the early stages of the disease. Positive Babinski signs and other evidence of an associated upper motor neuron lesion have been reported rarely. Pseudohypertrophy affects the calf muscles in 80 percent of cases, is uncommon in the hamstrings and glutei, and involves the deltoid and triceps rarely. Contracture and wasting of the muscles lead to atrophy and deformity of the skeleton, and obesity is a common complication of the resultant immobility. A moderate degree of mental retardation is not unusual. The essentially progressive nature of the disease is evident in the rarity of survival beyond the age of 20 years.

The Becker variant of pseudohypertrophic muscular dystrophy begins at a later age and has a slower rate of progression. Survival into late adult life is not uncommon with this form of muscular dystrophy.

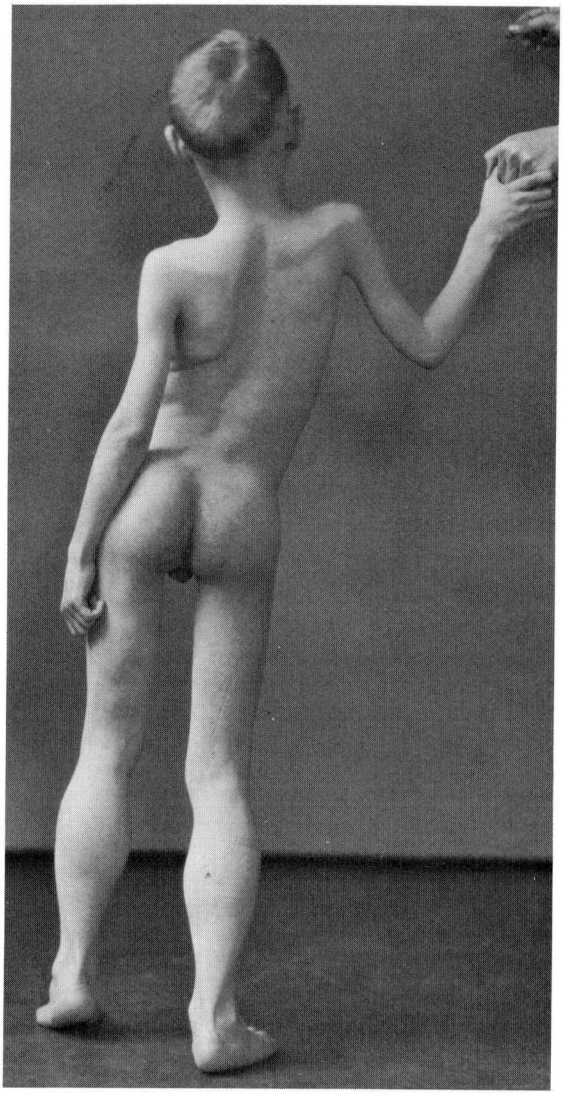

Fig. 78. Progressive muscular dystrophy: Duchenne type. A boy aged 10 years with weakness and atrophy of the proximal musculature, pseudohypertrophy of the calves and buttocks, scoliosis, lordosis of the lumbar spine, and a tendency to walk on the toes. (Courtesy of the Mayo Clinic, Rochester, Minnesota.)

The facioscapulohumeral dystrophy of Landouzy and Dejerine is a slowly progressive myopathy which begins at any age from early childhood until adult life, is sometimes familial, and affects both male and female with equal frequency. It is usually transmitted by an autosomal dominant, rarely by an autosomal recessive gene. Inability to close the eyes completely may be noted from early childhood, and pouting of the lips and immobility of facial expression characterize the myopathic facies. The first symptoms usually include drooping of the shoulders with difficulty in raising the arms above the head and generally occur between 6 and 20 years of age. The deep ten-

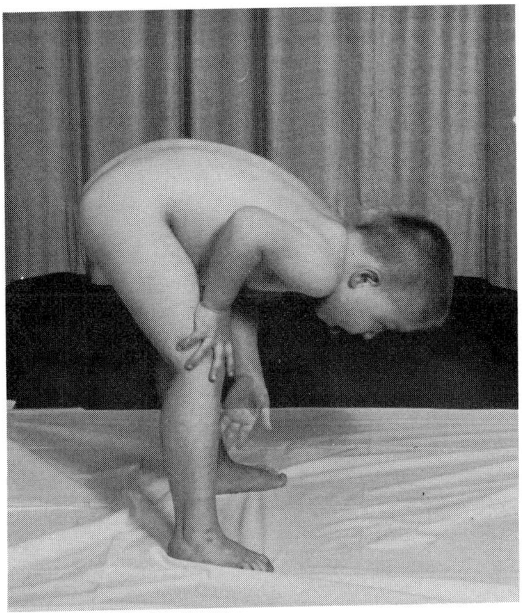

Fig. 79. Gower's sign in a boy with Duchenne pseudohypertrophic muscular dystrophy. The necessity to "climb up the legs" when rising from the floor.

don reflexes are depressed or absent in affected muscles. Weakness of the lower limbs is often delayed for 20 to 30 years, and pseudohypertrophy of muscles is uncommon. The disease may become arrested for prolonged periods, and most patients survive and remain active to a normal age. Contractures and skeletal deformities develop less frequently and constitute a less prominent clinical feature than in the Duchenne form of dystrophy.

Limb-girdle muscular dystrophy commences late in the first or in the second or third decade. It progresses more slowly than the Duchenne type but more rapidly than the facioscapulohumeral type of dystrophy. It is usually transmitted as an autosomal recessive, but occasionally by a dominant gene. Those cases which begin with muscular weakness in the shoulder girdle are classified traditionally as juvenile scapulohumeral muscular dystrophy of Erb. Those in which the pelvic girlde and thigh muscles are first affected are examples of the atrophic pelvifemoral dystrophy of Leyden and Möbius. The course of the disease, though relatively slow, nevertheless leads to severe disablement and death before the normal age. Pseudohypertrophy is rare, but prominence of the deltoid and gluteal musculature commonly occurs as a compensatory physiologic hypertrophy in the early stages of the disease.

Other less common forms of muscular dystrophy include Gower's type, in which the distal rather than the proximal limb muscles are affected first, and dystrophic ophthalmoplegia, which is very slowly progressive and is limited to the levators of the eyelids and the external ocular muscles. In the ophthalmoplegic type, ptosis of the eyelids, the first symptom, presents at any age from infancy to adult life and is associated later with weakness of lateral and vertical movements of the eyes. A history of similar symptoms in the family is obtained in half the cases.

In about 10 percent of patients with progressive muscular dystrophy the electrocardiogram shows nonspecific abnormalities. Cardiomegaly is not uncommon, and cardiac failure due to dystrophic disease of heart muscle is sometimes the cause of sudden death.

Determination of certain serum enzymes may be a useful diagnostic aid. Elevated enzyme levels are observed only during the period when muscles are actively undergoing change. Late in the disease, these enzyme levels are often normal.

A marked increase of creatine kinase activity in the serum has been reported in patients with the Duchenne type of muscular dystrophy and in their female relatives (heterozygotes), and lesser degrees of abnormal activity occur in patients with other types of dystrophy. Also, elevations of glutamic oxalacetic transaminase and aldolase are observed. Reduction in the transformation of creatine to creatinine, the most constant biochemical abnormality, reflects only a decrease in total effective muscle mass and is not pathognomonic of dystrophy. Administration of vitamin E is followed by reduction in creatinuria but does not result in objective improvement of muscle function.

In treatment, physical rehabilitation may help to maintain residual function. Frequent but not violent activity is advisable, and all limb joints should be moved regularly both actively and passively through a full range to prevent contractures. Confinement to bed must be avoided. When possible, school attendance or occupation with tasks and hobbies should be encouraged. A cheerful and optimistic attitude of physician and parent is important in the psychologic management.

The Myotonias

Congenital Myotonia

Congenital myotonia (Thomsen's disease) is an anomaly of muscular contraction manifested by muscular spasms or cramps and hypertrophy. It presents during infancy, early childhood, or adolescence and is inherited as a Mendelian dominant or occasionally as a recessive factor. Muscular contraction is strong, but relaxation is delayed and normal motor function is impeded. The infant may be slow to stand and walk. The disease may affect most of the skeletal muscles but seldom involves the muscles of respiration or swallowing. Muscular hypertrophy, especially prominent in the lower limbs, may also affect the upper limbs and face. The child may have a Herculean appearance. Percussion of the surface of the muscle results in a sustained contraction and localized dimpling. Muscles of the thenar eminence, forearm, and tongue are especially susceptible. Tendon reflexes are normal or slightly exaggerated. On shaking hands the patient's grip is relaxed slowly and awkwardly in a manner pathognomic of myotonia; after tight closure the eyes are opened slowly. With repetition of muscular effort movement becomes more rapid, and relaxation following contraction is more prompt.

Symptoms of myotonia are relieved by quinine, calcium, and procaine amide; they are exacerbated by cold.

Dystrophia Myotonica

Dystrophia myotonica, or myotonic dystrophy, is a steadily progressive, familial disease in which a myopathy is complicated by myotonia. Cataracts, baldness, and testicular atrophy are frequently associated defects, and mental retardation is not uncommon. The disease is usually transmitted as a mendelian dominant character, and the phenomenon of anticipation is observed; the children are affected at an earlier age than the parent and are more likely to exhibit the fully developed syndrome.

Muscular weakness and wasting may begin at any age. The symptomatic infant has difficulty in sucking owing to bilateral facial weakness. Muscle weakness, hypotonia, and delay in attaining motor milestones are other manifestations during infancy. Rarely, pure myotonia may be the only feature of this disorder in early childhood. In contrast to most myopathies, the distal rather than proximal muscles of the limbs are affected primarily. The tendon reflexes are often depressed or lost. Ptosis of the eyelids and weakness and atrophy of the facial muscles may be early manifestations; in the older child, wasting of the sternomastoids and the development of a swan-neck posture occur later. Weakness of laryngeal and pharyngeal muscles is apparent later in the monotonous and nasal character of the voice and the dysphagia. Myotonia, the most striking characteristic feature, does not involve all skeletal muscles but is particularly evident in the hands, face, and tongue. Electrocardiographic abnormalities point to involvement of the heart, and acrocyanosis is indicative of changes in peripheral blood vessels.

Electromyography is useful in confirming the diagnosis.

Quinine and procaine amide control the myotonia to some extent, but otherwise treatment is of no avail.

Paramyotonia

This term is used to describe a syndrome of myotonia which usually is restricted to the tongue and which spreads to involve the muscles of the face and extremities only on exposure to cold. Unlike dystrophia myotonica, paramyotonia is nonprogressive and not complicated by muscular wasting; it differs from myotonia congenita in the lack of hypertrophy and the restricted involvement of muscles. The disorder is inherited by a single autosomal dominant gene and is not transmitted by unaffected members of the family. Originally described by Eulenberg, paramyotonia has been reviewed more recently by Drager and co-workers, who reported a family with 30 members affected. These patients complained of cramping of the muscles of the face in cold weather and slurred speech asociated with stiffness of the tongue after drinking cold liquids. Weakness of the extremities may occur in some attacks and may be associated with elevation of the serum potassium. The relation of paramyotonia to familial hyperkalemic paralysis is discussed elsewhere (p. 186).

Myositis

Infectious Mysositis

Acute suppurative myositis may occur with bloodstream infection or in association with infectious arthritis. Staphylococci and streptococci are the most common causative organisms. Gas gangrene due to *Clostridium perfringens* develops only in traumatized or necrotic muscle. Tuberculous infection in striated muscle may be due to local extension from a neighboring joint or cold abscess or rarely may result from hematogenous dissemination.

Trichinosis is the most frequent parasitic infection of muscle in the Western Hemisphere; cysticerosis commonly involves muscle in infected patients in India and other Asiatic countries. Toxoplasma may invade muscle but causes no specific symptoms; the demonstration of the protozoan parasite in a biopsy of muscle is sometimes of value in the diagnosis of acquired toxoplasmosis.

Polymyositis

Polymyositis is an acute, subacute, or chronic disorder of muscle characterized by symmetric weakness predominant in the shoulder and pelvic girdles. Polymyositis is associated with cutaneous lesions in dermatomyositis and may also occur as a feature of scleroderma or rheumatoid arthritis.

Muscular pain, tenderness, atrophy, and depression of deep tendon reflexes are inconstant and appear late in the course of the disease. Dysphagia occurs in more than half the patients. The electromyographic and histologic abnormalities are characteristic but not pathognomonic of the disease. Nonspecific clinical features include fever, arthralgia, loss of weight, Raynaud's phenomenon, edema, and heliotrope erythema of the eyelids and face. The sedimentation and basal metabolic rates are frequently elevated, and examination of the blood may reveal

TABLE 28. *The Clinical Differential Diagnosis of Polymyositis and Duchenne Muscular Dystrophy**

Clinical Features	Polymyositis	Duchenne Muscular Dystrophy
Sex incidence	females > males	males only
Rate of progress	rapid	slow
Muscular weakness	symmetric and proximal	proximal
Dysphagia	common	unknown
Muscular atrophy	mild	marked
Pseudohypertrophy	rare	common
Muscle pain and tenderness	common	uncommon or rare
Deep tendon reflexes	absent, normal, or brisk	depressed or absent
Muscle biopsy	inflammatory cell infiltration	no inflammatory cells
Dermatomyositis, scleroderma, or rheumatoid arthritis	sometimes associated	not associated
Spontaneous remission	occasional	never
Response to cortisone	remission	none

*Modified from Walton and Adams. *Polymyositis*, London, E. & S. Livingstone, Ltd., 1958.

leucocytosis and eosinophilia. High levels of creatine phosphokinase and aldolase in the serum are indicative of persistent activity of the disease.

Most cases appear to be related etiologically to the collagen group of diseases, but some may result from unknown toxic and metabolic factors. In the absence of skin and joint involvement, the acute forms of the disease may bear a close clinical resemblance to idiopathic myoglobinuria while chronic forms may resemble progressive muscular dystrophy. The differentiation from muscular dystrophy (Table 28) is often difficult but is important in prognosis and therapy.

Some patients with polymyositis improve or recover spontaneously, but treatment with corticosteroids is advisable in those with evidence of progressive weakness.

Myositis Fibrosa

Generalized myositis fibrosa is a slowly progressive disease which begins in early life and is characterized by replacement of muscle with fibrous connective tissue. The muscles are firm and woody to palpation, their elasticity is lost, and in the final stages of the disease movement becomes impossible. The sternomastoids and muscles of the legs, neck, chest, and back are among those first affected. With the development of muscular contractures the joints become fixed in abnormal postures. Myositis fibrosa is sometimes classed as a chronic progressive form of dermatomyositis, since the histologic changes in the muscle may be similar to those of polymyositis. A therapeutic trial of corticosteroids may be considered.

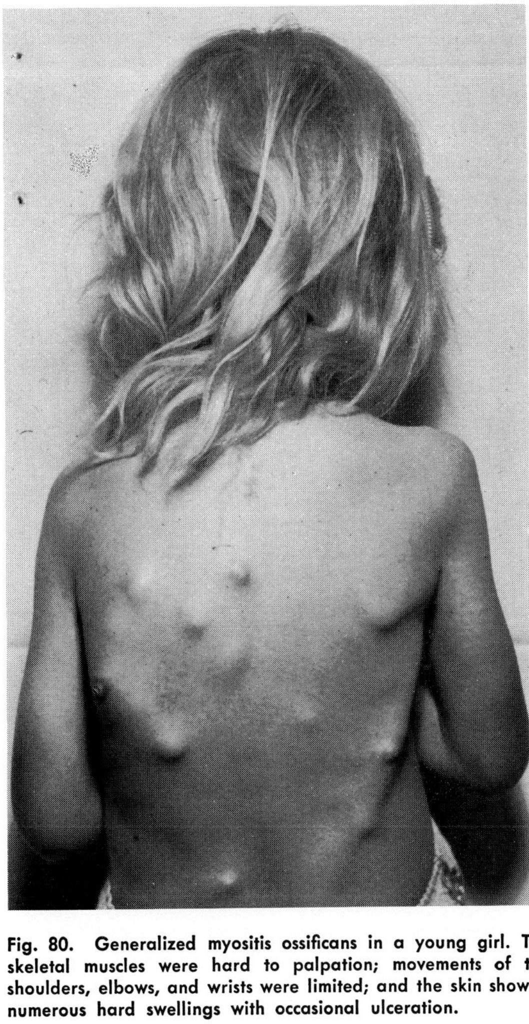

Fig. 80. Generalized myositis ossificans in a young girl. The skeletal muscles were hard to palpation; movements of the shoulders, elbows, and wrists were limited; and the skin showed numerous hard swellings with occasional ulceration.

Myositis Ossificans

Generalized progressive myositis ossificans is an uncommon disease of unknown cause which is characterized by the formation of soft, fluctuant, or hard swellings in the interstitial tissue of the muscle and related structures. The masses are of variable size and shape and consist at first of fibrous tissue, often with subsequent formation of bone; they sometimes shrink before ossification occurs. Usually they are painless, but the overlying skin is often reddened and occasionally ulcerated. The disease generally gegins before 10 years of age, and the muscles of the neck and back are affected first (Fig. 80). The swellings develop spontaneously or follow minimal trauma; they appear in succession over a period of months or years. The muscle fibers are not involved primarily but undergo atrophy and destruction secondary to pressure and inactivity as the result of disease in the interstitial tissue. Congenital anomalies, the most frequent of which is underdevelopment of the great toes or thumbs, are associated in about three-fourths of the cases.

The prognosis is grave, and survival beyond puberty is rare. Treatment is usually ineffectual, although it is claimed that remissions have been induced by corticosteroids.

Generalized myositis ossificans must be differentiated from a localized traumatic form and from calcinosis universalis, in which calcium is deposited in the subcutaneous tissues.

Metabolic Myopathies

Familial Periodic Paralysis

This hereditary and familial disease is characterized by intermittent attacks of flaccid paralysis with complete absence of deep tendon reflexes and electrical inexcitability of the muscles. The onset is usually before puberty, and attacks may recur for many years. The sexes are affected equally.

An attack generally begins with weakness in the muscles of the back and pelvic girdle, and flaccidity gradually spreads to involve the lower limbs, shoulder girdle, upper limbs, and neck. The respiratory muscles and muscles innervated by the cranial nerves are usually spared. Dysphagia may occur in severe attacks, and death, though rare, has been reported. Smooth muscle is not affected, but cardiac enlargement and a slow and irregular pulse are present in some cases. Attacks occur at any time but most commonly during sleep or inactivity. They may be preceded and accompanied by excessive perspiration and thirst and are precipitated by the ingestion of excess carbohydrate, exposure to cold, muscular exertion followed by inactivity, or the injection of insulin or epinephrine. Attacks are usually of two to three hours' duration but may last as long as seven days. Recovery is gradual and usually complete, though slight weakness may persist in some cases. The presence of vacuoles in muscle is characteristic.

The paralysis is associated with hypokalemia but is not related to the absolute concentration of serum potassium. The fall in the level of serum potassium is not reflected in an increased urinary excretion but may be related to a shift of potassium from the blood to the cells of the muscles and liver. An abnormal degree of binding of potassium by large protein molecules may occur.

In some cases, attacks have been preceded by an increase in the urinary excretion of aldosterone and retention of sodium. An abrupt fall in the level of potassium is serum and urine has been observed. As the attack subsides, there are diuresis of sodium, an increase in the urinary excretion of potassium, and a return to normal of the level of aldosterone in the urine. Attacks appear to be precipitated by retention of sodium; they may be prevented by restriction of dietary sodium. Potassium chloride is given for the treatment of acute attacks.

The prognosis is excellent, and the episodes become less frequent and less severe in adult life.

Hypokalemic Paralysis

The association of a low concentration of serum potassium and weakness or paralysis of skeletal muscles may occur in diabetic acidosis, in Addison's disease following the administration of excess desoxycorticosterone (DOCA), and in some cases of renal insufficiency. Complete paralysis as observed in familial periodic paralysis is rare. The more usual findings are diffuse muscular weakness and apathy, with delirium, coarse muscular twitching, and tetany. The electrocardiogram is of value in the differentiation of hypokalemic and hyperkalemic states.

Hyperkalemic Paralysis

Muscular weakness and elevated levels of serum potassium may be associated in patients with renal insufficiency, especially after the administration of potassium, in untreated Addison's disease, and in crush syndrome and hemolytic reactions. The onset and evolution of paresis are rapid, and the distribution resembles that of familial periodic paralysis. The legs, trunk, and arms are affected in an ascending sequence. The administration of 5 to 15 g of potassium by mouth to healthy individuals will often produce paresthesia, but muscular weakness is exceptional.

Hereditary Episodic Adynamia

As described by Gamstorp, this condition is characterized by attacks of spontaneously abating paralysis, affecting particularly the muscles of the extremities and the trunk and generally accompanied by an elevation of the serum potassium. The disease is inherited as a single, autosomal, dominant gene with complete or almost complete penetrance. The incidence is the same in both sexes.

The onset of episodic symptoms is usually before the age of 10 years. Attacks invariably occur during rest which follows exertion, and at least once a week; they last at most one hour. The extent and severity of the paresis vary from slight weakness of a single extremity to severe states in which the patient is unable to turn over or sit up. Respiration is seldom involved, and the muscles innervated by cranial nerves are affected only mildly. Deep tendon reflexes may be weak or absent, and Chvostek's sign is sometimes positive during attacks. Percussion myotonia may be elicited, and the disease is more troublesome in cold, damp weather. The clinical manifestations of adynamia episodica resemble those of paramyotonia. Nevertheless, Gamstorp maintains that the term adynamia episodica hereditaria should be retained for those patients who, in response to a small dose of potassium, have elevated serum levels and react with muscular weakness, regardless of the presence of myotonia.

As a general rule, paresis is accompanied by an increase in the level of serum potassium without change in the urinary excretion of potassium. Electrocardiographic changes are consistent with hyperkalemia. Attacks may be precipitated by oral administration of potassium in doses insufficient to produce symptoms in normal persons. Symptoms are prevented by glucose with or without insulin administered before, or simultaneously with, a provocative dose of potassium. Acetazolamide orally, calcium administered intravenously, the intake of food, especially bread, or gentle exercise may shorten the duration of attacks; but sooner or later the symptoms abate spontaneously. Improvement occurs, and attacks are less frequent after 30 years of age.

Other descriptions of a form of periodic familial paralysis resistant to or exacerbated by the administration of potassium have been given by Wyllie and Watkins.

Myohemoglobinuria

Myohemoglobin may appear in the urine spontaneously and without known cause or following crush injuries, extreme muscular activity, or the ingestion of eels or fish poisoned by resinous waste products of factories (Haff disease). In the cryptogenic cases (Meyer-Betz), paroxysmal attacks of myohemoglobinuria are associated with weakness or paralysis of skeletal muscles. The onset of illness is usually sudden and sometimes accompanied by nausea, fever, and vomiting. The affected muscles are swollen and painful. The disease may be familial, occur at any age, and vary greatly in severity. The patient may die from uremia or respiratory paralysis in the first attack or may recover and suffer repeated episodes of muscle weakness. Cardiac and smooth muscles are unaffected. The diagnosis of myohemoglobinuria is established by electrophoresis or spectroscopic examination; it may be suspected in a patient who shows no evidence of hemolytic anemia when the urine is dark and gives a positive reaction for occult blood in the absence of red blood cells. Serum enzymes are markedly elevated.

Glycogen Myopathies

Of five different types of glycogen storage disease described, two (Types II and V) have significantly increased amounts of glycogen in the skeletal muscle associated with weakness.

TYPE II: CARDIOMUSCULAR GLYCOGEN DISEASE (POMPE). This is the commonest variety of glycogen storage disease with generalized muscular weakness and hypotonia. Inherited as an autosomal recessive trait, it is associated with an absence of the enzyme α-1-4 glucosidase (acid maltase). Clinically it closely resembles Werdnig-Hoffmann disease in that the child often is asymptomatic at birth and manifests progressive hypotonia, areflexia, and muscle weakness at a few months of disease. Macroglossia and cardiomegaly are additional features. Diagnosis is based on the characteristic clinical findings, the presence of glycogen vacuoles in the muscle biopsy, and the absence of acid maltase activity upon enzymatic assay. The infant usually dies at 1 year of age from cardiac or respiratory failure. A late infantile variety, also associated with acid maltase deficiency, closely resembles Duchenne's pseudohypertrophic muscular dystrophy. It is manifested by either a delay in acquisition of motor milestones or by regression of previously acquired motor skills. Differentiation from Duchenne's muscular dystrophy may only be possible by electromyography, muscle biopsy, and appropriate biochemical studies.

TYPE V: McARDLE'S DISEASE. In this variety of glycogen myopathy, excessive amounts of muscle glycogen are associated with a total absence of muscle phosphorylase. The synthesis of glycogen is normal, but the degradation of glycogen to glucose-1-phosphate is deficient. The accumulation of pyruvic and lactic acids expected in the venous blood after exercise of ischemic muscle is lacking. The disease is familial and is transmitted by a recessive, rare, autosomal gene. Symptoms begin in childhood and occur only after moderately severe exercise. Muscular weakness, stiffness, and painful cramps develop with effort and disappear rapidly with rest. Between attacks, the physical examination, including deep tendon reflexes, is normal. The diagnosis is confirmed by the failure of venous lactate to rise after ischemic work and lack of phosphorylase activity in muscle. Symptoms may be prevented by limiting exercise.

TYPES I, III, AND IV. In Type I (Von Gierke's disease) skeletal muscle is not involved. Types III and IV, rare varieties, involve the liver mainly, and the myocardium and skeletal muscles to a lesser extent.

Endocrine Myopathies

Disorders of muscles may occur with a wide variety of diseases of the endocrine glands. In the majority of these myopathies, morphologic changes have been slight or absent, and a derangement of some enzyme system necessary for contraction of muscle has been invoked as a possible explanation for the muscle weakness.

Hyperthyroidism in association with a chronic form of myopathy has occasionally been reported, and an acute thyrotoxic myopathy which sometimes progresses to a form of bulbar paralysis may also occur. Treatment of the hyperthyroidism alleviates the muscle weakness. Thyrotoxicosis and myasthenia gravis may occur concomitantly, but the association of the two diseases is unexplained. About 5 percent of all patients with myasthenia gravis develop thyrotoxicosis at some time during their illness, and an inverse relation between the two diseases is occasionally observed. Symptoms of myasthenia may be aggravated by administration of antithyroid drugs and alleviated on their withdrawal. The frequency of abnormalities of the thymus gland and the occurrence of focal collections of small lymphocytes, or "lymphorrhages," in striated muscles in both myasthenia gravis and thyrotoxicosis point to some common factor of posisble significance in etiology.

Hypothyroidism may be complicated by true generalized hypertrophy of muscles. The Debré-Semelaigne syndrome, characterized by enlarged muscles, weakness, early fatigue, and slowness of movements, is one of the clinical manifestations of cretinism. The symptoms are relieved by thyroid medication.

In hyperparathyroidism, symmetric weakness, fatigability, and atrophy of limb muscles, with discomfort on muscular effort, are prominent symptoms which may be related to the disorder of calcium metabolism. Hypopituitarism is associated with muscle weakness and atrophy. Flexion contractures of the limbs observed in Addison's disease may be related to an excessive accumulation of sodium in the tendons and their consequent shortening. The deformities have been relieved following treatment with ACTH.

Myasthenia Gravis

Myasthenia gravis is characterized by undue weakness and fatigue following maintained contraction of voluntary muscles and a tendency to recovery with rest. Ocular movements, facial expression, mastication, deglutition, and speech are affected primarily. Muscles of the neck, trunk, and limbs may be involved, and respiratory embarrassment occurs in severe cases. Cardiac and smooth muscles are spared. The disease may develop at any age, but in children the first symptoms occur most commonly at or soon after birth or in relation to puberty. Three forms of myasthenia gravis of infancy and childhood are distinguished: (1) neonatal transient form; (2) neonatal persistent (or congenital) form; and (3) juvenile myasthenia gravis.

Myasthenic symptoms may occur with diseases other than myasthenia gravis, and a myasthenic syndrome has been described in association with muscular dystrophy, polymyositis, ocular myopathy, and thyrotoxicosis.

Neonatal transient myasthenia occurs in infants born to mothers with the disease. The majority of infants of myasthenic mothers are unaffected, symptoms developing in only 10 to 20 percent. There is no correlation between the severity of the infant's symptoms and the duration or severity of the mother's illness and her treatment during pregnancy.

At birth, or within a few hours thereafter, the infant becomes limp, his cry and movements are feeble, he is unable to suck, and swallowing and breathing are impaired. Muscular weakness and hypotonia are generalized and symmetric, and the Moro and deep tendon reflexes are absent or depressed. External ophthalmoplegia and ptosis occur relatively infrequently.

A newborn infant of a myasthenic mother whose previous pregnancy resulted in a neonatal death of undetermined cause should be carefully observed for signs of myasthenia. The diagnosis is established by the intramuscular or intravenous injection of edrophonium chloride (Tensilon) in a dose of 1 mg or neostigmine methylsulfate 0.1 to 0.2 mg. Symptoms should be relieved almost immediately (Fig. 81A and B). In moderate and severe cases and especially those with bulbar symptoms, a positive Tensilon test should be followed by continuous therapy with anticholinesterase drugs. In the milder forms of the disorder the infant may recover completely without specific therapy, but treatment must be instituted immediately should respiratory difficulty, choking, dysphagia, or inability to suck supervene.

Pyridostigmine bromide (Mestinon) and neostigmine bromide (Prostigmine) have a less rapid but more prolonged effect than Tensilon and may be effectively used in treatment. Mestinon is preferred because it is less toxic, having fewer muscarinic side effects. The required dosage differs in each patient and must be adjusted according to the individual response. The following have been found satisfactory as initial doses, to be given every four hours at the time of each feeding: oral doses, Mestinon bromide, 5 mg (5 drops of syrup of Mestinon, containing 60 mg per 4 ml); Prostigmine bromide, 1 mg. Parenteral preparations are approximately 30 times as potent as the oral: intramuscular doses, Prostigmine methylsulfate, 0.05 to 0.1 mg. When a dose level sufficient to relieve bulbar symptoms has been determined, further increments in dosage are unnecessary and may be hazardous.

Overdosage with anticholinesterase medication

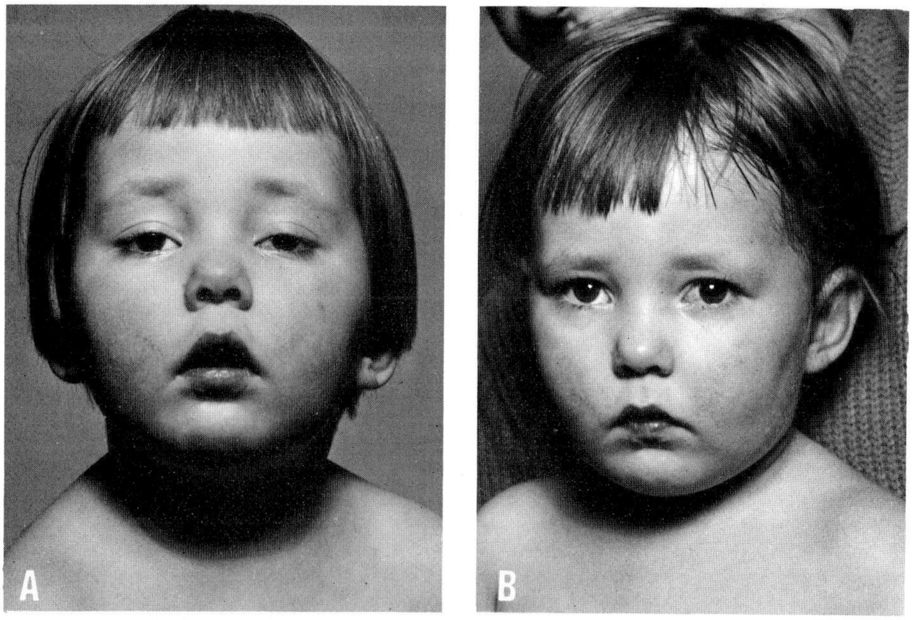

Fig. 81. *A.* A 3-year-old girl with myasthenia gravis. Ptosis, bilateral and asymmetric, was most marked at the end of the day and not apparent on waking. A right-sided exophoria was variable in degree. *B.* After Tensilon, 5 mg intravenously, the ptosis cleared within 30 seconds and the beneficial response lasted about 10 minutes. The patient was treated with regular doses of Mestinon, 7.5 mg three times a day.

(cholinergic crisis) is manifested by the following signs: increase in muscle weakness and worsening of respiratory difficulty and dysphagia after each dose of drug, muscular fasciculations, and prominent muscarinic side effects, which include excessive salivation, vomiting, diarrhea, pallor, sweating, and bradycardia. Tensilon, 0.05 ml (0.5 mg) given intravenously, will cause a mild and transient exacerbation of cholinergic weakness and may be used to differentiate the crisis due to excessive medication and that associated with a worsening of myasthenia. Atropine may be administered for anticholinesterase overdosage. The oronasopharyngeal secretions should be suctioned repeatedly and oxygen administered when indicated.

After the first week of treatment the gradual withdrawal of medication may be attempted. If symptoms increase, the original dosage is reinstituted, and the effects of withdrawal are observed again after two or three days. The duration of the illness is short, and the natural course is from a few hours to seven weeks. With efficient therapy recovery is complete.

Congenital myasthenia gravis occurs in infants born to mothers who are unaffected by the disease. In contrast to the transient neonatal type, involvement of bulbar musculature is unusual, and generalized muscle weakness is not severe. Ptosis relieved by sleep is the commonest presenting sign, and external ophthalmoplegia and diplopia occur frequently during childhood and later life. Other less common symptoms include weakness of the facial muscles and limbs, a weak and nasal voice, and some difficulty in chewing and swallowing. A family history of myasthenia in brothers, sisters, and cousins is obtained occasionally.

In contrast to the late form, congenital myasthenia affects both sexes equally, is rarely complicated by acute myasthenic crises, and symptoms are only moderately severe but persistent. Ophthalmoplegia is largely resistant to anticholinesterase medication, and complete remission of the disease is rare.

In juvenile myasthenia gravis the onset may be in early childhood, but in the majority of cases symptoms begin after 10 years of age. The disease is occasionally familial; before puberty females are affected six times more frequently than males. The most common first symptom is intermittent and asymmetric ptosis which later becomes bilateral. Weakness of the legs which follows exertion as in swimming, generalized muscle weakness, and nasal voice also occur as frequent initial symptoms. Facial weakness, difficulty in chewing and swallowing, ophthalmoplegia, and diplopia are less common at the onset but frequently develop later. In young children, walking may be delayed, and the gait is awkward and interrupted by frequent stumbling. Older children are incapable of sustained activity, they tire easily, and their shoulders droop. As the disease progresses, muscles weakened by use take longer to recover, and some additional exertion or intercurrent infection may precipitate a paralytic failure of the respiratory musculature.

The primary lesion in myasthenia gravis is believed to involve defective transmission of impulses at the neuromuscular synapse, the exact nature of which is unknown. The motor nerve fibers conduct normally, and the response of skeletal muscle to direct stimulation is normal. The neuromuscular block and the symptoms of myasthenia are similar to those of curare poisoning, and an abnormal metabolite with a curarelike action has been postulated as a possible factor in etiology. Other popular theories of the mechanism of the neuromuscular block include a deficient synthesis of acetylcholine due to overactivity of the enzyme cholinesterase or an abnormal structure of the synapse.

The general character of myasthenia gravis is suggestive of an endocrine or metabolic disorder. The onset is often in relation to puberty, and remission or relapse is frequently associated with menstruation, pregnancy, or changes of thyroid function. At autopsy the central and peripheral nervous systems show no gross or microscopic abnormalities; focal collections of small lymphocytes, or "lymphorrhages" present in affected skeletal muscles cannot be considered causative. That the thymus may play a significant role in the mechanism of myasthenia is suggested by the coincidence of thymic hyperplasia in 50 percent of cases and the apparent beneficial effect of thymectomy in some patients. It has been suggested that myasthenia is an autoimmune disease in which the thymus reacts against protein antigens in the motor end-plate. Thyoma has been found in almost one-third of the reported cases in adults but is rare in childhood.

The differential diagnoses include bulbar poliomyelitis, diphtheritic paralysis, polyneuritis, intracranial tumor, and hyperthyroidism. The initial illness is commonly misdiagnosed as hysteria or laziness. Diagnosis is confirmed by the intravenous injection of Tensilon (Figs. 81A and B), which relieves the presenting symptoms within a few minutes. In children weighing up to 34 kg, the dose is 0.2 ml (2 mg); in those over 34 kg, 0.5 ml (5 mg) may be given. If Prostigmine is employed, the intramuscular dose is 0.25 to 1.0 mg of Prostigmine methylsulfate, dependent upon the weight or surface area of the child; the patient is examined for signs of improvement at 5- or 10-minute intervals for a period of 45 minutes, and Atropine may be required for the relief of muscarinic side effects.

Treatment with anticholinesterase drugs is instituted and controlled as outlined for neonatal myasthenia. Mestinon is given orally in initial trial doses of 5 to 10 mg at intervals of two to four hours, or Prostigmine in doses of 1 to 5 mg orally. Mytelase (ambenonium chloride) is prescribed occasionally; it causes less bronchial secretion than do other anticholinesterase drugs, and its use may be indicated in patients with respiratory paralysis. Five milligrams of Mytelase chloride are equivalent to 15 mg of Prostigmine bromide or 60 mg of Mestinon bromide.

Thymectomy may be followed by improvement and sometimes by complete remission. It is considered of particular value in young female patients who have had the disease for less than five years, and is indicated especially in patients with generalized muscle weakness and bulbar symptoms resistant to therapy.

The prognosis in children is variable but relatively good compared with adults. The case fatality rate is approximately 5 percent. The course is generally prolonged, and complete remission following drug therapy or thymectomy may be expected in less than 25 percent of cases up to six years from the onset; complete remission after this time is rare. Ptosis and ocular palsies are often refractory to treatment, and relapse and failure of response to medication are frequently related to systemic or upper respiratory infection and to menstruation.

References

DISEASES OF THE MUSCLES

Adams, R. D., Denny-Brown, D., and Pearson, C. M. Diseases of Muscle. A Study in Pathology, 2nd ed. New York, Paul B. Hoeber, Inc., 1962.

Swaiman, K. F., and Wright, F. S., Neuromuscular Diseases of Infancy and Childhood. Springfield, Ill., Charles C Thomas, Publ., 1970.

Walton, J. N., ed. Disorders of Voluntary Muscle. Boston, Little, Brown and Co., 1964.

——— and Nattrass, F. J. On the classification, natural history and treatment of myopathies. Brain, 77:169, 1954.

LIMP INFANT SYNDROME

Banker, B. Q., Victor, M., and Adams, R. D. Arthrogryposis multiplex due to congenital muscular dystrophy. Brain, 80:319, 1957.

Batten, F. E. The myopathies or muscular dystrophies; critical review. Quart. J. Med., 3:313, 1910.

Bing, R. Ueber angeborene Muskeldefecte. Virchow Arch., 170:175, 1902.

Brandt, S. A case of arthrogryposis mulitplex congenita anatomically appearing as foetal spinal muscular atrophy. Acta Paediat. Scand., 34:365, 1947.

Debré, R., and Semelaigne, G. Syndrome of diffuse muscular hypertrophy in infants causing an athletic appearance. Its connection with congenital myxedema. Amer. J. Dis. Child., 50:1351, 1935.

DeLange, C. Congenital hypertrophy of the muscles, extrapyramidal motor disturbances and mental deficiency: A clinical entity. Amer. J. Dis. Child., 48: 243, 1934.

Dodge, P. R. Congenital neuromuscular disorders. Res. Publ. Ass. Res. Nerv. Ment. Dis., 38:479, 1959.

Dubowitz, V. The Floppy Infant. Clinics in Developmental Medicine No. 31. London, National Spastics Society, 1969.

Engel, W. K., Wanko, T., and Fenichel, G. M. Nemaline myopathy. Arch. Neurol., 11:22, 1964.

Greenfield, J. G., Cornman, T., and Shy, G. M. The prognostic value of the muscle biopsy in the "floppy infant." Brain, 81:461, 1958.

Schreier, K., and Huperz, R. Über die hypoplasia musculorum generalisata congenita. Ann. Paediat., 186: 241, 1956.

Shy, G. M., and Magee, K. R. A new congenital nonprogressive myopathy. Brain, 79:610, 1956.

Tizzard, J. P. M. Neuromuscular disorder of infancy. *In* Walton, J. N., ed., Disorders of Voluntary Muscle. Boston, Little, Brown and Co., 1964, pp. 369-388.

Turner, J. W. A. Relationship between amyotonia congenita and congenital myopathy. Brain, 63:163, 1940.

Walton, J. N. The limp child. J. Neurol. Neurosurg. Psychiat., 20:144, 1957.

MUSCULAR DYSTROPHIES

Jackson, C. E., and Carey, J. H. Progressive muscular dystrophy; autosomal recessive type. Pediatrics, 28:77, 1961.

Mabry, C. C., Roeckel, L. E., Munich, R. L., and Robertson, D. X-linked pseudohypertrophic muscular dystrophy with a late onset and slow progression. New Eng. J. Med., 273:1062, 1965.

Milhorat, A. T. The diagnosis of muscular dystrophy. Proc. 3rd Med. Conf. Muscular Dystrophy Ass. Amer., Inc. Amer. J. Phys. Med., 35:103, 1955.

Murphy, E. G., and Charniak, M. M. Glutamic oxalacetic transaminase activity in the serum in muscular dystrophy and other neuromuscular disorders in childhood. Pediatrics, 22:1110, 1958.

Pearce, J. M. S., Pennington, R. J., and Walton, J. N. Serum enzyme studies in muscle disease. Part II. Serum creatine kinase activity in muscular dystrophy and in other myopathic and neuropathic disorders. J. Neurol. Neurosurg. Psychiat., 27:96, 1964.

Walton, J. N. Muscular dystrophy and its relation to the other myopathies. Res. Publ. Ass. Res. Nerv. Ment. Dis., 38:378, 1959.

Zellweger, H., and Hansen, J. W. Slowly progressive X-linked recessive muscular dystrophy (type IIIB). Arch. Intern. Med. (Chicago), 120:525, 1967.

THE MYOTONIAS

Adams, R. D., Denny-Brown, D., and Pearson, C. M. Diseases of Muscle, A Study in Pathology, 2nd ed. New York, Paul B. Hoeber, Inc., 1962.

Bastron, J. A. Myotonia and other abnormalities of muscular contraction arising from disorders of the motor unit. Res. Publ. Ass. Res. Nerv. Ment. Dis., 38:534, 1959.

Dodge, P. R., Gamstorp, I., Byers, R. K., and Russell, P. Myotonic dystrophy in infancy and childhood. Pediatrics, 35:3, 1965.

Drager, G. A., Hammill, J. F., and Shy, G. M. Paramyotonia congenita. Arch. Neurol. Psychiat., 80:1, 1958.

Hirsch, D. R., Dancis, J., and Ward, R. S. Myotonia congenita. J. Pediat., 35:760, 1949.

MYOSITIS

Adams, R. D., Denny-Brown, D., and Pearson, C. M. Diseases of Muscle, A Study in Pathology, 2nd ed. New York, Paul B. Hoeber, Inc., 1962.

Barwick, D. D., and Walton, J. N. Polymyositis. Amer. J. Med., 35:646, 1963.

Blau, A. Primary generalized myositis fibrosa; report of 2 cases with histopathology. J. Mount Sinai Hosp. N.Y., 5:432, 1938.

Eaton, L. M. The perspective of neurology in regard to polymyositis, study of 41 cases. Neurology, 4:245, 1954.

Pearson, C. M., and Rose, A. S. Myositis: the inflammatory disorders of muscle. Res. Publ. Ass. Res. Nerv. Ment. Dis., 38:422, 1959.

Riley, H. D., Jr., and Christie, A. Myositis ossificans progressiva. Pediatrics, 8:753, 1951.

Rowland, L. R. Muscular dystrophies, polymyositis and other myopathies. J. Chron. Dis., 8:510, 1958.

Walton, J. N., and Adams, R. D. Polymyositis. Baltimore, Williams and Wilkins Co., 1958.

METABOLIC MYOPATHIES

Buchanan, D., and Steiner, P. E. Myoglobinuria with paralysis (Meyer-Betz disease). Arch. Neurol. Psychiat., 66:107, 1951.

Conn, J. W., Fajans, S. S., Louis, L. H., Streeten, D. H. P., and Johnson, R. D. Intermittent aldosteronism in periodic paralysis. Lancet, 1:802, 1957.

Danowski, T. S., and Tarail, R. Potassium metabolism and dysfunction of the nervous system associated with hyper- and hypokalemia. Res. Publ. Ass. Res. Nerv. Ment. Dis., 32:372, 1953.

Debré, R., and Semelaigne, G. Syndrome of diffuse muscular hypertrophy in infants causing athletic appearance; its connection with congenital myxedema. Amer. J. Dis. Child., 50:1351, 1935.

Engel, W. K. Muscle biopsies in neuromuscular diseases. Pediat. Clin. N. Amer., Vol. 14, Nov. 1967.

Gamstorp, I. Adynamia episodica hereditaria. Acta Paediat. Scand., 45(Suppl.):108, 1956.

Gass, H., Cherkasky, M., and Savitsky, N. Potassium and periodic paralysis. Medicine, 27:105, 1948.

Hers, H. G. α-Glucosidae deficiency in generalized glycogen storage disease (Pompe's disease). Biochem. J., 86:11, 1963.

McArdle, B. Myopathy due to a defect in muscle glycogen breakdown. Clin. Sci., 10:13, 1951.

——— Metabolic myopathies. Amer. J. Med., 35:661, 1963.

Rowland, L. P., Fahn, S., Hirschberg, E., and Harter, D. H. Myoglobinuria. Arch. Neurol., 10:537, 1964.

Schmid, R., and Mahler, R. Chronic progressive myopathy with myoglobinuria. Demonstration of a glycogenolytic defect in muscle. J. Clin. Invest., 38:2044, 1959.

Shy, G. M. Some metabolic and endocrinological aspects of disorders of striated muscle. Res. Publ. Ass. Res. Nerv. Ment. Dis., 38:274, 1959.

Smith, H., Ameck, L. D., and Sielbury, J. Type II glycogenosis. Amer. J. Dis. Child., 111:475, 1966.

——— Zellweger, H., and Afifi, A. K. Muscular form of glycogemosis type II (Pompe): report of a case with unusual features. Neurology, 17:537, 1967.

Swaiman, K. F., Kennedy, W. R., and Sauls, H. S. Late infantile acid maltase deficiency. Arch. Neurol., 18:642, 1968.

Wyllie, W. G., and Watkins, A. G. Periodic familial paralysis. Proc. Roy. Soc. Med., 41:861, 1948.

MYASTHENIA GRAVIS

Keynes, G. The results of thymectomy in myasthenia gravis. Brit. Med. J., 2:611, 1949.
Kibrick, S. Myasthenia gravis in the newborn. Pediatrics, 14:365, 1954.
Millichap, J. G., and Dodge, P. R. Diagnosis and treatment of myasthenia gravis in infancy, childhood, and adolescence; a study of 51 patients. Neurology, 10: 1007, 1960.
Osserman, K. E. Myasthenia Gravis. New York, Grune and Stratton, Inc., 1958.
Rowland, L. P., Hoefer, P. F. A., and Aranow, H., Jr. Myasthenic syndromes. Res. Publ. Ass. Res. Nerv. Ment. Dis., 38:548, 1959.
Schwab, R. S., and Viets, H. R. Myasthenia gravis. Res. Publ. Ass. Res. Nerv. Ment. Dis., 38:624, 1959.
Simpson, J. A. An evaluation of thymectomy in myasthenia gravis. Brain, 81:112, 1958.
Strauss, A. J. L., Seegal, B. C., Hsu, K. C., Burkholder, P. M., Nastick, W. L., and Osserman, K. E. Immunofluorescence demonstration of a muscle-binding complement-fixing serum globulin fraction in myasthenia gravis. Proc. Soc. Exp. Biol. Med., 105:134, 1960.
Walker, R. P. Congenital myasthenia gravis. Amer. J. Dis. Child., 86:198, 1953.
Wyllie, W. G., Bodian, M., and Burrows, N. F. E. Myasthenia gravis in children. Arch. Dis. Child., 26: 457, 1951.

Chapter 13
DISORDERS OF THE NERVOUS SYSTEM SPECIFIC TO CHILDREN

ARNOLD P. GOLD and SIDNEY CARTER

Spasmus nutans, familial dysautonomia, and acute cerebellar ataxia are disorders specific to patients of the pediatric age group. Though rare, they present with a typical clinical picture which distinguishes them from other neurologic entities.

Spasmus Nutans (Head Nodding)

This disorder characteristically presents with a triad of signs; intermittent nystagmus, head nodding, and tilting of the head. The condition is self-limited, generally disappearing by 3 years of age.

The syndrome has its onset in infancy most often between the ages of 4 and 16 months. There is no particular sex incidence and it is more common in Negroes. The cause is unknown; there is no evidence to support vitamin deficiency and inadequate illumination as contributing factors. Spasmus nutans is seen more frequently during winter months.

Nystagmus may be the initial sign. It is often either unilateral or more marked in one eye and is characterized by rapid movements of a small amplitude in any direction. The abnormal eye movement disappears on covering the eyes and during sleep. The head nodding, which occurs in any direction, is typically slow and inconstant with a series of nods usually lasting but a few seconds. This movement is increased by placing the child in a vertical position and is abolished when supine. Head tilt is the least common finding and is often a compensatory posturing for the impaired vision secondary to the nystagmus.

Spasmus nutans must be differentiated from congenital nystagmus which tends to be familial, involves both eyes and fails to improve with time. Head movement when present is in the same direction as the nystagmus.

The condition is self-limited, and there is no specific therapy.

Familial Dysautonomia

RALPH E. MOLOSHOK

Familial dysautonomia, a congenital heritable syndrome, was first described in 1949 by Riley and coworkers. Although autonomic dysfunction is predominant, the striking features of this syndrome indicate the presence of a diffuse disturbance of function of the entire nervous system. The incidence in families is compatible with the hypothesis that it is transmitted by a recessive autosomal gene which is generally limited to persons of Jewish extraction.

Features which have been present in all cases are: reduced or absent tear production during crying, postural hypotension, coldness of the hands and feet, excessive perspiration, usually with transient blotching of the skin with excitement or during eating, relative indifference to pain, and emotional lability. Muscular coordination is impaired as manifested by difficulty in swallowing and chewing during infancy, prolonged drooling, dysarthria, and a delay in reaching the milestones of motor development. There is a general retardation of body growth, and pubescence is usually delayed. Scoliosis occurs in about half of the children who have survived past the age of 10 years. Deep tendon reflexes are either hypoactive or more frequently absent. Impairment of autonomic homeostatis is manifested by erratic regulation of body temperature with hypothermia, particularly during infancy, and periods of unexplained hyperpyrexia. Hypertension occurs with excitement or in association with febrile crises, while other patients are unable to maintain the upright position because of severe postural hypotension. Corneal anesthesia and defective lacrimation predispose to ulceration and scarring with impaired vision.

Severe life-threatening episodes are experienced in the course of the disease. Acute pulmonary crises occur as a result of bronchial hypersecretion, aspiration, and bronchopneumonia. Periodic bouts of intractable vomiting may be associated with bizarre self-destructive schizoid behavior. Severe hyperpyrexia may be accompanied by hypertension and diminished renal function or by a convulsive state. In a few instances sudden deaths have followed a shocklike state. Cardiac arrest and shock have been experienced during anesthesia.

The cause of this syndrome is unknown. No consistent anatomic findings have been seen at autopsy. It has been postulated that an inborn error of metabolism exists which affects the synthesis of a neurohumoral substance of importance to the transmission of nervous impulses. The studies of Smith, Dancis, and co-workers support this concept and have provided more precise means of diagnosis. Measurement of the urinary excretion of the metabolic products of the catecholamines has revealed that there was a uniform elevation of the ratio of homovanillic acid (a product of dopamine metabolism) to vanillyl mandelic acid (a product of epinephrine and norepinephrine metabolism).

A valuable diagnostic test is the response to the intradermal injection of 0.02 ml of a 1:10,000 dilution of histamine. The reaction of denervation is observed in patients with dysautonomia. Normally a wheal about 1 cm in diameter is produced and is surrounded by a red flare measuring 3 to 5 cm in diameter. The flare is dependent upon an axon reflex along sensory fibers; it has been uniformly absent in tests performed on patients with dysautonomia.

Hypersensitivity to the intravenous infusion of norepinephrine is another diagnostic feature in patients with dysautonomia, in whom a rise in blood pressure greater than 50 mm Hg is seen. While the normal pupil does not respond to the intraconjunctival instillation of a 2.5 percent solution of methacholine, in dysautonomia miosis occurs.

The absence of taste buds on the tongue, similarly a reaction of denervation, provides an objective anatomic diagnostic sign. Physiologic studies of respiration in dysautonomic children have revealed a relative insensitivity to hypoxia and to elevated carbon dioxide levels in the blood.

Prognosis for life must be guarded, as death has occurred in about 25 percent of the known cases, especially during the early years of life. These deaths have resulted from the acute crises described. The survivors have been handicapped by psychomotor difficulties although, with age, adaptation to stress appears to improve.

Treatment is strictly symptomatic. Guidance for the parents in the management of difficult behavior patterns in these children is most important. Vomiting attacks can often be controlled by the use of chlorpromazine in combination with phenobarbital. Inasmuch as these children adjust poorly to environmental change and stress, a stable routine of daily activity may prove helpful. The use of tranquilizing drugs has been of benefit to some children.

Acute Cerebellar Ataxia

STUART WEISS

Acute cerebellar ataxia, an unusual neurologic syndrome peculiar to the pediatric age group, is characterized by the sudden or subacute onset of ataxia of trunk, extremity, and ocular movement without other specific neurologic involvement or systemic symptoms. Complete recovery occurs within a few weeks to months in a high percentage of patients. Children between the ages of 1 and 4 years are most often affected; however, older children are occasionally seen with this syndrome. Sexes are equally susceptible.

ETIOLOGY AND PATHOLOGY. Frequently, a history of preceding nonspecific upper respiratory illness or gastrointestinal disturbance is obtained; however, most children develop ataxia without prior illness. Although some clinicians consider acute cerebellar ataxia as a transient sensitivity or inflammatory reaction in the cerebellum or cerebellar tracts to a nonspecific viral or systemic illness, others regard the syndrome as a viral cerebellitis, especially in the few severely involved patients.

Occasionally inborn errors of protein metabolism have been discovered in children with acute ataxia. Recurrent acute ataxia often precipitated by the stress of minor infections has been inherited in several families as a Mendelian dominant. No information as to the specific location or type of pathologic change is available to support any specific etiologic entity.

Recently, some children with acute cerebellar ataxia have been shown to have an associated often occult neuroblastoma.

CLINICAL MANIFESTATIONS. The major clinical feature of the syndrome is the rapid development of truncal ataxia with a lesser degree of extremity ataxia, which is less marked in the arms than in the legs. In the child more severely involved, there may be complete inability to support the body in a sitting position or to keep the head erect. Muscles of the trunk and extremities are hypotonic. Often an irregular, jerky tremor of the head and body is present.

Some children with severe ataxia may also develop jerky, irregular ocular activity with volitional eye movement (ocular dysmetria), others, involuntary darting multidirectional conjugate ocular movement (opsoclonus) and a few, a nystagmus with rhythmic fast-slow components. Isolated cranial nerve involvement, particularly the facial and less often the vagus, may occur in association with cerebellar ataxia. A specific viral infection (polio I) has been documented as the etiologic factor in the latter patients.

Vague systemic abnormalities such as lethargy, irritability, photophobia, and mild nuchal rigidity may accompany the neurologic deficit.

LABORATORY DATA. The patients who are usually afebrile at the time of hospitalization have normal peripheral blood counts, urinalysis, and serologic tests for syphilis. Erythrocyte sedimentation rates, heterophil agglutination, and total serum proteins are normal. Abnormalities of serum and urine amino acids by chromatographic analysis may be found in rare instances. Electroencephalographic abnormalities of major degree are uncommon. Lumbar puncture reveals a normal pressure, an occasional mononuclear pleocytosis to 50 cells, and normal protein, gamma globulin, and sugar values.

Viral cultures of throat, stool, and cerebrospinal fluid in a small number of children with acute ataxia have grown poliomyelitis virus type I and ECHO virus types 6 and 9. Confirmation of a specific viral infection with neutralizing and complement-fixing antibodies is desirable through acute and convalescent phase sera. Demonstrable acute changes in antibody titers and positive viral cultures are rare except in those cases of ataxia discovered during large-scale viral epidemics.

Roentgenograms of the chest and the vertebral spines as well as an intravenous pyelogram should be made to exclude an associated neuroblastoma.

DIAGNOSIS. A variety of diagnostic possibilities should be considered in a child with acute cerebellar ataxia. Posterior fossa tumors may produce ataxia abruptly. This ataxia is usually asymmetric in the degree of involvement of extremities and associated at the time of examination with evidence of increased intracranial pressure, cranial nerve palsies, head tilt, and nystagmus with preponderance in one direction. Active infection with poliomyelitis virus I, ECHO virus types 6 and 9, and influenza A virus has been demonstrated in occasional patients with acute ataxia. Classical acute ataxia in the course of varicella is of sufficiently frequent occurrence to be recognized. Infrequent association of acute ataxia without evidence of diffuse encephalitis has also been reported with rubella, rubeola, mumps, typhoid fever, and infectious mononucleosis.

Acute ataxia associated with myoclonic jerking and opsoclonus has been the initial manifestation of an occult neuroblastoma in several patients. These nonmetastatic neurologic abnormalities may antedate the discovery of the tumor by days to months. With removal of the tumor, the trunk and ocular ataxia may gradually improve.

Acute ataxia with a photosensitive pellagralike skin rash is the major clinical manifestation of Hartnup disease. Urinary screening for indican and indole acetic acid and characteristic blood and urinary chromatographic patterns of amino acids indicate this diagnosis in suspected patients.

Recently hyperpyruvic acidemia, hyperalanemia, and hyperalanuria have been discovered in one child with acute ataxia. Endogenous deficiencies of niacinamide and thiamin have been considered to be partly responsible for the above metabolic errors.

Certain exogenous toxins can produce a syndrome of acute ataxia. Excessive ingestion of drugs, such as diphenylhydantoins and barbiturates, or inhalation or ingestion of DDT (diphenyltrichloroethane), and lindane, causes ataxia as an early sign of toxicity. Lead ingestion and thallium poisoning produce acute ataxic syndromes which may not be readily reversible.

Demyelinating disease such as juvenile multiple sclerosis may be considered in the differential diagnosis if a previous history of neurologic deficit is present. The absence of a fluctuating course with successive exacerbations makes this diagnosis a rarity.

Acute labyrinthitis is characterized by positional vertigo, nausea, and vomiting in association with acute imbalance together with the absence of other distinguishing features of acute ataxia such as extremity incoordination and ocular dysmetria. Labyrinthine function is depressed on caloric stimulation.

PROGNOSIS. Most patients with acute cerebellar ataxia have a rapid recovery of extremity coordination and gait stability within periods of one week to six months following the onset of illness, emphasizing the benign prognosis with which this syndrome is identified. Some patients, as high as 33 percent in one series, have persistent neurologic deficit with ocular dysmetria, truncal and extremity ataxia, and lesser degrees of intellectual impairment. However, even in this group of patients gradual improvement has taken place over periods of several years.

Factors such as age of onset, sex, race, presence of prodromal symptoms, and specific laboratory data seem to have little significance in predicting the degree of recovery of the less fortunate children. There has been some correlation between the severity of the initial neurologic manifestations of the disease and a less favorable prognosis.

THERAPY. In the absence of a specific treatable cause of the syndrome, therapy of acute cerebellar ataxia is symptomatic, being directed toward maintenance of fluid and nutritional requirements, nursing supervision for general body care, and physical rehabilitation after the acute phase of illness is past.

The child should be kept at bed rest until the active progression of ataxia has ceased. Bed sides and rails should be protected with padding, as the children are often irritable and may strike their ataxic extremities against metal bed surfaces. Barbiturates or other sedatives should be used judiciously if the irritability or agitation is sufficiently severe to exhaust the child.

Nursing personnel and physicians should be careful to support the patient completely during care or treatment, as the ataxia may not allow normal muscular control of the head or trunk. Attempts at standing or walking the child should be withheld until the ataxia has sufficiently improved to avoid injurious falls. Similarly, excessively rapid attempts to achieve physical rehabilitation should be avoided lest the child become fearful and apprehensive because of inability to control the extremities or trunk during convalescence. In patients with unusually severe and persisting problems in balance, football helmets may be worn during rehabilitation.

Physical therapy to children over 3 years of age is aided by their ability to understand rehabilitation direction and to help themselves to develop functional balance in attempting ambulation.

Parental anxiety is best contained by guarded reassurance by the physician and a clear, simple explanation of the course and usual prognosis of the illness.

References

SPASMUS NUTANS

Herrman, C. Head shaking with nystagmus in infants; a study of sixty-four cases. Amer. J. Dis. Child., 16: 180, 1918.

Norton, E. W. D., and Cogan, D. Ct. Spasmus nutans; a clinical study of twenty cases followed two years or more since onset. Arch. Ophthal., 52:442, 1954.

FAMILIAL DYSAUTONOMIA

Moloshok, R. E., and Moseley, J. Familial dysautonomia: pulmonary manifestations. Pediatrics, 17:327, 1956.

Moses, S. W., Rotem, Y., Jagjagoda, N., Talmor, N., Eichhorn, F., and Levin, S. Clinical, genetic and biochemical study of familial dysautonomia in Israel. Israel J. Med. Sci., 3:358, 1967.

Riley, C. M. Familial dysautonomia. Advances Pediat., 9:157, 1957.

——— and Moore, R. H. Familial dysautonomia differentiated from related disorders. Pediatrics, 37:435, 1966.

Smith, A. A., and Dancis, J. Physiologic studies in familial dysautonomia. J. Pediat., 63:838, 1963.

——— and Dancis, J. Response to intradermal histamine in familial dysautonomia; a diagnostic test. J. Pediat., 63:889, 1963.

ACUTE CEREBELLAR ATAXIA

Berglund, G., Mossberg, H. O., and Rydenstam, B. Acute cerebellar ataxia in children. Acta Paediat. Scand., 44:254, 1955.

Blaw, M. E., and Sheehan, J. C. Acute cerebellar syndrome of childhood. Neurology, 8:538, 1958.

Bray, P. F., Ziter, F. A., Lahey, M. E., and Myers, G. G. The coincidence of neuroblastoma and acute cerebellar encephalopathy. Trans. Amer. Neurol. Ass., 1969, p. 28.

Cottom, D. G. Acute cerebellar ataxia. Arch. Dis. Child., 32:163, 1957.

Curnen, E. C., and Chamberlain, H. R. Acute cerebellar ataxia associated with polio virus infection. Yale J. Biol. Med., 34:219, 1962.

Dyken, P., and Oldrich, K. Dancing eyes, dancing feet: infantile polymyoclonia. Brain, 91:305, 1968.

Goldston, A. S., Millichap, J. S., and Miller, R. H. Cerebellar ataxia with pre-eruptive varicella. Amer. J. Dis. Child., 106:197, 1963.

Goldwyn, A., and Waldman, A. M. Acute cerebellar ataxia in children, report of three cases. J. Pediat., 42:75, 1953.

Hill, W., and Sherman, H. Acute intermittent familial cerebellar ataxia. Arch. Neurol., 18:350, 1968.

James, T. Acute ataxia of cerebellar type in children. Report of a case with rapid and complete recovery. Glasgow Med. J., 33:455, 1952.

Keller, J. J., and Karelitz, S. Acute ataxia in a 20-month old female. Pediatrics, 1:754, 1948.

King, G., Schwartz, G. A., and Slade, H. W. Acute cerebellar ataxia. Pediatrics, 21:731, 1958.

Klingman, W. O., and Hodges, R. S. Acute ataxia of unknown origin in children. J. Pediat., 24:536, 1944.

Lasater, G. M., and Jabbour, J. T. Acute ataxia of childhood: A summary of fifteen cases. Amer. J. Dis. Child., 97:61, 1959.

Lonsdale, D., Faulkner, W. R., Price, W., and Smeby, R. R. Pyruvic acidemia with hyperalanemia: vitamin B dependency. J. Pediat., 74:827, 1969.

McAllister, R. M., Hummeler, K., and Coriel, L. L. Acute cerebellar ataxia. Case report with isolation of type 9 ECHO virus from cerebrospinal fluid. New Eng. J. Med., 261:1159, 1959.

Mendez-Cashion, D., Sanchez-Longo, L. P., Valcarcel, M., and Rosen, L. Acute cerebellar ataxia in children associated with infection by polio virus 1. Pediatrics, 29:808, 1962.

Shanks, R. A. Notes on cerebellar ataxia in childhood. Arch. Dis. Child., 25:389, 1950.

Solomon, G. E., and Chutorian, A. M. Opsoclonus and occult neuroblastoma. New Eng. J. Med., 279:475, 1969.

Walcher, D. N., and Ross, A. T. Acute cerebellar ataxia of undetermined origin in childhood. Amer. J. Dis. Child., 96:278, 1958.

Weiss, S., and Carter, S. Course and prognosis of acute cerebellar ataxia in children. Neurology, 9:711, 1959.

INDEX

Page numbers in *italic* refer to figures or tables.